TREATING FAMILY OF ORIGIN PROBLEMS

TREATING
FAMILY OF ORIGIN
PROBLEMS
A Cognitive Approach

RICHARD C. BEDROSIAN
GEORGE D. BOZICAS

FOREWORD BY
Aaron T. Beck

THE GUILFORD PRESS
New York   London

© 1994 The Guilford Press
A Division of Guilford Publications, Inc.
72 Spring Street, New York, NY 10012

Printed in the United States of America

This book is printed on acid-free paper.

Last digit is print number: 9 8 7 6 5 4 3 2

Library of Congress Cataloging-in-Publication Data

Bedrosian, Richard C.
    Treating family of origin problems : a cognitive approach /
Richard C. Bedrosian, George D. Bozicas.
        p.   cm.
    Includes bibliographical references and index.
    ISBN 0-89862-178-X
    1. Adult children of dysfunctional families—Rehabilitation.
2. Cognitive therapy.   I. Bozicas, George, D.   II. Title.
    [DNLM: 1. Family.   2. Cognitive Therapy—methods.   3. Child of
Impaired Parents—psychology.   4. Mental Disorders—therapy.   WM
425 B413t 1993]
RC455.4.F3B43   1993
616.89'142—dc20
DNLM/DLC
for Library of Congress   93-33386
                                                                    CIP

Acknowledgments

I wish to express gratitude to all my clinical supervisors over the years, particularly Peter Urquhart, Marion Lindblad, Stuart Cohen, and, of course, Aaron Beck. Throughout my professional career, I have worked with many talented and supportive colleagues. Almost from the first day we started graduate school together, Steve Kagel helped me to become more flexible and inclusive in my therapeutic orientation. During my years at the Center for Cognitive Therapy in Philadelphia, Gary Emery, Jeffrey Young, David Burns, and Arthur Freeman were among those who exerted significant influence on my work. Likewise, my colleagues at the Herbert Lipton Mental Health Center taught me a great deal about all aspects of the mental health field. In my role as a clinical consultant to various local agencies and individual clinicians, I have encountered innumerable professionals who have also served in turn as role models for me. Since 1983, a number of truly remarkable individuals have come to work in my clinical practice. I wish to thank all the former members of Bedrosian Associates for their contributions, particularly my "soul sisters," Patricia Waldeck and Nanci Pradas, whose many words of wisdom continue to echo in my thoughts. Finally, I would like to acknowledge the current members of our staff, Lynn Brennan, Barbara Clark, Deborah Kelly, Cheryl Steinberg, and, of course, George Bozicas, my talented co-author. They are all dear to me. The caring, the insight, the forthrightness, and the self-honesty that characterize both their clinical work and their personal lives serve as a daily inspiration for me.

Without a strong and supportive family behind me, I could never have devoted three years of weekends to the preparation of this volume. My wife, my children, my parents, and my sisters all made sacrifices so that I could have the time necessary to complete the book. I am blessed beyond measure to have all of them in my life. During this self-imposed ordeal, I have often missed the laughter and the companionship that have always been such a special part of our lives together. I pray that we all will have an opportunity to make up for lost time now.

Finally, I would like to offer a special word of thanks to my friend and former colleague, Dorothy Bozicas, the Greek Lady. She lovingly pored over our manuscript at various stages, offering us invaluable feedback on both style and content. More importantly though, she offered us inspiration, through the courage and commitment she manifests in her own life.

RICHARD C. BEDROSIAN, Ph.D.

I would like to express my appreciation to several individuals who have played various roles in my professional development: Lawrence Grebstein, James Prochaska, Philip Kleespies, Mitchell Bornstein, Richard Weisblatt, and Charles Streff. I would also like to acknowledge my Bedrosian Associates colleagues: Nanci, Cheryl, Debbie, Lynn, and Barbara. Their integrity and professionalism have inspired me, and I thank them for their insights and support. Also special thanks to my friends and colleagues, Robert Stern and Robin Gibbs, for their consistent availability and encouragement.

I thank my wife Julie for her patience and understanding. I thank my brother Paul and my sister Tina for their love and support. I thank my father, James, for his humor, his caring, and his pride. I miss him. And lastly, I thank my mother, Dorothy, for her love of knowledge and for her spirit and determination.

Finally, I would like to thank Richard Bedrosian. I have been enriched beyond measure through our association.

GEORGE D. BOZICAS, Ph.D.

Foreword

During the past 30 years I have watched a process of evolution occur within the cognitive therapy movement. As training and supervision in cognitive therapy has become available to successive cohorts of mental health professionals, it was inevitable that new generations of practitioners would enhance the scope and the clinical sophistication of the treatment techniques practiced under the cognitive umbrella. Likewise, it was to be expected that some practitioners would bring with them concepts and stategies associated with other schools of treatment, approaches that they would attempt to integrate with a cognitive framework. This volume presents the integrative work of two such practitioners.

Although this book reflects a unique synthesis of ideas and treatment interventions, it has its roots firmly embedded in the cognitive therapy movement. Richard Bedrosian was trained at the Center for Cognitive Therapy in 1977, fresh from a year of training in family therapy at the Philadelphia Child Guidance Clinic. As a supervisee of mine, he eagerly embraced the cognitive model of treatment, finding it particularly applicable to work with depressed and suicidal individuals and their families. I believe he was one of the very first writers who attempted to translate family systems concepts into cognitive terms. Dr. Bedrosian went on to train and supervise some of the outstanding cognitive therapists in the country, including his co-author, George Bozicas.

Much of the published work on adult children of dysfunctional families, while well intended, has failed to provide clinicians with a clear model for the assessment and treatment of such individuals. This volume translates the concept of "dysfunctional family" into cognitive terms which should be readily understood by therapists from a variety of orientations. The cognitive framework emphasizes the crucial role of information processing for understanding the coping strategies developed by individuals who grow up in troubled families.

Drs. Bedrosian and Bozicas also offer a model for assessing the current manifestations of family of origin problems so that, despite a historical focus, treatment can still be geared toward the individual's present-day complaints. This practical orientation should make the book invaluable to mental health professionals who must work under the short-term mandates of managed care. Throughout, the authors illustrate how traditional cognitive therapy techniques such as Socratic dialogue can be utilized to promote awareness of the impact of family of origin problems on the individual's thinking and behavior. They demonstrate how some of the typical features of cognitive therapy, such as the use of structured sessions and the emphasis on repetition and practice, can help to make each treatment session a powerful learning vehicle for the client who is working on family of origin material.

I am pleased to see the way in which Drs. Bedrosian and Bozicas tackle some of the most complex subjects confronting all practitioners of psychotherapy. Their discussions of sensitive topics such as the maintenance of boundaries in the therapeutic relationship, and the impact of the therapist's personal issues on the treatment process, are probing, honest, and thought-provoking.

Although the book is filled with numerous practical suggestions and many lists of specific techniques, the authors manage to keep the reader aware at all times of the complex set of considerations which underlie their choice of particular interventions. Through their vivid, detailed case descriptions, they bring the multilayered reality of clinical work to life. Along with other recent publications in a similar vein, this volume should help to counteract criticisms that cognitive therapy is overly simplistic or mechanistic in its approach to treatment.

AARON T. BECK, M.D.

Contents

TREATING FAMILY OF ORIGIN PROBLEMS

Introduction

PURPOSE OF THE BOOK

This volume is aimed at an audience of mental health professionals from a variety of disciplines and theoretical backgrounds. It shows how the clarity and discipline associated with cognitive therapy can be brought to bear on the treatment of family of origin issues such as alcoholism and incest without compromising depth and clinical sophistication. Clinicians who have had little or no exposure to the cognitive therapies will find the book to be a guide to formulating an active treatment plan, one that can be sustained over time, despite the inevitable vicissitudes of the therapeutic process. Therapists with cognitive backgrounds should also find the volume helpful, in that it illustrates how the therapy approach developed by Beck and his colleagues can be expanded to embrace significant concepts from other treatment orientations, that is denial, boundaries, enabling, and so on.

When compared to other books on the treatment of adult children of dysfunctional families, our volume is unique in its use of an integrative cognitive model, its utilization of structured cognitive therapy techniques, and its emphasis on repetition and practice as essential components of the recovery process. We show how issues typically highlighted by practitioners from other orientations, such as "denial," can be reconceptualized and effectively treated within a cognitive framework. We find that other volumes on the treatment of family of origin material tend to overemphasize the *descriptive* level, by presenting the target psychological deficits in rich detail, while they neglect the *prescriptive* level, by failing to convey adequately the complex nature of the treatment process. In preparing our book, our overriding goals have been to operationalize the diverse elements involved in successful treatment of family of origin issues and to present them to the reader, not as a set of narrow, rote strategies, but as a set of *concepts* that can be applied to a variety of cases.

The major goals of cognitive approaches to treatment involve the identification and modification of maladaptive cognitions. Although practicing clinicians may implicitly assume that such cognitions develop in childhood as a result of conditions in the family of origin, the cognitive-behavioral literature still retains a decidedly ahistorical bias. Typically, orthodox cognitive therapists have avoided direct exploration of the historical roots of dysfunctional thinking. Our treatment approach involves a purposeful, structured exploration of historical material, aimed at generating hypotheses about basic beliefs, information- processing styles, and acquired coping strategies. Through clinical examples, we illustrate how the cognitive therapist can integrate family of origin material into the assessment and treatment process, while he or she preserves the simplicity and the power of the cognitive model. The use of a family of origin focus need not result in repetitive, unproductive historical review in treatment sessions. Throughout the volume, we try to illustrate repeatedly how the cognitive therapist can bring historical material alive by integrating it with the patient's current experiences.

Unlike other texts on cognitive therapy, our book also includes close examination of the *therapist* and of certain unique elements of the therapeutic relationship. We explore how the therapist's *own* family of origin issues influence the treatment process. We describe treatment cases in which the therapists *themselves* first needed to confront fears, self-doubts, and other personal demons *before* they could effectively address the difficulties of the particular clients. We also discuss ways of utilizing the clinician's affect to enhance the treatment process. In our sections on the therapist's posture, we address various metacommunicative elements in the therapeutic relationship which can affect the client's ability to use treatment constructively. Throughout the volume, we provide examples in which the clinician was able to utilize embedded messages and other techniques to circumvent resistance and facilitate the examination of threatening material by the client. Many of our case vignettes also illustrate how the therapist can confront various types of acting out behaviors, while remaining in a supportive, collaborative posture. We strive to show that the therapist can provide a consistent focus in treatment, despite substantial shifts in material offered by the client. A number of cases we present will demonstrate how the clinician can continue to highlight the underlying mechanisms that cause distress, without becoming trapped in an exclusive, unproductive focus on the client's symptoms.

Therapists from other theoretical backgrounds sometimes complain that cognitive treatment approaches tend to be presented in a pat, mechanistic manner, with little appreciation for or recognition of the real vicissitudes of clinical practice. The treatment orientation presented in this volume evolved directly from the clinical experiences of the authors, and, as such, reflects our efforts to deal with the day-to-day struggles of clinical work. Readers will not find simplistic, "cookbook" answers in this volume, nor will they be made to feel inadequate by wildly successful case examples in which profound changes occur overnight. As fellow veterans of the "psychotherapy wars," we want our readers to be aware throughout the volume that we fully appreciate the frustrations and the complexities of clinical work.

The style of treatment presented in this volume evolved through many years of clinical experiences with hundreds of clients. Prior to the actual writing of the book, the authors spent many months reviewing a variety of successful and unsuccessful cases, all of which had involved family of origin material as part of the treatment process. We continually asked ourselves a number of questions: What did treatment really involve? What elements distinguished successful cases from the unsuccessful ones? What did we learn from serial therapeutic contacts with certain clients? Which clients seemed to experience recurring difficulties? What kind of changes seemed to produce long-term symptom relief in our clients? What type of cases did we typically have difficulty treating, and why? How did our *own* family of origin experiences affect how we approached certain cases?

Going into the project, we were committed to the belief that we could describe our activities as therapists *clearly, directly,* and *comprehensively,* without glossing over the complex realities of clinical work. Most importantly, we wanted to articulate a *mindset* for the reader to adopt in his or her clinical work, not merely to provide a set of treatment techniques. To that end, we knew it would be crucial to describe with some accuracy the inner experience, or cognitions, of the therapist. Although our clinical work had expanded over the years to include an explicit focus on family of origin issues, we believed that it still reflected a strongly cognitive orientation. In our view, the approach to assessment and treatment, as outlined in succeeding chapters, remains highly compatible with the basic cognitive model employed by Beck and his colleagues over the past 15 years. Let the reader be the judge.

The authors are full-time, private practice clinicians, not psychotherapy researchers or personality theorists. Although we have tried to incorporate relevant research findings into the text wherever possible, we are well aware that we cannot offer empirical support for the majority of our observations and recommendations. We apologize in advance for any inaccurate generalizations or unwarranted inferences we might make. No doubt our clinical observations have been biased by any number of factors. We have attempted, however, to keep our terminology and our basic operating assumptions as simple as possible. We hope we have stuck fairly close to the clinical data, as impressionistic as they might be. We also have included a description of the history of our clinical practice, and the population of clients we serve, so that the reader can better judge the degree to which our treatment approach might be applicable in his or her current professional work. We have tried to avoid embarrassing ourselves by refusing to address some rather broad and significant theoretical questions (e.g., Is there an unconscious?) which have puzzled greater minds than ours for decades. We hope that the clinical strengths of this volume will enable the reader to assume a forgiving attitude toward our theoretical shortcomings.

THE CLINICAL POPULATION

This volume is based on clinical experiences with a population of clients who were treated primarily in a private practice setting, in central Massachusetts, from 1980 to the present. Most of the clients had some form of health insurance, which generally meant that they were employed. However, we estimate that over half of the clients who were employed held jobs of a blue-collar variety. Likewise, a substantial percentage of our clients had no more than a high school education. Moreover, the typical health insurance plan in Massachusetts will pay out only $500 for outpatient psychotherapy per calendar year, the minimum mental health coverage mandated by state law. Low-income clients of modest educational attainment may be quick to discontinue treatment as soon as any significant reductions in distress occurs. They may not be able to pay for psychotherapy once their insurance benefits have been exhausted, or they may choose to invest their limited resources in more valued priorities, such as consumer goods. Nonetheless, we have experienced some of our most satisfying treatment outcomes with low-income or blue-collar clients, many of whom have engaged in serial therapeutic contacts spanning several years. On the other hand, we have also seen a variety of clients who came from the upper ranges of the educational, social, and economic spectra. Some of these clients have been quite compliant with the typical norms of psychotherapy, despite their other psychological difficulties, whereas others, not surprisingly, have not been as cooperative. As our practice has become better known among the mental health community, we have been privileged to treat an increasing number of our fellow therapists, for a variety of difficulties and at various stages in their professional careers.

The central Massachusetts area is home to a number of well-established ethnic communities. The Irish, Italians, French-Canadians, Poles, Finns, Swedes, Lithuanians, Greeks, Armenians, eastern European Jews, Lebanese, and more recently hispanic peoples of various national backgrounds, all settled in the region in substantial numbers. There is a small but stable African-American population in the area, which has not grown substantially since the early decades of this century. Asian-Americans are only just arriving in sufficient numbers to establish their own ethnic communities in the area.

Catholicism is probably the most common religious identification among our clients. Many of the adults we treat are products of parochial schools, which are quite numerous in the area. Our client base also contains substantial numbers of Jews and Protestants, including many members of a nearby Seventh Day Adventist community. Although the more fundamentalist Christian sects are nowhere as popular as they are in other areas of the country, a number of our clients from neglectful or abusive families of origin seem to have gravitated toward cult-like, authoritarian religious involvements.

From the end of World War II until the late 1970s, the central Massachusetts area was hit again and again by the loss or relocation of key industries, ranging from shoe factories to steel plants. Along with many other negative effects, the inevitable economic decline probably eroded the level of family functioning in the area. Often the region's "best and brightest" were prone to leave the area for an education, or a first professional job, never to return. New residents in the area during the period joined a labor force increasingly devoted to menial jobs. Fort Devens, an Army base in North Central Massachusetts, brought large numbers of single young men to the area, many of whom remained because they had married and/or impregnated local young women. It seems as if a disproportionate share of the dysfunctional families we have seen were created in this fashion.

Beginning in the 1970s, the burgeoning computer industry began to revolutionize the economy of central Massachusetts. Opportunities for training and occupational advancement proliferated, while salaries escalated rapidly. Unlike the experience of earlier decades, many individuals who had been trained in prestigious Massachusetts colleges and universities remained in the local labor force following graduation. Engineers and a variety of other professionals migrated to the area from around the country and the world. Real estate values soared, particularly in communities closest to Boston and around the Route 128 and 495 beltways. The increased demand for affordable single-family housing resulted in large-scale development in once sleepy, semirural towns. Cities such as Worcester, Leominster, and Fitchburg, which had re-

mained stagnant and blighted for decades, experienced a flurry of upscale commercial development.

The area's largest employer, Digital Equipment Corporation,
seemed to produce a zeitgeist in the 1980s that encouraged employee
involvement in psychotherapy. Every major Digital site had an active
Employee Assistance Program that arranged referrals for psychological
services. Moreover, for much of the decade, the health care insurance
plan chosen by most Digital employees provided them with nearly
open-ended psychotherapy benefits, in contrast to the $500 yearly cap
on outpatient mental health services imposed by most other insurers in
the state. We were fortunate to be able to work with many Digital
employees before the health insurance situation began to erode. Consequently, some of our clients were able to participate in uninterrupted
treatment for relatively long periods of time, an arrangement that unfortunately is becoming more of a rarity with each passing year.

As this volume was being prepared, the central Massachusetts area
again faced the symptoms of severe economic decline. Between March,
1990 and March, 1991, the New England area lost over 240,000 jobs.
Layoffs, which have even occurred at Digital for the first time, continued to disrupt thousands of households in the area. Real estate values
have plummeted 25% and more over the past 2 years, resulting in the
erosion of the primary source of wealth in most families. Coupled with
the rise of restrictive managed care practices in health insurance, the
current economic woes have severely hampered the ability of many
individuals to receive even modest amounts of psychological services.
It remains unclear to what degree such developments in the economy
and in the insurance industry will affect the kind of therapeutic work
we describe in this volume. However, it seems certain at this point that
the health insurance carriers will fund less and less of the recovery
process of our clients as time goes on, particularly in the absence of
serious symptomatology.

HISTORY OF THE CLINICAL PRACTICE

Our clinical practice, Bedrosian Associates, first opened in Leominster,
Massachusetts in 1980. A second office, now located in Northboro,
opened in 1981. The practice quickly became fairly well known, primarily because of the hands-on, active treatment techniques it offered to
the public. At the time, practitioners with training in behavior therapy,
cognitive therapy, structural family therapy, and other more direct
forms of treatment were still relatively hard to find in the area. The
majority of the local mental health professionals had been trained in the

psychodynamic therapies. Clients and referral sources both looked to the practice to provide a short-term, largely ahistorical treatment approach that produced quick relief from a variety of symptoms. In many instances, clients drove from far off corners of New England to be treated at the practice because it had been recommended to them by Aaron T. Beck or David Burns. Needless to say, their expectations regarding the potential efficacy of cognitive treatment techniques were often unrealistically high. Psychoanalytically oriented colleagues often referred clients to the practice, typically males, whom they judged to be unsuitable for a more intensive, insight-oriented approach. Initially, the bulk of the referrals involved depression, anxiety, marital difficulties, or adolescent adjustment problems. As the staff grew in size and breadth of expertise, so did the range of referring problems being treated in the practice.

The opportunity to observe a large number of clients longitudinally forced us over the years to contemplate the limitations of symptom oriented treatment approaches. We also gained an appreciation for how hard it really can be to produce changes in basic beliefs and relationship patterns. Some individuals simply did not improve on a symptomatic level. On the other hand, it seemed that a number of individuals whom we had treated successfully for symptoms such as anxiety and depression kept returning to the practice with the same difficulties, or additional ones. Often such clients would experience symptoms in connection with significant life transitions, such as parenthood. In many instances, clients would use treatment to extricate themselves with relief from one problematic relationship, only to become involved with an equally troubled individual a year or two later. Despite initial improvements in mood and transient increases in self-esteem, it was clear in retrospect that their basic patterns of thinking and behavior had not changed, particularly in intimate relationships. More and more, it seemed as if such chronically symptomatic clients reported histories of physical and/or sexual abuse. Likewise, addictions, particularly to alcohol, seemed omnipresent in the lives of these clients, both in their families of origin and in their current relationships.

Somewhat hesitantly, we began to utilize historical material in our work with clients, particularly those with chronic or recurring symptoms. We found ourselves sailing in uncharted waters, since the cognitive therapy publications available in the early 1980s generally assumed a decidedly ahistorical stance. On the other hand, the psychotherapy literature on subjects such as the addictions, sexual abuse, and adult children of alcoholics (ACOA) generally espoused concepts that seemed either inaccurate or were difficult to translate clearly into cognitive terms. Although it seemed likely that a cognitive model could be useful in understanding phenomena such as the effects of child sexual abuse, the connections among thinking, emotions, and behaviors were not always easy to identify in certain clients, particularly incest survivors. The need to conceptualize and treat historical issues in cognitive terms only intensified as the mass media began to present material on dysfunctional families to the public at large. It seemed that more and more clients entered therapy explicitly identifying themselves as incest survivors or ACOAs, searching for ways to reduce the negative impact of historical events on their currents lives.

Nearly all of the clinicians who have worked in the practice had professional roots in the local community mental health system, dating as far back as 1977. The length and breadth of our involvement in the communities in which we practice often provide us with an extensive knowledge of the backgrounds of the individuals and families we treat. With a sense of tragic inevitability, we have often been forced to watch dysfunctional family processes continue on into succeeding generations, as troubled teenagers grow up with significant psychological deficits, find impaired or otherwise unsuitable partners, and bear children who will also suffer the effects of a disturbed family environment. Not surprisingly, we may deal with various subsystems of a particular family at different times, perhaps over a period of five or ten years. Often one individual who has had a positive therapy experience will end up referring several siblings or cousins, and their families, to us over the succeeding years. Consequently, we have been able to observe and to treat a number of extended family systems, each from a variety of perspectives, and in a number of configurations.

It still amazes us how often we end up already knowing information about the other individuals, not related by blood, with whom our clients become involved. Some of the coincidences that occur seem quite remarkable. It is still a shock, however, to hear our client discussing a boss, a friend, or a lover and to realize that we have clinical knowledge of the individual in question. We suspect that these coincidences happen nonrandomly. We believe that many of our clients gravitate toward individuals with complementary psychological issues. Is it an unreasonable inferential leap to assume that communities contain dysfunctional interpersonal *networks* as well as dysfunctional families? Unfortunately, we think not.

One more aspect of sustaining a practice for many years in the same location deserves mention—the issue of both personal and professional boundaries. We point out again and again how so many of our clients, particularly survivors of incest, have difficulties maintaining appropriate interpersonal boundaries in a variety of relationships. In subsequent chapters, we emphasize that in order to facilitate the recovery process with such individuals, the therapist must maintain secure, explicit boundaries. The longer one practices in a given area, the harder it may become to avoid uncomfortable entanglements with clients. Likewise, it becomes harder and harder to go out in public without seeing current and former clients. Even conducting one's leisure business outside of one's "catchment area" offers little security. One of the authors has seen clients, among other places, in Boston Garden at Celtics' games (40 miles away), in a tiny seafood restaurant on Cape Cod (100 miles away), on the beach in Ogunquit, Maine (105 miles away), and in the airport at Bangor, Maine (300 miles away)! As the therapist's reputation leads to referrals that may present dual relationship difficulties, as the therapist begins to be badgered by friends and neighbors to treat their spouses or family members, as the therapist begins to feel current and former clients turn up simply everywhere he or she goes, then does the role of consultation and support from professional colleagues in handling boundary problems become crucial.

Many of the clients we discuss in this book have perplexed us, some for long periods of time. We have made countless errors and have sustained many wounds ourselves in our therapeutic encounters with them. Perhaps other therapists might have been more effective with them, and sooner. In many instances, it took time and persistence for us to get to know them, and more importantly, for them to get to know themselves. Fortunately both we and our clients persevered, until slowly, new attitudes and behaviors began to emerge. Looking back on the process, we can see that they led us nearly as often as we guided them. As much as the tales of human misery we hear deplete and disappoint us, the resiliency and the forward movement of our clients continue to inspire us. The opportunity to participate in their growth makes being a psychotherapist a joyous experience for us, despite the daily hardships involved.

1

Characteristics of Dysfunctional Families

When can a therapist legitimately conclude that an adult client is the product of a dysfunctional family of origin? Does a dysfunctional family truly differ from so-called normal families? Aren't all families dysfunctional to one degree or another? Are we teaching our clients to blame their parents for their own failings, their own choices in life?

The majority of our clients are not the "worried well." The cases we present in this volume involve family histories that would be identified by even a casual observer as pathological on a number of dimensions. In addition to being frequently appalling or horrifying, the tales of childhood and adolescence we hear from our clients invariably involve not one or two, but multiple severe stressors in the early environment. We seldom if ever agree inwardly with our clients when they say, "It wasn't that bad." Indeed, it probably *was* that bad—and worse. We continue to believe (or is it hope?) that the families from which our clients come are not representative of the population at large, perhaps because the alternative view only fills us with a sense of helpless despair.

Below we list a number of factors which in our opinion, define dysfunctional family functioning. Although we may emphasize certain elements in our own unique way, our selection of variables closely parallels those employed by others to describe families in which incest and other problems have occurred (e.g., Brown, 1988; Calof, 1987; Courtois, 1988). Perhaps each factor by itself is not sufficient to cause enduring difficulties for the developing child. We speculate, however, that when combinations of the following factors are present in a child's life, they work in concert to thwart the development of strong self-esteem, flexible coping strategies, and constructive relationship patterns.

IMPAIRED PARENTING

Parenting is probably by far the most complex, demanding task any individual will undertake over the course of his or her lifetime. It should be a humbling experience for anyone, especially for therapists who work extensively with children prior to becoming parents themselves. The list of what children need from their parents in order to achieve ultimate competency as adults grows longer and more involved with each succeeding developmental stage.

In the early stages of prenatal and postnatal development, it is comparatively difficult for parents to botch the job, unless of course they either neglect or actively sabotage the health of the baby. Soon, however, the child must be taught meanings and interpretations rather than specific skills. Now the parent's performance as a teacher will be affected by his or her own neurological or psychological deficits, if they are present. Likewise, the ongoing emergence of the child as an independent being with desires and interests of his or her own requires not only limit setting from the parent but a sense of relative detachment as well. The role of disciplinarian will expose the parent's difficulties with frustration tolerance and conflict resolution. The child's increasing level of socialization in the extrafamilial world may be complicated by the parent's own difficulties with shame or alienation. The onset of adolescence introduces new and even more threatening elements to the parent–child interaction, particularly the emergence of the youngster's sexuality. Once again, the demands of raising an older child will expose the parent's deficiencies in judgment and self-esteem. Finally, any parent, let alone an impaired one, will be sorely tested by the demands of raising a child with special physical or psychological needs. An individual with significant psychological deficits of his or her own will find it inordinately difficult to cope effectively with a child who suffers from problems such as chronic illness, mental retardation, attention deficit disorders, learning disabilities, and so on. In dysfunctional families, such children may be more likely to experience scapegoating or abuse, crippling infantilization, or emotional neglect.

Let us review some of the common circumstances that could impair the ability of an individual to parent children effectively:

- Physical illness or severe physical disability
- Substance abuse, either episodic or continuous
- Organic or biochemically based mental illness (e.g., schizophrenia, bipolar disorder, and so on)
- Neurological malfunction
- Severe learning disability or attentional disorder
- Mental retardation

- Extreme stress or trauma (e.g., war, genocide, violent crime)
- Sexual perversion or obsession
- Recurrent depression, including suicidal wishes
- Severe anxiety disorder
- Severe eating disorder
- Severe personality disorder
- Single parent with multiple stressors, limited physical and/or psychological resources

Other writers (e.g., Black, 1981; Brown, 1988; Courtois, 1988; Glass, 1985; Thurman, Whaley, & Weinraub, 1985) have discussed disruptions in family structure and functioning that result from the presence of an impaired parent. At the extreme, impaired parents cannot even respond to the most basic physical needs of the developing child. They may be unable to provide a minimal level of organization and leadership, leaving the family in a chaotic state. Their children may experience severe neglect and/or abuse which becomes obvious to the point that community agencies intervene. However, in our experience, many seriously impaired parents are not neglectful or abusive in ways visible to the community at large. Their families may never draw the scrutiny of social service agencies or the law enforcement system. In fact, on superficial inspection, the parents may appear to be typical, hard-working citizens, whereas the actual family dysfunction takes place behind closed doors.

We assume that family pathology can be multigenerational in scope. We also assume that both genetic and environmental factors contribute to the continuation of parental impairment from one generation to the next. Many of our clients were raised in large extended family systems, and in some cases entire neighborhoods or communities, that were riddled with alcoholism, sexual abuse, and other symptoms of severe psychopathology across multiple generations. During their formative years, these clients may have been continually exposed to impaired and/or abusive grandparents, uncles, aunts, cousins, and neighbors. The parents may have been unable or unwilling to protect their children from being victimized by members of the extended family, stepparents, adults or older children from the neighborhood, or abusive authority figures from the community at large.

PARENTIFICATION OF CHILDREN

Parental impairment creates a leadership vacuum in a family. In such instances it is often natural for one or more of the children to step in and fill the vacant parenting role. In addition to assuming responsibility for themselves and their siblings, these children may also function as caretakers for their own parents or other adults in the family. Unfortunately, parentified children also function as impaired parents themselves, because of a number of factors. First of all, they generally have responsibility, but ultimately no authority, no real power to execute their "duties," and they are probably doomed to failure from the outset. They have little or no chance of succeeding in providing a better life for anyone else in their families, yet they are sure to blame themselves, and may be blamed by others as well, if they fail. They may be consumed with anxiety as they ponder the enormity of their responsibilities, and be overwhelmed by feelings of worthlessness when things go badly. It is no wonder that although parentified children often grow into extremely competent adults, they also continue to experience feelings of intense anxiety and low self-esteem despite the level of their accomplishments.

Second, although they make tremendous sacrifices of time and energy for their "wards," probably forsaking their own interests and social development in the process, parentified children are still children, intellectually and emotionally. They cannot handle the cognitive complexity parenting demands, nor do they have the insight or the foresight that only adult experience can bring to the task. Consequently, they are apt to enact a caricatured, monochromatic version of the parental role. In other words, a parentified ten-year-old can only enact a ten-year-old's conception of what a mother's or father's role should be. Given their overall level of intellectual and psychological maturity, it is not surprising that parentified children may be overly punitive and controlling on the one hand, yet too indulgent and inconsistent on the other. Later in life, they may it find it equally difficult to parent their own offspring without being controlling or enabling. They also are likely to reenact the parenting role in a wide range of inappropriate contexts (e.g., marriage or career) as adults, often with same limitations and performance problems they had experienced in childhood.

Third, children are wont to develop superstitions in order to manage the anxiety they experience regarding their families. They tend to be egocentric and grandiose in the degree to which they think they can influence events around them (Elkind, 1974). Consequently, they may develop unwarranted faith in the power of certain strategies to remedy dysfunctional conditions in the family (compulsively cleaning the house, for example). Like all of us, they tend to stick with what works, or what they think works. The coping strategies and interpersonal behaviors of parentified children may become overly rigid and stereotyped, often with long-term negative consequences for themselves and possibly their siblings as well. For many of our clients, obsessions and/or compulsive behaviors in adult life appear to be clear legacies of parentification in childhood.

As discussed above, parentified children are at risk for a range of psychological and relationship difficulties in adult life, despite their high level of responsibility and apparent self-sufficiency. Parentified children may grow up to marry impaired individuals much like their parents, thereby perpetuating dysfunctional family processes into the next generation. They may find it hard to sustain intimate relationships without somehow sacrificing major portions of their own identities in the process. Parentified children may gravitate toward the helping professions (Fussell & Bonney, 1990; Guy, 1987). In our experience, adults who played parental roles in childhood seem overrepresented in vocations such as nursing and clinical psychology. Not surprisingly, it may be quite challenging for such individuals to maintain a consistent sense of professional detachment when dealing with their patients or clients.

BOUNDARY VIOLATIONS

Boundaries delineate physical and psychological space between individuals, generations, and/or subsystems within a family. We assume, as do others (Minuchin, 1974), that the establishment and maintenance of effective boundaries are crucial to the developmental processes of families and individuals. As they establish a committed intimate relationship, two young adults must separate to some degree from their respective families of origin. In order to communicate successfully on the multiple levels required in a marriage, the young couple needs to exclude other family members from a variety of transactions. Otherwise, communications between the intimate dyad tend to become re-routed through third parties, particularly in-laws, who may form destructive coalitions with one spouse against the other. On the other hand, despite the need for psychological and physical intimacy within the marriage, the spouses also need "space" from each other in order to pursue independent interests, relationships, and areas of competency. Spouses who engage in "codependent" patterns of interaction are unable to achieve sufficient psychological distance from the thoughts, feelings, and behaviors of the other.

Couples who bear children must face another set of boundary challenges. They have a responsibility to nurture and protect developing children, yet they must find a way to sustain a sense of connectedness as a dyad. They must monitor the child's medical status, academic progress, and peer relationships outside the family without violating his or her dignity and privacy. In the process, they must learn to restrain children without inflicting harm, and to protect them from dangers in the extra-familial environment without thwarting the development of independence. Parents also must learn to distance themselves from their children's thoughts, feelings, and behaviors at times, particularly when offspring need to learn some of the more painful lessons of life through direct experience. On the other hand, they need to shield their children from unnecessary exposure to problems in the marriage or in the extended family.

In dysfunctional families, we often observe a disrespect for children's boundaries that goes back several generations. Parents may directly victimize children in a number of ways, as described below, or they may fail to prevent them from being victimized by others inside the family or in the community at large. Children thereby learn a style of relating that fails to acknowledge the normal physical and psychological barriers around individuals and between generations. Coupled with a basic sense of worthlessness, such an interpersonal style sets up the individual for recurrent abuse, exploitation, manipulation, and other relationship problems throughout his or her lifetime.

Let us briefly review some of the common types of boundary violations that occur in families. These include:

Recurrent physical abuse of children or other family members.
Incest.
Recurrent inappropriate sexual or seductive behavior.
Recurrent exposure to sexual relations between other family members.
Recurrent, intrusive medical procedures, possibly unjustified on medical grounds, for example, repeated enemas.
Recurrent intrusive parental involvement in children's personal hygiene long past the age when they are capable of caring for themselves.
Severe parental restrictions on children's diet, schedule or activities probably not justified on medical or psychological grounds.
Recurrent, persistent messages that parents or other authority figures know the inner thoughts or experiences of children.
Persistent violations of the child's privacy by parents or caretakers with minimal or no justification.
Unreasonable and unjustified interference with the developing child's contact with peers and other elements of the extrafamilial world.
Inability or unwillingness of parents to protect children from victimizing experiences outside the nuclear family.
Chronic cross-generational coalitions, for example, persistent use of children or adolescents as confidantes by parental figures.

✓Unnecessary exposure of children to details of parent's finances, sexual behaviors, infidelities, marital conflicts, and so on.

Extreme parental emphasis on and intrusive involvement in the child's achievement-oriented activities, particularly in athletics and the arts.

Research findings on adult survivors of incest illustrate the wide-ranging effects of severe boundary violations in childhood on adjustment later in life. According to Courtois (1988), the long-term effects of incest reveal themselves in the adult's emotional reactions, self-image, physical/somatic perceptions, sexual functioning, and interpersonal relationships. Common emotional effects include: symptoms of generalized anxiety; trauma-specific phobias such as fears of the dark or of enclosed spaces; chronic depression, including feelings of helplessness; self-mutilating behaviors and suicidal thoughts; and feelings of detachment and emotional deadness.

The self-perceptions of incest victims typically reflect powerful feelings of badness and shame. Survivors often see themselves as disgusting, freakish, and unworthy. Consistent with their shame, survivors frequently view their bodies as disgusting. As a consequence, they may neglect themselves through poor self-care habits. Survivors may suffer from a variety of nonspecific, anxiety-based physical symptoms such as gastrointestinal disturbances, chronic muscle tension, and respiratory difficulties. They may also experience abuse-specific reactions such as gagging, vomiting, rectal discomfort, constipation, and genitourinary pain or infections. A high proportion of incest survivors develop sexual difficulties of many types. Problems often manifest themselves in the areas of sexual emergence, sexual orientation and preference, and sexual arousal, response, and satisfaction (Maltz & Holman, 1987). Interpersonal markers of incest include: difficulties with trust; problems committing to relationships; perpetuation of relationships experienced as empty, one-way, superficial, idealized, conflictual; and relationships characterized by caretaking of an immature partner. Finally, incest survivors evidence a variety of social effects ranging from isolation to compulsive social interaction. Victims also may develop patterns of rebellious and antisocial behaviors.

CHRONIC REJECTION

Parents in dysfunctional families are unable to validate children in healthy ways. Children may be blamed repeatedly for their parents' difficulties, perhaps by grandparents or other family members. Parents may scapegoat children because they resemble hated spouses or members of the extended family. In blended families, a passive biological parent may allow the child to be abused or driven from the home by a stepparent. The biological parent may also accuse the child of deliberately causing problems in the new marriage. Recurring physical or verbal abuse communicate to the child that he or she is unlovable and unacceptable. In other families, children may simply be ignored, neglected, or abandoned. Of course, these parental sins of omission also communicate rejection and thereby undermine the development of self-esteem. In families characterized by extreme forms of denial, children who express themselves directly may be repeatedly punished and labeled as "spoiled," "too emotional," or even "crazy".

We assume that, if left to their own devices, children will internalize the blame for any rejection they experience at the hands of parents or other caretakers, largely because they tend to perceive causation in egocentric terms. Moreover, the rejecting or abusing adult may make it clear again and again that his or her actions were directly caused by the child's unacceptable personality and/or behavior, thereby assuring that the youngster will develop a sense of intrinsic badness. Both children and adolescents can become locked in endlessly repeating cycles of misbehavior and rejection that are extremely difficult to interrupt, as any family therapist knows.

Children in dysfunctional families may also be rewarded by caretakers for the wrong attributes and the wrong actions, thereby cementing into place self-esteem issues and skewed coping strategies that can produce a range of negative effects for years to come. A parentified child, for example, may receive praise only when she comes to mother's rescue by taking care of her siblings. In a disengaged, emotionally distant alcoholic family, the children may secure a greater degree of involvement from the parents only when they draw unwanted attention to the family by acting out in the community at large. Children in such families who conform, or who act up in a less obtrusive manner, may simply be ignored.

When incest or sexual abuse occurs in the home, the child may receive some scant nurturance or approval from the perpetrator, but the positive elements come wrapped in a degrading package. Children may continue to participate in sexually abusive activities, motivated solely by a desire for the rudimentary sense of closeness or approval the experiences offer, thus setting the stage for powerful feelings of worthlessness and self-blame later in life. In highly punitive and/or physically abusive families, parents may tend to favor certain children over their siblings, or at least spare them from the most severe forms of discipline. Like their abused siblings, these "favored" children also pay a price later on in life. Having been rewarded with relative safety from physical abuse in exchange for their compliance and their silence, these children may become chronically avoidant of conflict and confrontation later in life. Moreover, they may experience chronic feelings of worthlessness that stem from "survivor guilt." As adults, they may report having felt responsible for the abuse their siblings had received.

Some children from dysfunctional families are fortunate enough to find people outside the home who will take a sincere interest in them. A teacher, a coach, a therapist, or even a friend's parent may attempt to provide the kind of validation lacking in the home. Although we would agree that a caring person can make a real difference in a youngster's life, it is rare, in our opinion, to encounter such surrogate parents who truly wish to serve the *child's* interests, without an underlying agenda of a more selfish nature. Further, the child's ability to benefit from nurturance outside the family may be limited by feelings of disloyalty, as well as by outright interference from the family. Parents may deeply resent any of the child's relationships outside the home, particularly those that involve positive interactions with other authority figures. If there are shameful secrets in the family such as incest or physical abuse, the parents may strongly censure and actively sabotage children's efforts to bond with alternative caregivers. The child who continues to pursue relationships with surrogate parental figures under such circumstances will do so at the cost of ongoing criticism, punishment, and even abuse in the home, along with the feelings of disloyalty and worthlessness that inevitably result.

TRAUMATIC EXPERIENCES

The typical client we treat comes from a family background that any sensible observer would describe as inordinately stressful for the developing child. Our clients are not the type who find themselves in treatment because they were denied violin lessons or summer camp as children. Their stories characteristically involve severe psychopathology on the part of one if not both parents, with a range of resultant disturbances in the childrearing functions. A large percentage of our clients are apt to recall not one, but many, instances from childhood in which they were *afraid for their own lives or the lives of various loved ones.* These individuals were forced to adapt to "chronic emergencies" in their families, in which basic physical and/or psychological survival was a daily issue. Consequently, they learned basic patterns of thinking and behavior under conditions of extreme threat.

As described in a thought-provoking paper by Martin Seligman

(1971), the concept of prepared learning rests on the assumption that each particular species will be preprogrammed or primed to learn responses to certain classes of stimuli during the lifespan, primarily in situations where a threat to survival exists. Episodes of "one-trial classical conditioning," in which, for example, an individual may develop a lifelong phobia as a result of a single experience, may reflect the organism's biologically based readiness to respond to certain basic dangers. Seligman argues that in evolutionary terms, a species that is "prepared" to identify and avoid recurring sources of danger in the environment will have a greater ability to survive. In our view, the concept of prepared learning may be extended to help explain how traumatic experiences can alter the trajectory of a youngster's development. Perhaps repeated exposures to dangerous situations, particularly those that involve parents or caretaking adults in the environment, keep children more or less permanently oriented to the avoidance of fearful stimuli. As we discuss in Chapter 3, once avoidance responses are acquired, they are extremely robust, almost to the point of being irreversible. When continued exposure to feared stimuli is unavoidable, such as when individuals with whom the child has constant contact are involved, then the youngster must develop increasingly sophisticated cognitive and behavioral strategies to avoid harm, or at least the expectation of harm. As a result, complex, fear-based modes of thinking and behavior begin to dominate the child's adjustment to the world at large.

In objective terms, how threatening do conditions have to become, or how often do they have to occur, in order to make a lasting impact on the developing child? Surely every child who experiences corporal punishment, for example, does not become scarred for life as a result. Likewise, we are certain that children can and do recover psychologically from events such as loss of a parent, or sexual molestation by someone outside the nuclear family, without the benefit of professional help. It should be noted, however, that typically our clients report *multiple* episodes of trauma or victimization of *varying types* at the hands of *multiple perpetrators*. Along with Brown (1988), we would have reservations about asserting that all adult survivors of families with pathology such as alcoholism suffer from posttraumatic stress disorder. On the other hand, like other clinicians (Courtois, 1988; Ochberg, 1988; Walker, 1991), we have found it helpful to conceptualize and to treat certain clients as victims of trauma. We fear that some clients with whom we have worked successfully in such a manner would have been labeled as personality disordered by other therapists, resulting in far more negative implications for prognosis and treatment.

Let us return to the literature on sexual abuse for some further clues as to the impact of traumatic experiences on the developing child. Browne and Finkelhor (1986), in a comprehensive review of research on the impact of child sexual abuse, including incest, found that victims as a group showed greater short-term and long-term psychological impairment than nonvictims. They noted that although extreme effects were not inevitable, the risk of initial and lasting effects is significant and should be taken seriously.

In a well-designed study of female incest victims drawn from a randomly selected community sample, Russell (1986) found considerable variability in subjects' reports of experienced trauma. Approximately one-fourth of subjects reported serious lasting effects, one-fourth some effects, one-fourth little effects, and one-fourth no lasting effects. Russell's data also suggested that the most serious aftereffects occurred when the abuse: (1) was of longer duration and greater frequency; (2) was perpetrated by closer relatives (e.g., fathers); (3) involved a greater age difference between the victim and perpetrator; (4) was perpetrated by males; (5) involved coercion or force; and (6) involved penetration.

It seems reasonable to assume that children who experience some sort of victimization in the extrafamilial world have a reduced risk of subsequent psychological problems when compared to youngsters who have been victimized by members of their own families, particularly parents or caretakers. When parenting functions are more or less intact, the child who has been victimized outside the home has an opportunity to receive the nurturance, validation, and if necessary, the psychological help, necessary to resolve the trauma. The parents do not repeatedly blame the child for the trauma, nor do they have difficulty protecting him or her from further abuse. They are willing to take any steps necessary to insure the safety of their child. Moreover, the child does not feel responsible for assisting the parents to resolve *their* feelings about the traumatic episode.

Russell (1986) noted, however, that her results may have been affected by a tendency on the part of many of her subjects to minimize the effects of their abuse. Indeed, the tendency for victims to minimize or deny a history of abuse is a thorny problem for researchers and clinicians alike, one that we discuss at length in Chapters 6, 7, and 9. Courtois (1988) writes eloquently of the denial processes that can stimulate historical revisionism on the part of incest survivors:

> In order to survive their experiences of repeated and progressive abuse and to cope with the double binds found in many incestuous families, incest victims deny, dissociate, and repress the abuse and their reactions to it. This disconnection or blunting is a survival strategy which often persists into adulthood. It may be quite functional in allowing the victim

to cope, but it also masks reactions to the trauma and prevents resolution. Additionally, it causes incest survivors to appear asymptomatic or less injured when in reality they are emotionally deadened as part of the trauma response. (p. 94)

In our practice, we are no longer surprised when clients are unable to recall childhood episodes of physical or sexual abuse on intake, only to report vivid intrusive memories of such traumatic experiences during subsequent treatment. Consequently, we cannot place total faith in the histories we initially obtain from our clients, particularly if they are newcomers to the intensive self-exploration associated with psychotherapy. Moreover, we suspect that the available research probably underestimates the incidence of child abuse and neglect in our society.

In our clinical experience, isolated incidents of a traumatic nature in childhood may not, in and of themselves, necessarily produce the kinds of recurring life difficulties experienced by our typical clients, particularly if the youngster is fortunate enough to live in a supportive family environment. However, it is important to remember that for many of our clients, the *entire interpersonal context,* including nuclear family, extended family, neighborhood, and in some cases even the subculture in which they spent their formative years, included multiple traumatic and/or victimizing elements. In many instances, the structure and functioning of the nuclear family were not adequate to shield the developing child from the effects of ongoing stress and recurring victimization outside the home. Thus, the effects of trauma or victimization on the child would only be amplified by rejection or other destructive processes within the family.

In the course of treatment, some of our clients will rediscover instances of childhood trauma, particularly sexual abuse. Often these clients will recall some of the physical details of the sexual abuse before they can identify the perpetrators. In their attempts to identify the perpetrators of sexual abuse, clients will begin to think back to the kinds of individuals they encountered regularly in the neighborhood, at extended family gatherings, and at religious or civic observances. It can be quite shocking to hear a client report that the childhood milieu contained not one or two, but as many as a dozen or more potential perpetrators.

DISTORTED COGNITIONS

As Beck (1976) and others (Beck & Emery, 1985; Beck & Freeman, 1990; Guidano & Liotti, 1983) have described, many forms of psychopathology are associated with distortions in thinking. We assume that impaired parents suffer from a range of cognitive distortions, including mistaken perceptions of self and others, maladaptive notions regarding marriage and family life, and superstitious beliefs about the world around them. Not surprisingly, impaired parents facilitate the development of similarly distorted thinking patterns in their offspring, directly, through explicit communications and modeling, and indirectly, through the style of relationships they establish within the family. Later in this chapter we discuss in considerable detail the impact of the dysfunctional family on the youngster's beliefs about the self, others, the world, and interpersonal relationships.

Clinicians from various orientations have described in considerable detail the ways in which attentional processes can be misdirected in dysfunctional family systems (Black, 1981; Brown, 1988; Courtois, 1988; Minuchin, 1974; Satir, 1967). That is, family members may habitually, and perhaps obsessively, focus on certain topics, such as the misbehavior or messiness of the children, while denying or minimizing other problems of a serious nature, such as alcoholism or severe marital conflict. Parents stimulate the development of maladaptive information-processing habits in children directly through explicit injunctions ("Just put your worries about Dad out of your mind"), reinforcement contingencies, and modeling, and indirectly, through the style of relationships they establish within the family. In Chapter 3 we discuss information-processing difficulties, including maladaptive patterns of overvigilance and denial, in considerable detail.

DISTORTED COMMUNICATIONS

Parents in dysfunctional families may model a lack of appropriate assertive skills, as they find themselves victimized again and again by their spouses, their children, and others outside the home. On the other hand, some family members may communicate directly, but in an aggressive, destructive manner, with negative consequences for all involved. Needless to say, the child who follows the path of either the extremely unassertive or the highly aggressive parent will experience severe relationship problems later in life.

Many family systems theorists and therapists (e.g., Bowen, 1966; Minuchin, 1974; Satir, 1967, 1972; Watzlawick, Beavin, & Jackson, 1967; Wynne, Jones, & Al-Khayyal, 1982) have described a range of communicational difficulties that characterize dysfunctional families. Parents who engage in cross-generational coalitions, recruiting their children into alliances against spouses, grandparents, or other family members, will characteristically burden youngsters with too much information of an anxiety-provoking, highly personal nature. Moreover, such triangulation inducts the child into a labyrinthine communicational world, routinely characterized by secrets, deception, and manipulation. These children learn backstage strategies for orchestration and control, not direct methods for confronting issues. Likewise, although some clinicians have vastly overestimated the role of double-binding family communication patterns in the etiology of mental illness (Bateson, Jackson, Haley, & Weakland, 1956), it is also clear that such interactional styles severely tax the psychological resources of children and adolescents, let alone adults. For example, a youngster may be told by her mother that since her father is a hopeless gambler and a philanderer, a divorce is imminent. A day or two later, she may see her parents behaving amorously with one another, while the mother indicates nonverbally that she does not wish to be reminded of their previous discussion. Similarly, a young boy might be told indignantly by his parents that he is loved on the one hand, whereas on the other hand, he experiences criticism and rejection at every turn. It seems reasonable to assume that children who consistently receive such contradictory messages from their parents may well grow up with a few communicational deficits of their own. Moreover, they might also experience understandable difficulty trusting their judgments when, as adults, they encounter mixed messages and questionable motives in significant relationships.

As other clinicians have noted repeatedly (Black, 1981; Brown, 1988), members in dysfunctional families are apt to collude with one another to avoid open discussion of critical topics, particularly those that concern parental impairment such as alcoholism. Children may receive severe rejection or punishment if they violate the family norms of denial and secrecy by raising forbidden topics within the household or worse, by disclosing information to outsiders. In families where denial processes are particularly strong, children may find that their complaints of ill health, emotional distress, academic difficulties, or even physical or sexual abuse are minimized, disbelieved, or simply ignored by the parents. Some children may learn under such circumstances that the safest course is merely to withdraw, whereas others may learn to "turn up the emotional volume" by acting out one way or another, in order to elicit a response from the parents.

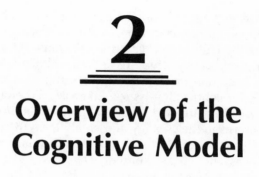

2

Overview of the Cognitive Model

This chapter reviews components of the traditional cognitive model that have remained central in our thinking. In outlining the basic theoretical framework, we define "cognitions" and describe the relationships among cognitions, emotions, and behaviors. We familiarize the reader with the concept of cognitive distortions, and illustrate how underlying schema guide patterns of thinking, feeling, and behaving.

GENERAL PROPERTIES OF COGNITIONS

In our usage, the term "cognitions" refers to any aspect of the stream of mentation. Under the rubric of cognitions, we include schemas, which are basic beliefs about the self, others, and relationships. Basic schemas, along with rules for processing information, may not be readily identifiable during the early stages of treatment, either to the client or to the therapist, but may be embedded or implicit in the behaviors the individual presents.

Like other cognitive therapists, we characteristically work with the client's "self-talk." However, we are well aware that most of our clients do not think in an orderly, grammatical sequence of phrases, sentences, or paragraphs. *We assume that each client's inner dialogue is a highly idiosyncratic mix of symbols, images, telegraphic phrases, personal abbreviations, quotations from significant others, and so on, all moving rapidly in and out of the perceptual foreground.* Consequently, we are vitally interested in gaining access to multiple modes of thought on the part of our clients. Any good cognitive therapist will inquire about the spontaneous, idiosyncratic imagery the client experiences, as well as the symbols or metaphors he or she characteristically uses. The client's responses to novels, films, music, and other artistic works may be far more informative at times than more direct responses to the therapist's questions. Likewise, the cognitive therapist should be willing and able to utilize dream and fantasy material with certain clients, particularly during periods of trauma revelation, as we discuss in Chapter 11.

Most cognitions are associated with a certain *degree of belief*. The individual's level of belief in a particular idea will often determine his or her openness to alternative points of view. When degree of belief is at or near 100%, as is the case with delusions, for example, the individual will remain impervious to any and all competing ideas. Therapists who work with schizophrenics learn quickly not to challenge delusions. To our knowledge, no one has ever used cognitive restructuring to change the content of a delusion. In our clinical work, we find that clients who are far from psychotic will also reveal important beliefs that are every bit as rigid and immutable as delusions. When the cognitions in question are central to the client's distress, the clinician may not be able to address the accuracy or appropriateness of the ideas in a direct manner without arousing defensiveness or otherwise damaging the therapeutic collaboration. Instead of confronting the *validity* of certain beliefs, the therapist may choose to focus on their *utility*, their impact on the client. The therapist may also back off the topic entirely in favor of addressing less strongly held beliefs.

As our clients regularly demonstrate, individuals are capable of holding contradictory or incompatible beliefs simultaneously. The client who states, "I believe it intellectually but not emotionally," is really saying that he or she has a relatively low degree of belief in one set of cognitions and a much higher level of belief in a competing set of ideas. Another example that illustrates the presence of competing belief systems within the individual involves suicide attempters, the majority of whom reported the presence of *both* a wish to live and a wish to die at the time of their self-destructive actions (Kovacs & Beck, 1977). We consistently find that the belief systems of our clients are both complex and multidimensional, as we discuss below.

The therapist needs to assess carefully the *consistency* (or inconsistency) of the client's thinking. The individual's degree of belief in certain cognitions may fluctuate sharply from one situation to another depending on a variety of contextual factors, including degree of emotional arousal, perception of threat, level of interpersonal conflict, and so on. Likewise, the relative strengths of two or more competing belief systems may change, so that one mode of thinking may appear to gain ascendency in one situation, whereas another set of ideas may influence the individual more strongly in a different context. It is vital for the therapist to gain an understanding of the client's thinking not only during times of distress but also during any periods of more successful functioning, as some of our clients with the lowest self-esteem may still experience a sense of personal worth, however fleeting, in certain situations. By monitoring situational fluctuations in the client's thinking and emotional arousal, the therapist may determine the optimal timing for interventions aimed at particular beliefs. During sessions when the client's thinking is more rational or realistic, the therapist should take the opportunity to review material that might have elicited defensive reactions in the past or to anticipate cognitive distortions that may occur in the future.

Clinicians need to remember that interpersonal transactions, including those that occur in the therapeutic relationship, can exert a powerful influence on belief systems. Many of our clients exhibit patterns of thinking that emerge only in specific relationships (e.g., intimate relationships or authority relationships) or during certain types of interactions (e.g., situations that involve conflict or being blamed). We assume that in the process of therapy events within the treatment situation itself can (and usually do) trigger dysfunctional cognitions that are characteristic of the client in other relationships. Moreover, the therapist may inadvertently stimulate the client to *increase* his or her degree of belief in certain self-defeating ideas. As Brehm (1966) outlined in his theory of psychological reactance, an individual who feels as if his or her *right* to hold a particular belief is being attacked will respond by clinging even more strongly to that belief.

RELATIONSHIPS AMONG COGNITIONS, EMOTIONS, AND BEHAVIORS

Cognitions and Emotions

According to Lazarus (1991), there is no hard evidence that emotions, including those commonly assumed to be produced by physical or drug-induced conditions, occur in the absence of mediating cognitions. He contends, therefore, that there is clarity and parsimony to the position that cognitive mediation is necessary and sufficient for emotion to occur. The opposing view, which argues for the primacy of affect over cognition, is best represented by Zajonc (1980, 1984). According to Greenberg and Safran (1989), however, the traditional distinctions among cognitions, emotions, and behaviors are rapidly breaking down, replaced by more integrative information-processing models of human behavior (e.g., Buck, 1985; Lang, 1985; Levanthal, 1979, 1984). These models emphasize the adaptive nature of emotional responses and regard emotion as a biologically wired-in form of information about the self in interaction with the environment. Emotional responses provide continuous feedback about the organism's preparedness to engage in particular actions.

While ongoing research efforts attempt to clarify the precise nature of the cognition–emotion–behavior relationships, we continue to find it clinically useful to assume that emotional and behavioral responses to situations are mediated by perceived meanings or cognitions (Beck, 1976). However, we believe that therapists will regularly find exceptions to the rule, exceptions that *do* involve physiological or neurological problems on the part of their clients. Individuals who suffer from biologically based mental disorders, such as schizophrenia and manic–depressive illness, may show emotions without the expected precipitating cognitions. Alcoholics and other substance abusers alter their moods regularly through the chemicals they ingest. It is not always possible to determine exactly what an intoxicated person is thinking, although his or her emotions might be all too obvious. Likewise, a host of purely medical problems, such as endocrine malfunctions, seem to produce and maintain dysphoric emotional states independent of cognitive processes. Therapists must be wary of postulating a psychological etiology for every client's symptoms, including dysphoric emotions. In fact, an apparent lack of connection between emotion and meaning, between affective symptoms and current psychological stressors, should alert the therapist to the possibility that something may be medically wrong with the client.

In order to understand the individual's emotional response in a given situation, we must understand the accompanying cognitions or, in other words, the idiosyncratic personal meaning of the event to the individual. As we discussed in the preceding section, the designation "personal meaning" refers to the entire range of the individual's mentation, including symbolism and imagery. When an individual appears to overreact emotionally to a situation, we generally assume that the personal meaning of the experience contains distorted components. Beck and his associates (Beck, 1976; Beck & Emery, 1985; Beck, Rush, Shaw & Emery, 1979; Beck & Freeman, 1990; Bedrosian and Beck, 1980; Burns, 1980) have described in great detail the typical cognitive distortions that accompany problematic affective responses such as depression and anxiety (see sections on cognitive distortions below). Why the distortions in meaning take place is a separate issue, one that is crucial to the long-term prevention of psychological distress. We typically assume that basic schemas and information-processing strategies acquired in childhood often must change in order to produce durable changes in the cognitive distortions in adult clients.

The cognitive model explicitly disavows a "hydraulic" viewpoint of emotion. In our opinion, emotions do not accumulate in some sort of reservoir inside the individual, nor do they invade the musculature or the internal organs. Unexpressed affect does not "back up" on the individual, like sewage in an obstructed septic system. The symptoms associated with individuals who fail to experience or express normal emotions result from defective reality testing, poor self-esteem, problematic relationships, and the like, not *from an* absence *of* affect per se. For example, from our perspective, chronically unassertive individuals will experience depression as a result of the recurring victimization and chronic helplessness that characterize their lives, not as a result of "retroflected rage."

Other than those exceptional instances that involve the kind of biochemical difficulties we discussed previously, emotions occur only as a consequence of the individual's experience of a given situation. If an individual continues to relive a situation in exactly the same way, we assume that he or she will continue to experience similar emotional responses to it. Certain experiences in our lives will always be painful or tragic, even though we may have diminished their impact on our day-to-day functioning. Not surprisingly, the authors have little faith in the curative powers of catharsis or abreaction, particularly in the absence of explicit learning on the part of the client. Moreover, the effects of powerful experiences, such as incest, or the loss of a loved one, are too complex to be understood or digested, let alone accepted, "on the first pass." From a cognitive perspective, affective responses to major life events, such as the loss of a loved one, persist over time because the bereaved individual continues to process additional meanings and implications long after the precipitating event. As we discuss in Chapter 11, clients who experience "flashbacks" or "anniversary reactions" in response to losses or traumatic experiences may find it reassuring to know that there is a rational explanation for their intense, potentially disruptive emotional responses.

The basic cognitive model assumes that changes in cognitive distortions and underlying schemas will produce relief from dysphoric affect and other psychological symptoms. The typical cognitive therapist probably tends to gravitate toward the affective *excesses* of the client, as he or she works with the individual to identify and change the ideation which accompanies the unpleasant emotions in question. As our treatment model has evolved, we have found ourselves focusing more and more on those instances when the dysphoric affect one would normally expect in response to a distressing situation fails to occur. We believe that affective *deficits*, like affective excesses, often reflect significant distortions in thinking on the part of our clients. *In the cognitive model, the absence of the expected or appropriate emotional response to a particular stimulus reflects information-processing difficulties and/or distortions in meaning, rather than the direct repression or blockage of affect.* Affective deficits often provide important clues about the cognitive foundations of the individual's current distress, particularly in the area of interpersonal relationships. As we illustrate with a variety of case examples, many of our clients consistently fail to process vital data, information that would typically elicit anger, anxiety, and other powerful emotional responses from less impaired individuals. Consequently, these clients may make themselves unduly vulnerable to various forms of victimization in relationships. We shall spend considerable time is Chapters 3, 6, 7, 9, and 11 discussing the assessment and remediation of such denial processes in our clients.

Once stimulated through any means, emotions may then exert secondary influences on the individual's cognitive processes in a number of ways (Beck & Emery,1985; Easterbrook, 1959). Beck & Emery (1985) use the term "tunnel vision" to describe the manner in which anxiety narrows the individual's perceptual field. Although anxiety may increase vigilance to certain classes of stimuli, it also hampers performance on more complex intellectual tasks (Korchin, 1964). Anxiety begets narrowly focused attention to feared stimuli, which in turn begets more anxiety. The more the panic-prone person attends to the palpitations or the hyperventilation, the worse the symptoms and the accompanying fear become. In the meantime, the individual fails to process information that might reduce anxiety or, in some cases, might indicate other legitimate sources of danger that requiring attention. Even moderate amounts of anxiety or tension may produce similar effects on cognitive performance, particularly when complex, intellectually demanding activities are involved. For example, as therapists, we consistently find that we make unexpected errors in treating clients when we become so anxious about potential negative developments, such as premature termination, that we ignore other potentially important considerations.

The *occurrence* of affect also gives rise to significant perceptions and interpretations on the individual's part, which in turn affect subsequent feelings and behaviors. Anxiety again provides an obvious example of the continuous feedback loop between cognitions and emotions. Once the individual begins to feel the symptoms of anxiety, particularly the signs of autonomic arousal, he or she will make inferences about the experience (e.g., "I won't be able to tolerate this," "I will have a heart attack," "I will go crazy," and so on.). Understandably, such cognitions serve to perpetuate, and perhaps even intensify, the feelings of anxiety. Clients who have been exposed to a mentally ill parent, or one with a history of violent behavior, may be particularly frightened when they experience intense anxiety, anger, or sadness primarily because they have vivid and disturbing images of the actions such emotions might stimulate. Likewise, some clients develop a sense of guilt or worthlessness, when they experience intense emotions, particularly anger, directed at spouses or family members. They may see themselves as disloyal to their families for even having certain thoughts and emotions, and may be fearful that their angry feelings will inevitably lead to destructive interactions with important people in their lives. Similarly, some of our clients have no concept of the normal role of affect in everyday life. Consequently, they may view a totally normal emotional experience, such as grief over the death of a loved one, as a sign of pathology or personal weakness. As we detail in Chapter 3, such clients may utilize denial mechanisms as a means of preventing the occurrence of troubling negative emotions, only to lose additional vital information in the process.

For many of our clients, emotions, particularly the negative ones, seem to occur as if they were unrelated to either meaning or context. Early in treatment, such individuals may not readily identify either cognitions or situations that trigger certain troublesome emotional responses. This is not surprising, for a few significant reasons. *First of all, we assume that the human mind is capable of extremely rapid internal transmission of information and ideas, particularly when the relevant concepts have been encoded in symbolic form.* Our clinical experiences have led us to conclude that personal imagery and symbolism, rich in meanings and implications, have the capacity to produce *almost instantaneous changes* in the individual's emotions and behaviors. Many of our clients have never learned to observe or articulate their most basic inner experiences, let alone those that occur in a rapid-fire sequence. Moreover, if the chain of cognitions or imagery culminates in other compelling thoughts, powerful emotions, and/or impulsive behaviors, the individual may be so distracted by the results that he or she cannot even attend to ideational precipitants. However, just as repeated listenings enable us to grasp the subtleties of a fast-paced piece of music, so does practice in self-observation enhance the ability of our clients to recognize rapid sequences of dysfunctional thoughts and imagery.

Cognitions and Behavior

Many of the statements we made in the previous section regarding the connections between cognition and affect also hold true for the relationship between thinking and behavior. We assume that cognitions, particularly basic schemas, form the foundation of the individual's behavior in all areas of life.

We do concede, however, that it may be hard at times to believe that the behavior of our fellow human beings is connected to thinking of any kind!

Cognitions and Family Systems

The authors maintain that there is virtually no conflict between a cognitive perspective and a family systems orientation when it comes to understanding the lives of our clients. We insist that the clinician needs to utilize *both* levels of conceptualization in order to assess the impact of family of origin dysfunction on the client. Further, as we illustrate in succeeding chapters, individual treatment should be conducted with systems dynamics and goals in mind, while family and marital therapies need to include close attention to the cognitive barriers that impede systemic change. Because of space limitations, the present volume focuses primarily on individual treatment. However, the authors find that couples therapy, which usually addresses many of the same issues targeted in our individual treatment model, provides a unique and powerful recovery vehicle for adults who grew up in dysfunctional families. Many, in fact perhaps the majority, of the cases we present in this volume were involved in both individual and marital or family sessions at different times in the course of treatment.

In our view, every relevant parameter of family structure or dynamics (e.g., scapegoating, boundary violations, coalitions, sibling roles, and so on) directly influences the development of basic beliefs about the self, others, the world, and relationships. Likewise, we assume that pathological relationship patterns in the client's current life are maintained by distorted belief systems and deficiencies in information processing. Once acquired, basic patterns of thinking and behavior determine the manner in which the individual develops relationships outside the nuclear family. As we discuss later in greater detail, schemas and information-processing styles "tune" the individual to receive and resonate with certain stimuli in the environment, particularly in the arena of relationships. The individual may be most strongly attracted to others who will participate in relationship dynamics reminiscent of certain features of the family of origin. Many of our clients put themselves in painful or victimizing relationships again and again throughout their entire lives, while others become victims in relationships they did not necessarily choose (e.g., supervisor–supervisee) but fail to take appropriate actions to protect themselves.

Our clients often engage in repetitive cycles of interaction with the significant people in their lives which resonate with the cognitive distortions and basic issues of each participant. The process of *resonance* in a marital or family system keeps threat high and behavioral flexibility low, so that individuals continue to participate in the same dysfunctional transactions again and again, in a stereotyped fashion, with the same distressing results. Moreover, the basic belief systems and information-processing styles of spouses, close friends, and other participants in significant relationships may interlock in a complementary, but ultimately destructive, fashion. Consequently, ongoing relationship problems often only serve to reinforce cognitive distortions on the part of everyone involved, while basic assumptions tend to remain unchallenged. For example, many of our clients who habitually assume excessive responsibility for the behavior of others often seem to pair up with individuals who characteristically externalize blame for their actions. When problems occur in their intimate relationships, these clients become so easily preoccupied with trying to determine what *they* did wrong that they never successfully confront the behavior of their partners.

As we discuss in greater detail in Chapter 3, the escalating demands of developing families, particularly those with young children or adolescents, increase the pressure on individuals and relationships, often resulting in the symptoms that lead to a referral for mental health services. Since we draw strongly on a family systems perspective at all times, no matter what treatment modality we are working in, the authors generally expect to find family systems pathology when we encounter an individual client. At this point in our clinical practice we find ourselves pleasantly surprised on those occasions when we are able to conclude that the client's primary relationships are relatively positive ones. Many of our clients can benefit from marital or family therapy, if not at the time of the initial presentation for treatment, then at some time in the future. Often, one of the most significant functions of individual therapy is to move the client to a point of readiness for family or marital treatment. In succeeding chapters, we discuss how effective cognitive work will often provide the client with the ability to articulate and sustain a posture that facilitates more effective confrontation of marital or family problems. The resultant destabilization in the family system may then culminate in prodding hitherto resistant spouses or other family members into participation in treatment.

THE ROLE OF SCHEMA

The concept of *schema* has been used in diverse contexts and with considerable variation in meaning in developmental and cognitive theory. According to Stiles et al. (1990), a schema is "a familiar pattern of ideas, a way of thinking to which new experiences can become assimilated. It is a generic term that may refer to a tightly organized theory, a metaphor, a narrative or script, or a more loosely organized network of associations, incorporating both mental content and patterns of action" (p. 412). Drawing from Piaget (1962, 1970), Stiles and colleagues explain that when a schema assimilates a new experience, it integrates, explains, and incorporates the novel data into a system of associations. Experiences that are disequilibrating, inconsistent, or incongruent, however, may remain partly or wholly unassimilated depending on the degree of psychological pain associated with the events in question. Similarly, the more painful the event, the more powerful and rigid the coping strategies designed to avoid it. On the premise that such avoidance strategies contribute to the maintenance of symptoms, Stiles and colleagues view the optimal treatment situation as one that can *sustain the client's attention* on such negative experiences so that they can be explained, understood, and ultimately mastered.

If successful treatment ultimately involves mastering negative experiences, how does the clinician know which of an often vast array of bad experiences to focus on? A recent trend in the cognitive therapy literature has begun to address this question by exploring the distinctions between core, or central, and peripheral cognitive processes or schemas (Safran, Vallis, Segal, & Shaw, 1986). According to Safran et al. (1986), core cognitive processes are those that relate directly to the individual's definition and experience of the self. These processes can be distinguished from cognitive operations of a peripheral nature by their ability to predict an individual's reactions to a wide range of situations. Changes in the perception of reality that do not affect one's basic self-attitude (but might result in temporary symptom relief) are said to be "surface" in nature. Enduring therapeutic change, or "deep" change, is hypothesized to occur only when the individual's core of tacit self-knowledge has been altered (Guidano & Liotti, 1983). Although our model certainly stresses the primary importance of beliefs about the self, we would assert that long-term therapeutic benefits also result from specific changes in beliefs about others, the world, and relationships, as well as from alterations in the individual's information-processing strategies.

We find that the basic beliefs of our clients reveal themselves in unique, multidimensional configurations. From our clinical experiences, it would appear that the actual structure and overlapping organization of thought are exceedingly complicated and most certainly complex beyond global descriptive terms such as "shame" or "codependency." True, there are consistent themes that seem to appear again and again, but we are continually fascinated by the cognitive complexity of our clients, even those who have major difficulties in life functioning. Although many of our clients tend to view matters in rigid, all-or-nothing terms, they are nonetheless capable of holding mutually contradictory beliefs about a range of important matters, for example, suicide (Kovacs & Beck, 1977). Even clients with the worst self-esteem difficulties have isolated pockets of competency and self-worth, pockets we can find if we take the time and effort to map out the territory. We admire any behavioral scientist who attempts to define the content and/or structure of schemas (e.g., Young, 1990), but we readily acknowledge that undertaking or evaluating such efforts is far beyond our capabilities. Not surprisingly, we never think in terms of one "central conflict" in our assessment of clients, and we seldom, if ever, address just a single cognitive mechanism at any given time in treatment. As our clinical examples indicate, we find it useful to work with many different domains of the individual's belief systems in the course of treatment, often simultaneously and in varying combinations over time.

Beliefs about the Self

Beliefs about the self serve as the foundation for everything the individual seeks to accomplish in all areas of life. We assume that the strongest determinants of the child's view of the self will always be his or her interactions with parents or other caretakers. Needless to say, school adjustment, peer relationships, and interactions with other authority figures in the community will also influence the child's self-image, but, in our opinion, to a much smaller extent. We have found that beliefs about the self are idiosyncratically organized and articulated by each individual. Moreover, the self-schema of each individual will present a unique combination of themes, each of which may deserve consideration in treatment.

Let us describe a number of important themes addressed by the individual's basic beliefs about the self:

- Identification, both positive and negative, with parents or other family members
- Sex-role identification
- Sexual identity
- Body image and physical attractiveness
- Sexual desirability and/or sexual performance
- Social or interpersonal desirability
- Academic or vocational ability and/or performance
- Perceptions of affective responses and one's affective response tendencies, particularly regarding anger and/or anxiety

- Assessments and expectations of the reliability or validity of one's judgments and interpretations
- Assessments of one's normalcy, in physical, psychological, emotional, and/or social terms
- Perceptions of locus of control over significant life events
- Perceptions of responsibility for the behaviors of self and others
- Evaluations of moral or ethical track record
- Perceptions of sin, wrongdoing, or blameworthiness

Beliefs about Others and the World

We assume that early experiences in the family constitute the primary data base for the child's beliefs about other persons as well as the world at large. Parents and caretaking figures pass along their own superstitions and religious or philosophical beliefs to their children, perhaps much more effectively than do churches, schools, and other institutions.

Let us describe a number of important themes addressed by the individual's basic beliefs about others and the world:

- Perceptions of victimization at the hands of others
- Perceptions of the judgments and evaluations of the self made by others
- Expectations regarding the potential for rejection at the hands of others
- Expectations of physical and/or psychological harm at the hands of others
- Expectations regarding the effects of the emotional reactions of others
- Expectations regarding the competency, maturity, reliability, and/or psychological health of others
- Expectations regarding changes in the thoughts, feelings, and behaviors of significant others, and the manner by which such changes will occur
- Interpretations of the motivations, desires, and/or moral values of others
- Causal attributions for the thoughts, feelings, or behavior of others
- Idiosyncratic stereotypes regarding sex roles, sexual preference, race, ethnicity, religious affiliation, age, socioeconomic level, and/or authority status
- Perceptions of the forces of culture, economics, and/or sociopolitical institutions and their impact on the self and others

- Expectations of physical danger in the impersonal environment
- Perceptions of the "cosmic order" and its potential impact on the self and others

Beliefs about Relationships

Cognitions about relationships clearly dovetail with self-schemas and beliefs regarding others. Most of our clients probably could not articulate their basic beliefs about relationships if they were asked to do so on intake. The therapist generally must generate inferences about relationship schemas based on the client's history of interactions with significant others.

Let us describe a number of important themes addressed by the individual's basic beliefs about relationships:

- Norms regarding the appropriate expression of conflict and anger
- Norms regarding self-assertion
- Norms regarding the appropriate level of physical and/or psychological involvement in various types of relationships
- Norms regarding physical and/or psychological privacy
- Norms regarding self-disclosure in various types of relationships
- Norms regarding secrecy and coalitions in family or spousal relationships
- Norms regarding deception in relationships
- Norms regarding orchestration or manipulation, for any purpose, in relationships
- Expectations regarding equity or reciprocity of rewards in relationships
- Expectations that define the minimally acceptable treatment or degree of gratification in a relationship
- Expectations regarding the role and nature of sexuality in relationships
- Rules governing the assignment of culpability or responsibility in relationships
- Rules prescribing the proper maintenance of family or spousal loyalty
- Expectations regarding intergenerational relationships in families
- Expectations regarding the nature of hierarchichal relationships in the work setting

Cognitive Distortions

A series of seminal research studies by Beck (1963, 1964, 1967) and others (see Hollon & Beck, 1979 for a review) has illustrated how the phenomenology of a depressed individual is marked by an array of striking distortions in thinking. Based on his research findings, Beck went on to reconceptualize depression as a *thinking* disorder, rather than an affective one. As he described it, the phenomenology of the depressed person becomes dominated by the "cognitive triad," a negative view of the self, the world, and the future. Beck noted that depressed individuals selectively attend to data that support their negative ideas, while they ignore, minimize, or reject information discrepant with such viewpoints. Consequently, they can become trapped in a vicious cycle of negative thinking and depressed affect, a cycle that begins to appear self-perpetuating or "functionally autonomous" (Allport, 1961).

Later works by Beck and other writers examined the typical cognitive distortions associated with a range of psychological problems, including anxiety and panic disorders (Beck & Emery, 1985), eating disorders (Garner & Bemis, 1982), and marital violence (Bedrosian, 1982). Coming from a somewhat different perspective, Stephanie Brown (1988) and other writers (Black, 1981; Woititz, 1983) have noted the prevalence of cognitive distortions, particularly "black or white thinking" among adult children of alcoholics. David Burns (1980) provides some rather detailed descriptions of various types of cognitive distortions that are often useful for clients to read and digest.

Let us use a whimsical example to illustrate some of the typical kinds of cognitive distortions one might encounter in clinical practice. Suppose a psychologist in private practice delivers a presentation on cognitive therapy to the staff of a nearby psychiatric hospital. He stands at a podium in a small conference room. About 30 people are present, most of them seated. Those in the front of the room seem quite interested and attentive. In fact, a number of them take copious notes during the course of the presentation. A few minutes into his prepared remarks however, the psychologist begins to notice an older, well-dressed man, presumably a psychiatrist or a senior staff person, slouching in his chair in the back of the room. He appears to be absorbed in examining the tops of his shoes, with a bored expression on his face. As the presentation continues, his eyes begin to close. Later, his eyelids seem to flutter, suggesting the onset of REM sleep. Despite his efforts to focus on the more attentive members of the audience, the psychologist finds himself unable to ignore the sleeping man (see section on Overvigilance, in Chapter 3). His thoughts during the presentation reveal a number of typical cognitive distortions:

Personalizing/Assuming Excessive Responsibility

> My presentation is so boring, I put the man to sleep.
> If I were more competent or better prepared, he would still be awake.

Mind Reading

> He's probably an analyst.
> He thinks my treatment approach is shallow and superficial.
> He thinks I'm incompetent.

All-or-Nothing Thinking

> If I'm affecting him this way, my presentation must be a total failure.

Overgeneralization

> My presentations are always boring.
> I'm always boring.
> ✗ I bore everyone I know, even my wife and my kids.
> I'm a boring person.
> I'm an incompetent person with very little to offer.

Magnification/Catastrophizing

> Everyone here will realize my presentation is worthless.
> Everyone present will tell all their colleagues and friends how incompetent I am.
> Everyone will hear about this.
> Dr. Beck will find out that I tarnished the image of cognitive therapy.
> My professional reputation will be damaged irrevocably.
> I'll never overcome this humiliation.
> Referrals to my practice will dry up.
> My income will drop precipitously.
> I'll be ruined financially.
> My house will be repossessed.
> My wife and children will leave me.
> I will spend the rest of my days as a broken derelict.

As the previous example indicates, cognitive distortions consist of unwarranted inferences, errors of logic or reasoning, sweeping conclusions that fail to find support in data, and so on. In Chapter 3, we illustrate how core beliefs and cognitive distortions maintain a reciprocal relationship with the individual's basic style of information processing. Whenever the client uses *absolute terms* (e.g., everyone, no one, nothing, everything, always, never, and so on) to describe the self, relationships, or situations, the therapist should suspect the presence of significant distortions in thinking. The individual does not generally doubt the veracity of his or her inferences and conclusions but typically takes most cognitions at face value. Consequently, cognitive distortions may go unchallenged by the individual, while the negative impact on his or her emotions and behaviors continues unabated. We remind the reader that most, if not all, of the distorted ideas expressed by our worried psychologist in the previous example could have been experienced in the form of imagery, as opposed to self-verbalizations, with all the same emotional and behavioral consequences.

Many adult survivors of childhood trauma also reveal cognitive distortions which are more subtle in character. Often the irrational or distorted ideas are difficult to identify at first, partly because they may be deeply embedded in a network of interlocking assumptions on the part of the client. Moreover, as we suggested above, cognitive distortions do not all necessarily result in the experience of painful affect. In fact, the cognitive distortions may serve to prevent emotional distress, at least on a short-term basis. As we describe in Chapter 3, cognitive distortions may often spare the individual from experiencing pain, while they compromise reality testing in the process.

In our view, cognitive distortions are generally the direct outgrowth of dysfunctional schemas and deficiencies in information processing acquired by the individual in his or her family of origin. Schemas and information-processing strategies consistently "stack the deck," by orienting the individual toward stimuli which validate or resonate with basic beliefs about the self, the world, others, and relationships. Meanwhile, the person fails to perceive or process information that challenges the validity of basic assumptions, or simply reinterprets such data in a way that is consistent with core beliefs. For example, suppose a male client has learned in his family of origin that he is worthless or unacceptable in the eyes of his parents. For the rest of his life, he may be preoccupied or obsessed with flaws in his appearance, deficiencies in his personality, and/or defects in his performances in various areas of endeavor. He may attend carefully for signs that others also think he is worthless or defective in some way. He may be prone to personalize the actions of others, so that he may believe that his wife is rejecting him for being inadequate as a lover when, in fact, she truly *does* have a headache. Finally, he might consistently ignore or downplay the significance of his success experiences or instances of positive feedback from others. If pressed he might attribute his success to luck or his popularity to an ability to conceal his true self from others.

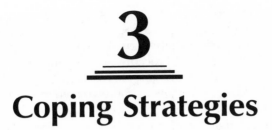

Coping Strategies

FOUNDATIONS OF COPING STRATEGIES: SOLOMON'S DOGS AND TRAUMATIC AVOIDANCE BEHAVIOR

We humans are survivors. We survive through an active process of cognitive and behavioral *adaptation* to those environments in which we find ourselves—however dangerous or threatening they may be. Indeed, the range of human adaptation throughout history speaks to the remarkable ability of our species to adjust to all sorts of adverse conditions when survival is at stake. Even the most helpless child in the most hopelessly victimizing circumstances finds a way to cope, a way to minimize pain and maximize feelings of well-being.

A series of experiments performed nearly 40 years ago by Solomon and his associates (Solomon, 1964; Solomon, Kamin, & Wynne 1953) provide some interesting perspectives on the nature of human coping strategies, particularly those based on trauma-driven learning. Solomon, Kamin et al. (1953) trained dogs in bifurcated metal cages. Once they were presented with a discriminative stimulus, such as a light, the dogs had 10 seconds to jump into the opposite section of the cage. Failure to do so resulted in the application of a very powerful electric shock through the metal grid of the cage. The researchers found that as soon as a single successful avoidance response occurred, the animal never again failed to avoid the shock. As time went on, the dogs continued to produce the avoidance responses more quickly, despite the fact that they no longer remained in the initial side of the cage long enough to receive the shock again. Although conditioned fear in its full-blown form was no longer being experienced by the animal, it clearly continued to "motivate" behavior in a powerful manner.

Not surprisingly, Solomon and his associates found that the dogs did not change their behavior when the electric shock was turned off. When presented with the discriminative stimulus (the light), the animals continued to jump across the cage as before, through hundreds of extinction trials, with the threat of shock no longer present. Elimination of the avoidance responses only occurred when the experimenter instituted special "therapeutic" procedures to retrain the dogs. The dogs stopped making the avoidance responses when they were physically prevented from doing so (e.g., by being restrained in a leather harness). While the dogs were restrained, they displayed many "emotional" behaviors when the light went on, such as urinating, defecating, and crying, until they "learned" that the shocks were no longer forthcoming. Likewise, when the experimenters blocked off the gate to the other half of the cage with a glass partition, the dogs repeatedly threw themselves against it until they "learned" that they were no longer in danger.

One more finding reported by Solomon and his associates should interest the reader. Once the dogs had learned the initial avoidance response, the investigators shocked the animals after they jumped to the other side of the cage. The researchers found that shocking the avoidance response actually resulted in the dog jumping faster and more vigorously into the other side of the cage. Moreover, once it was followed by shock, the avoidance response proved to be even more resistant to extinction than before. These findings should frighten anyone who thinks corporal punishment is a desirable socialization technique for children, as will be discussed below.

How does the research literature on traumatic avoidance learning help us to understand the acquisition of coping strategies on the part of children in dysfunctional families? First of all, the reader should recall our earlier discussion of "prepared learning." Just like the dogs in the cage, children in dysfunctional families often must learn survival strategies in the face of a high level of threat. Seligman (1971) speculates that various species, including humans, are primed biologically to learn how to avoid potentially dangerous stimuli. Solomon's research suggests that humans develop strategies to avoid pain, in part by learning to anticipate its occurrence in advance. We assume that with the advent of language, the child develops the ability to conceptualize the future and plan for various contingencies. The child learns ways to avoid pain, not only in the short term, but in the distant future as well. By remaining vigilant, the child learns to stay ahead of trouble, or at least learns how to maintain the *comforting illusion* of avoiding threat. As we discuss in subsequent sections, information-processing styles, such as overvigilance, are key elements in the individual's repertoire of coping skills.

We assume that as the child matures intellectually, he or she becomes capable of perceiving threat in increasingly abstract *or* symbolic terms through the operation of schemas. Consequently, an adult who has been physically abused in childhood may have transformed a fear of being beaten into a fear of making a mistake, or a fear of being criticized. The possibility of making an error or being criticized may provoke the same level of anxiety in the adult as the threat of being beaten originally elicited in the child. Not surprisingly, the individual may become overly fearful or defensive around authority figures in adulthood and may use coping strategies strongly reminiscent of, if not identical to, those he or she had employed in childhood.

Solomon's experiments help us to understand the genesis and re-markable durability of rituals, superstitions, and other responses the individual comes to associate with the reduction of anxiety or threat. Most of us find it comforting to believe that we can do something to influence the stressful conditions in our lives. We generally prefer to take *some* action, however ineffectual, rather than to remain helpless in the face of life's difficulties. Whereas actual control over stressful life events has been shown to mitigate the negative effects of such circum-stances (Dohrenwend, 1973), a mere belief in control over aversive events may also provide a stress-buffering effect (Glass & Singer, 1972). As we have noted earlier, children are apt to construct egocentric or otherwise distorted causal explanations for significant events in their lives (Elkind, 1974). Not surprisingly then, youngsters who grow up in dysfunctional families may develop active techniques for influencing the circumstances in their homes. These children may have as little power to alter their family dynamics as primitive tribesmen have to induce rain, yet they too may develop superstitions, rituals, or other coping strategies that *to them* seem to have the power to prevent bad things from happening. In our opinion, it is the *perceived efficacy* of an avoidance response or a coping strategy, not the objective outcome, that will determine its acquisition and continued utilization by the child. Although the superstitious behaviors may have little or no effect on the actions of others, they do help to relieve anxiety for the child. Con-sequently, it is not surprising that both the sources of anxiety and the strategies associated with reducing discomfort persist into adulthood. Superstitious behaviors often appear rigid and stereotyped. If the in-dividual is prevented somehow from engaging in the behavior, he or she may experience considerable anxiety, as well as tremendous hos-tility toward the thwarting agent.

An example that illustrates the persistence of superstitious avoid-ance responses into adulthood involves Marsha and Justin, the parents of two preschoolers, who sought treatment for marital problems. One of the presenting complaints involved constant bickering over the house-hold chores. Marsha acknowledged that Justin made sincere efforts to help, but she never felt satisfied with the finished product. Justin com-plained that Marsha was never happy unless things were done precisely her way. He also complained that she would become angry quite un-predictably over minor instances of untidiness on his part or on the children's part. At one point during treatment, Marsha recalled being 10 or 11 years old, alone in the house on a Saturday night, waiting for her alcoholic parents to return home after a night of drinking. She remem-bered meticulously cleaning the house, thinking that her parents would not abuse her or fight with one another if they returned to a clean, orderly home. Whether her strategy actually affected their behavior or not is irrelevant. Cleaning provided her with the *illusion of control* over the disruptive, potentially violent behavior of her parents. It became a ritual that enabled her to reduce her anxiety on Saturday nights, the most volatile and emotionally threatening time in the household. Mar-sha learned to associate the act of cleaning, and the end result of an orderly household, with anxiety reduction and a feeling of comparative safety. Conversely, Marsha learned to associate disarray in the home with the psychological bedlam fostered by her parents. The sight of a dirty or disorganized household was a stimulus to action that she simply could not ignore no matter how hard she tried. When she was thwarted in her attempts to keep a perfect house as an adult, she experienced a state of panic without knowing why. At these moments, she could quickly move from anxiety to agitation to intense anger, often verbally attacking her husband or children in the process.

As we discuss in greater detail in subsequent sections on informa-tion-processing styles, coping strategies are by no means exclusively behavioral in nature. In our view, *traumatic avoidance responses regularly occur on a cognitive level through the various types of denial mechanisms.* Like Solomon's dogs, our clients have learned that they can jump to safety by screening out painful stimuli, by minimizing the significance of threat-ening events, by constructing comforting rationalizations, and so on. Later in this chapter, we describe a number of ways in which denial strategies serve to protect the individual from a range of threatening consequences.

Solomon's research illustrates that once a traumatic avoidance re-sponse develops, the individual is going to keep using it, regardless of changes in contingencies that may have taken place. The individual works so hard to avoid the *occurrence* of punishment or negative con-sequences that he or she never has the opportunity to find out whether the dreaded aversive contingencies are still operative. Clearly many of our adult clients think and behave as if the stressors of childhood, and the fearfulness they may have experienced at that time, were still oper-ative.

On the other hand, the research on traumatic avoidance learning also suggests that fear can continue to motivate behavior in the absence of overt distress on the part of the individual. In response to threat, the individual may develop coping strategies, such as denial, that succeed in reducing anxiety in key situations or classes of situations. However, despite the relative absence of anxious feelings, the individual's outlook and behavior in many key areas of life may be conspicuously fear-based. It is sometimes more useful for the therapist to think in terms of avoidance *patterns* rather than discrete avoidance behaviors. Avoidance patterns can be discerned at times not by identifying specific behaviors but, rather by examining the client's entire life history. Such patterns may not necessarily include explicitly phobic components and may even be associated with areas of life in which the client has achieved great apparent mastery (e.g., career). In fact, the avoidance pattern may be so successful in warding off remote threats, that the individual no longer reaches the stage where he or she experiences any anxiety.

Two examples might serve to illustrate the way in which avoidance patterns endure in the absence of overt distress:

A man with a severe snake phobia relocates to a region where few species of the reptile live in the wild. Instead of moving to the suburbs, he purchases a high-rise condominium in the city, where he is surrounded by a reassuring sea of concrete. He may consistently avoid any outdoor areas he suspects might be the habitats of snakes. Backpacking trips, nature walks, dude ranch vacations, and so on, are all out of the question as leisure time activities as far as he is concerned. Moreover, he might routinely decline all social invitations between April and October, so as to avoid having to attend backyard barbecues. Unless the man unexpectedly finds a python coiled up in the bathtub, he might go for years, and perhaps decades, without ever actually *feeling* anxiety about snakes, despite the fact that he has allowed his phobia to influence many significant parts of his life.

Andy remembered people using terms like "child prodigy" and "boy wonder" to describe him when he was growing up. He began playing the piano before he entered grade school, and by the time he was in his early teens, he was performing as a guest soloist with well-known symphony orchestras. He could sing and act, and despite his heavy practice schedule, he regularly participated in school theatrical productions. He was apparently well-liked by peers of both sexes. Naturally, he was always a top student. Even when he attended a prestigious performing arts program at the university level, his musical abilities placed him head and shoulders above his contemporaries. Unfortunately, Andy's career never fulfilled the incredible promise of his early years. At the age of 30, he was still working in what he considered to be a second-rate orchestra, in a backwater location. He became severely depressed when a personality clash with his conductor led to a request for his resignation. In the course of treatment for his depression, Andy began to examine his history more carefully, particularly his relationship with his physically abusive father. He recalled how, in addition to the frequent and capricious beatings, his father had also rejected him in many ways, even to the point of ridiculing his artistic interests as unmanly. Andy recognized that throughout his childhood and adolescence he had used the piano and his other interests to escape from the verbal and physical violence in the family. His compulsive, perfectionistic work habits were driven not by a love of music, but by a fear that he would amount to nothing in the end, just as his father had predicted. He sought the adulation of an audience, not to feel special, but to fight off chronic feelings of worthlessness. Andy also realized that he had invested a great deal of effort hiding his real self, which he believed was truly unacceptable to others. Even with his closest friends, he always had to be "on"—witty, worldly, and entertaining at all times.

As the previous case example illustrates, the avoidance of a sense of worthlessness can lead to the evolution of complex coping strategies in the course of an individual's life. Among our clients are a number of high-level performers in various fields of endeavor, who are driven not by a deep affection for their work, but by a deep fear of failure. What is failure after all but an exposure of one's worthlessness?

Remember that in Solomon's experiments, even an electric shock, delivered after the animal had jumped, did not disrupt the original avoidance response. It was almost as if the dogs treated the shock delivered after jumping as an entirely separate event, unrelated to the initial traumatic avoidance response. In effect, the initial avoidance response preempted the dog's innate tendency to escape punishment. In order to achieve a sense of physical and/or psychological safety for themselves, our clients also encounter a range of negative consequences. It is important to keep in mind, however, that traumatic avoidance strategies involve driven, compulsive behavior. Like Solomon's dogs, who would throw themselves against an unyielding glass partition in order to jump to the other side of the cage, or were willing to tolerate a powerful electric shock once they got there, our clients are driven to escape threatening stimuli, and are heedless of the cost they may pay in doing so. For example, Marsha, whom we discussed earlier, often found herself engaged in destructive arguments with her husband and her children over housekeeping issues. She regularly felt guilty for the cruel way in which she treated her family during these conflicts, yet she found herself unable to stop the underlying compulsion, the need to keep the house in perfect order at all times.

Our clients may create profound difficulties for themselves through their coping strategies, but like Solomon's dogs, *their primary motivation is still to avoid pain.* In our opinion, it is perverse and entirely unnecessary to postulate that non-psychotic human beings "enjoy" pain or otherwise actively seek suffering as an end in itself. Even the teen-aged girl who repeatedly cuts her arms and legs with a dull razor blade is attempting, albeit in a twisted and destructive manner, to reduce her discomfort. While supervising the clinical work of one of the authors a number of years ago, Aaron T. Beck regularly observed that no one likes being depressed. He noted that when frustrated with a lack of results, some therapists would accuse clients of *choosing* or *wanting* to be de-pressed. Many of our clients wonder if they want or even enjoy the many difficulties in their lives. At times significant people in their lives also suspect them of harboring similar dark motivations. An under-standing of Solomon's research findings often helps such clients view their own motivations in a far more constructive light, thereby increas-ing their optimism about recovery in the process.

Solomon and his associates were able to produce extinction of the avoidance response, but at enormous cost to the animals, who had to suffer considerably before "learning" that the original phobic stimulus, the electric shock, was no longer operative. The parallel to psycho-therapy is perhaps obvious to the reader. As therapists, we often ask our clients to restrain themselves from executing coping strategies that they have associated with the avoidance of severe danger. Since many of these coping strategies have a driven, compulsive quality, it is not surprising that many clients are unwilling or unable to slow themselves down. In fact, just as people running for the exits during a fire are in danger of trampling others, the client may be prone to react destruc-tively to anyone, such as a therapist, who tries to prevent him or her from reaching safety. When clients are able and willing to restrain themselves from completing the usual coping strategies, they generally do not feel better immediately. In fact, they may feel considerably worse, since they now may experience intense anxiety and depression, without a clue as to how to deal with such emotional experiences. Consequently, it is not surprising that some individuals become more upset and/or symptomatic during the course of treatment. Likewise, it is understandable why some individuals also struggle with enormous resistance to the treatment process, as manifested by missed appoint-ments, premature termination, withholding of information, hostility toward the therapist, and so on.

We have discussed the example of Solomon's dogs, along with our interpretations of the experiments, with many clients. Such discussions nearly always yielded positive results in that we were able to provide our clients with a nonstigmatizing framework for understanding their own behaviors. Clients who had seen themselves as sick or crazy for engaging in a variety of compulsive and/or self-defeating behaviors were thereby able to perceive their actions in a new light, one that drew their attention back to those very stressors that had necessitated the avoidance responses to begin with.

As the preceding paragraphs suggest, we do view fear as the foundation of the driven, compulsive behaviors and, perhaps, even the entire life scripts exhibited by many of our clients. The reader should not infer from our discussion of coping strategies that we subscribe to a reductionistic, conflict oriented view of personality and behavior. Indeed, our conception of human personality and development as it unfolds throughout the life span of the individual probably comes closest to the self-actualization models of Rogers (1951) and Maslow (1962). However, we contend that the conditions in dysfunctional families obstruct normal growth and development in children and adolescents by undermining their sense of self-worth and keeping them preoccupied with issues of danger and safety. We seek to help our clients to understand and remove their obstructions, so that the "natural" process of growth and self-actualization can resume, this time unimpeded by victimization and fear.

INFORMATION-PROCESSING STYLES

In the normal course of development, every one of us will acquire rules for filtering and sorting stimuli of all sorts. Each person must find a way to order or prioritize information emanating from outside sources as well as data coming from within the organism itself (e.g., imagery and other spontaneous cognitions, pain and other bodily sensations, and so on). We assume that information-processing styles must be influenced to a great degree by individual variations in temperament, metabolism, neurochemistry, neuroanatomy, and the like, particularly in childhood. However, we also assume that as the child grows to adulthood, his or her actual learning history, as reflected in basic schemas, plays a progressively larger role in directing attentional processes. In contrast to their counterparts from normal families, children who are raised in dysfunctional home environments will develop schemas that are dominated by themes of physical and/or psychological threat. In turn, these basic schemas will organize and drive attentional processes around issues of threat. Information-processing styles are themselves coping strategies, but they also serve as building blocks for more complex coping mechanisms as many of the cases presented in this volume will illustrate.

Denial

In our usage, the term "denial" serves as an umbrella under which we group all operations that direct the individual's attention *away* from particular stimuli (or classes of stimuli). Denial involves a spectrum of cognitive and behavioral strategies that block recognition and processing of painful or threatening events. In the succeeding sections, we explore how denial operates on sensory/perceptual, conceptual, behavioral, and interpersonal/systemic levels. Our open-ended definition does not address the diverse underlying schemas that may stimulate denial. Denial may occur on a very basic sensory or perceptual level, as when the individual fails to acknowledge the very existence of certain stimuli. Denial may also involve an explicit conceptual process on the part of the client, often characterized by faulty logic, historical revisionism, mistaken causal attributions, and out-and-out distortion of reality. In our model, avoidant behaviors, such as procrastination, also reflect the operation of denial mechanisms. Lastly, denial may also include an interpersonal or systemic component, as when two or more family members collude to avoid acknowledgment of a mutually painful or threatening issue.

Denial processes ostensibly serve as a protective mechanism for the individual who grows up in a dysfunctional family. For the child who is exposed on a regular basis to destructive arguments, physical abuse, and/or sexual assaults over which he or she has no control, developing the ability to screen out painful or threatening stimuli is a sound coping strategy. Likewise, in adult life, strong denial mechanisms may come in handy when an individual must encounter painful, worrisome, or otherwise aversive situations over which no control is possible, such as while waiting for mammogram results or when allowing a teenager to take the family car for the first time. Unfortunately, however, for most aspects of adult life, the dictum that knowledge is power still seems to hold. Denial processes do not excise threatening stimuli with surgical precision. Although such strategies may prevent the occurrence of dysphoric affect, at least on a short-term basis, they also reduce the total amount and the scope of information available to the individual. Consequently, a person who has learned to rely excessively on denial mechanisms for handling potentially stressful matters may suffer the effects of such self-induced ignorance in many areas of life, particularly in relationships.

Signal Blocking: "Night of the Barely Living"

On the most basic, primitive level, denial involves signal blocking, the use of powerful mental filters, so that certain classes of information never become available for consideration, evaluation, or interpretation. Signal blocking shuts down the cognitive processing of potentially stressful situations, and with it, affect. The individual who relies on signal blocking as a primary coping strategy may present an extremely constricted range of emotion, or may appear totally unable to experience certain affective states (such as anger) at all, because the use of denial strategies has severely restricted information-processing capabilities. Such an individual has a deficiency in the ability to experience and process reality, a far more serious problem, in our opinion, than the inability to feel appropriate emotions. We consider the dissociation or "numbing out" experienced by incest victims to be a protypical manifestation of signal blocking.

The following cases reflect various clinical manifestations of signal blocking:

Gina and Spike, a couple in their late 30s, were involved in family treatment centered on their college-aged daughter, who had been the victim of long-term sexual abuse perpetrated by a former neighbor. In the presence of the daughter and the therapist, Gina relentlessly attacked her husband's lack of assertiveness and mediocre career accomplishments, even questioning his manhood itself in the process. His rambling, sometimes tangential monologues were frequently punctuated by Gina's exasperated sighs, eye rolling, and other theatrical nonverbal gestures. Gina's contemptuous attitude, expressed so overtly in front of the daughter, certainly pointed to issues in the marriage that sabotaged parenting functions in the family. In addition, her behavior made the therapist feel uncomfortable for Spike. On the other hand, Spike himself continually appeared relaxed and unruffled during the sessions. He seldom responded directly to Gina's verbal responses and ignored her nonverbal communications altogether. After a particularly bitter diatribe from Gina directed at the husband, the therapist turned to him and said: "Spike, I'd like you to help me with something. We both know that Gina gets pretty angry with you in here, not that she doesn't have valid reasons to at times. Session after session, I keep watching you for a response, thinking, 'This time the guy's going to get mad.' But you stay cool as a cucumber. How do you manage to do that?" Spike broke into a wide grin and replied, "Doc, I just let it go right over my head."

As a child, Donna had been physically abused by both parents and her older brother. It also appeared that she had been sexually abused as well, by two or more perpetrators. Despite a remarkable ability to recount many incidents in her life in a vivid, highly detailed manner, Donna often had great difficulty recalling the content of her treatment sessions. At times, the therapist would notice her eyes glaze over as he spoke to her. When asked what she was thinking about, Donna would shake her head as if awakening from a dream, making statements such as, "I think I lost you back there," or "I must have blocked you out, because I can't remember what we were talking about."

Teresa grew up in a large extended family rife with violence and addiction. She had been sexually abused on multiple occasions by a grown male cousin and had witnessed the rape of her older sister by a family friend. After a considerable period of time in treatment, Teresa discovered that her breasts were much less sensitive to touch than the rest of her body, even during sexual arousal. As a result of checking with her sister and a close friend, Teresa realized that under normal circumstances, her breasts should have been more sensitive to touch than other parts of her body, particularly during sexual relations. Her therapist had read about so-called "glove anesthesias" previously, but had never actually encountered such symptoms.

Like many clients who have difficulty articulating their inner experiences, Andre entered treatment as a result of his spouse's mounting frustration with him. He described his presenting complaints, such as they were, almost exclusively in terms of his wife's negative reactions to him. Andre did experience a vague sense of failure and inadequacy, particularly in regard to his marriage. However, when the therapist asked him directly what aspects of his wife's behavior made him angry or frustrated, Andre drew a complete blank. Incredibly, he could not recall ever yelling or otherwise behaving in an overtly angry manner toward his wife despite having been married for nearly 20 years! Although there had been no sexual component in the marriage for over 5 years, Andre seemed curiously tolerant of such a frustrating state of affairs. He and his wife had constructed their schedules so that they were able to avoid opportunities for intimacy, physical or otherwise. In addition to being unable to identify feelings of anger toward his wife, Andre also could not even verbalize what he might want from his wife or from his marriage. Indeed, when the therapist once asked him to dream up a perfect day for himself during which he could go anywhere in the world and do whatever he wanted, Andre drew a complete blank. Not only did he fail to complete the assignment, he never even figured out how to start it! When he was 3 years old, Andre's father had died in an auto accident. Andre could not recall anyone in the family ever having discussed his father in all the years that followed. In fact, there was not even a picture of his father in sight in the household.

Chronic and pervasive failure on the part of an individual to acknowledge large areas of experience produces a phenomenon the authors have dubbed, "Night of the Barely Living." These individuals are highly unresponsive to affectively-charged stimuli, giving them the appearance of being emotionally "dead." Although such people might appear quite personable in work or social contexts, they are chronically poor communicators at home. In fact, they may appear not to respond at all to crucial interactions with significant others. They often simply withdraw in the face of conflict in the family. The majority of the clients we have seen to date who seem to fit in this category have been male. Many of them have experienced physical abuse, extreme rejection, or a traumatic loss early in life. It may be coincidental, but among the career choices of such clients, the engineering, accounting, and law enforcement fields seem to be overrepresented.

Since they cannot easily identify issues or areas of discomfort, Night of the Barely Living types can be difficult to assess and to treat. Sessions with them can be long and boring for the therapist, who may in turn work too hard to bring issues to life. Since they do not experience great overt distress, let alone dissatisfaction with self, these individuals are at risk to miss sessions, resist paying bills, withdraw from treatment, and so on. Often their motivation for entering treatment comes not from within but from a disgruntled spouse who has made continuation of the marriage contingent on involvement in therapy. The spouse may turn out to be an emotionally overpowering individual, perhaps with a high level of anxiety and a correspondingly high need to control, who may communicate quite provocatively and aversively. Ironically, successful treatment of a Night of the Barely Living type may ultimately increase marital conflict. As the client begins to process events and their implications more thoroughly, he or she may begin to recognize and confront ongoing problems in the home.

Note that a psychodynamic model might assert that these Night of the Barely Living types have repressed their emotions, particularly anger. The cognitive model would counter that the emotions in question never occurred in the first place, because of the deficits in information processing. Because of signal blocking, which occurs reflexively or automatically, data regarding one's maltreatment or victimization never progresses beyond what learning theorists call the "buffer zone" into more active and complex modes of thinking and memory, where assignment of meaning can take place. Instead of being filled with repressed rage, the Night of the Barely Living Types are regrettably fairly empty inside, much as they appear on the outside. Their inner lives could best be described as "impoverished." Such highly constricted individuals will not be capable of feeling, let alone expressing, affect until they can learn how to process their experiences in a more deliberate, nonreflexive manner.

It is useful to introduce the subject of signal blocking by offering clients some examples that demonstrate the ability we humans have to "gate out" events on a basic neurological level. The use of hypnosis offers many compelling illustrations. In trance, some individuals are able to undergo major surgery or dental work without being anesthetized. Similarly, some hypnotic subjects can sit calmly while the operator sticks pins into their hands without experiencing pain. Another interesting example from hypnosis involves "negative hallucinations." The operator may instruct the hypnotic subject to respond only to his or her voice. Subsequently, a good subject will not react at all to the voices of others in the room. The subject may be able to screen out stimuli so effectively that he or she will not even blink if someone in the room yells out unexpectedly. After sharing such vignettes, the therapist may then simply ask the client, "If our brains are capable of screening out something as basic as pain or the sound of someone's voice, what other kinds of information might we be able to hide from ourselves?" "

"Positive Distortions": Denial Operating on the Conceptual Level

For many clients, denial processes go far beyond the gross level of signal blocking. These more complex denial operations do allow potentially threatening information to penetrate to higher cortical levels where processing occurs in accordance with basic schemas regarding the self, others and relationships. The individual's basic schemas prevent an accurate reading of various classes of critical situations, resulting in perceptions that are consistently and inappropriately skewed in a positive direction. We assume that the positive distortions occur because the consequences of a more negative viewpoint of a situation seem much too threatening for the individual to face. The positive distortions spare the individual from feelings of worthlessness or a sense of danger, preserve important relationships, sustain hope in the face of severe stress, and so on. Below are several examples of positive distortions expressed by our clients:

Kurt, a victim of severe physical abuse in childhood, recounted a day he spent with his 12-year-old nephew, during which he repeatedly teased and nagged the boy about his obesity. When the therapist expressed his concerns about the nephew's reaction to his insensitive comments, Kurt replied, "He wasn't upset by it. He knows I was just trying to help him out."

Unlike her siblings and her mother, Gina had always remained loyal to her institutionalized father, a paranoid schizophrenic who had traumatized the family with a series of violent episodes. Gina explained to her therapist that she regularly received a "special discount" from a merchant who sold her supplies for her catering business. Citing his civic and charitable involvements, she assured the therapist that his interest in her was merely a reflection of his altruistic character. "He's just a nice guy, that's all," she said. She was quite shocked when one day he suddenly engulfed her in his arms, pelvis to pelvis, and propositioned her.

As described earlier, Donna had experienced a number of traumatic events while growing up in an alcoholic family. When asked during the initial interview about her relationship with an older brother, she joined two fingers on her right hand and held them up to the therapist, saying, "We've always been this close." Subsequently during the same interview, she revealed that physical aggression and many other extremely abusive actions on her brother's part had been a regular occurrence in the household during her childhood and adolescence. Moreover, as an adult, her brother had rarely, if ever, initiated communications with her.

Readers who are familiar with the comic strip "Peanuts" will recall the oft-repeated story of Charlie Brown and the football. As football season begins every autumn, Charlie Brown enlists the aid of his chronic tormentor, Lucy, to help him practice his placekicking. Every year, the outcome of the interaction is the same. Charlie, remembering Lucy's behavior the previous year, distrusts her motivation, expressing his concerns that she will once again humiliate him under the guise of helping. Somehow Lucy always seems to convince Charlie that this year she is sincere in her desire to assist him and that she has no intention of letting go of the football before he can kick it. Charlie inevitably falls for the bait and runs excitedly to kick the football, only to land spectacularly on his backside when Lucy once again removes the target at the last instant.

Many of our clients play the role of Charlie Brown in their own lives as they allow themselves to be victimized again and again, often by the same individuals and in the same predictable ways. Clients who engage habitually in positive distortions often seem to have little appreciation of past history, particularly in their intimate relationships. In their interactions with significant others, they seem to react to each situation as if it were a novel one, without acknowledging the repetitive, predictable nature of certain behaviors and transactions. They prefer to attribute the abusive, exploitative, or otherwise disturbed actions of significant others to situational factors (e.g., "He's drinking more now because he's under a lot of stress at work") and are apt to become unduly optimistic about the future if they see evidence of even the most minimal changes in behavior. Often they will offer a skewed, revisionist history of the relationship with the individual in question, glossing over, minimizing, rationalizing, or even refusing to acknowledge past transgressions. They are able to sustain some very difficult relationships through the use of such denial strategies, but it is at tremendous cost to themselves and possibly other family members as well.

Avoidance: Denial Operating on the Behavioral Level

Many of our clients show a lifetime pattern of avoiding various types of stressful situations. They may consistently avoid confrontations or other affectively charged discussions with loved ones, or they may procrastinate chronically on projects for work, home, or school. Understandably, these behaviors can frustrate significant others, as well as therapists. The avoidant individual often experiences a chronic sense of worthlessness and helplessness, often suffering from a "low grade depression," perhaps spanning decades of his or her life.

David, a middle-aged lawyer, seemed to be late for almost everything in his life, including his therapy sessions. He let his bills pile up unopened for weeks and always carried a large stack of unanswered correspondence from his friends around in his briefcase. David kept other people, even his oldest friends, at arm's length, for fear that they might learn about his financial problems and other consequences of his chronic procrastination. An obviously intelligent, urbane man with a wide range of interests and abilities, David spent most of his evenings alone, in mindless communion with his television set. He always seemed to provide himself with reasons for why he could not take any steps to improve his lot in life. On the other hand, he was quite responsible and competent in his professional life. In fact, it was clear to the therapist that the senior partners at the law firm where he worked took advantage of David's diligence and eagerness to please.

David remembered first running away from home at age 8, when he had been anticipating yet another beating from his abusive mother. A few years later, he began to play hookey on a regular basis because of his fear of the harsh discipline employed at the parochial school he attended. David had been mistreated in other ways at home as well. Overweight from a young age, he recalled being referred to as "the Fat Boy" by his mother, who often predicted that other people would laugh at him and reject him because of his weight. When David expressed ambitions or interests, such as trying out for the basketball team in junior high school, his mother was apt to make derisive comments, such as, "What are you, some kind of big shot?"

Although chronically avoidant individuals may present a cordial, ostensibly open demeanor, they can be difficult to pin down and therefore frustrating to treat, particularly if the therapist unwisely invests time and energy in attempting to change the behavior pattern before understanding the cognitive processes that support it. As they become angry, therapists often label both the behaviors and the individuals as "passive–aggressive" perhaps without carefully pondering the implications for diagnosis and treatment.

Unfortunately, the passive–aggressive designation involves assumptions that not only appear to be wrong, but it also leads the therapist into a dead end with the client. If the therapist assumes that the client avoids risks, procrastinates on tasks, and frustrates others because of a deep-seated reservoir of anger, then the next logical step in treatment is to encourage him or her to acknowledge that anger. Unfortunately, as we indicated in the section on signal blocking, the client experiences neither the anger, nor the cognitions that support it. Moreover, there is no "reservoir" of angry affect for the client to tap into. Prodding, cajoling, or demanding such a client to acknowledge anger is analogous to attempting to squeeze blood out of the proverbial stone. No wonder therapists and clients find themselves confused and frustrated in such situations!

It should be clear to the reader from our discussion of Solomon's dogs that we generally view avoidant behaviors as fear-based, regardless of the amount of overt anxiety the individual experiences. Rather than press for behavior changes, we prefer to keep our chronically avoidant clients focused on the beliefs that induce helplessness and escapism as well as the denial mechanisms that short-circuit productive anxiety over unpaid bills, unfinished tasks, unresolved conflicts, and the like.

Collusion: Denial Operating on the Systemic Level

Family members may collude with one another in perpetuating denial regarding events and issues of great significance. In a collusive system, family members not only keep information hidden from the outside world, but they maintain silence with one another as well. Once again, we assume that denial in the family system constitutes an attempt to avoid a range of negative consequences. Below are several examples of collusion as it has occurred in our clients' lives:

Marsha and Justin were awaiting the arrival of her brother from the West Coast. A quarrel between Marsha and her brother during his last visit had occupied center stage for nearly two entire couples sessions afterwards. Although the siblings had barely spoken to one another for the previous 6 months, Marsha and Justin had told one another how excited they were about his arrival, each making statements such as, "It'll be great to see him," and "We'll all have a terrific time." Assuming that the brother's visit would be stressful, the therapist encouraged the couple to discuss in advance how they might respond if various difficulties were to recur. Marsha and Justin both looked surprised for a moment when the therapist alluded to the problems they had experienced with her brother the previous summer.

Over the course of several months of treatment, Peter and Sherry had never told their therapist that he slept on the couch in the living room every night, while she slept alone in the master bedroom. When the information finally surfaced, they assured the therapist that the arrangement existed only because Peter snored heavily and Sherry was a light sleeper. Both spouses denied any connection between the sleeping arrangements and the sexual problems they had acknowledged in the marriage. Likewise, both spouses denied feeling uncomfortable in any way about sleeping apart. Eventually Peter admitted that it was easier to sleep in the living room than to be rejected again and again by his wife, while Sherry ultimately acknowledged feeling lonely sleeping by herself every night.

It can be difficult to obtain validation for one's perceptions if they conflict with the "party line" in a collusive family system. Not surprisingly, children who grow up in such families may have trouble later in life trusting their own judgments, particularly in interpersonal situations. Clients from collusive marital or family systems who are in individual psychotherapy may feel quite guilty about the disclosures they make to their therapists. Moreover, they may have great difficulty sustaining constructive attitudes between sessions, succumbing instead to the tidal pull of family myths and cognitive distortions. In a collusive system, the bearer of bad news is always at risk for a range of punitive consequences. Family members who break the implicit code of silence may be labeled as crazy, disloyal, or overly emotional, and may even be abused or disowned. Likewise, therapists who challenge denial processes in the family too strongly, or without permission and support from key members, may be fired, or simply ignored.

Overvigilance

As was the case with denial, the term "overvigilance" serves as an umbrella term under that we group all operations which habitually turn the individual's attention toward certain stimuli or classes of stimuli. Our examination of overvigilance processes will focus on the sensory/perceptual, conceptual, behavioral, and interpersonal/systemic levels, analogous to the three domains of denial processes discussed earlier. At the most basic sensory or perceptual level of information processing, overvigilance produces what we term "signal sensitivity." That is, for a particular individual, certain stimuli or classes of stimuli automatically move to the perceptual foreground even when other data might legitimately compete for the person's attention. Once processed, these stimuli or classes of stimuli may then trigger habitual thought patterns in the individual, often with a markedly obsessive flavor. Together, signal sensitivity and obsessive thinking create a vicious cycle for the individual. Signal sensitivity produces an endless supply of raw data, whereas obsessive thinking creates fearful or dysphoric affect and provides the justification for continued overvigilance. For many of our clients, signal sensitivity and obsessive thinking serve as a breeding ground for compulsive behaviors. Finally, overvigilance shows up on the systemic or interpersonal level when family members remain chronically focused on the same narrow, but emotionally provocative, issues without a sense of closure or resolution.

The habitual use of overvigilance in adult life keeps the individual in a chronic state of tension and autonomic arousal. What begins as a mechanism to identify danger and prevent physical or psychological harm may end up producing needless worry, symptoms of anxiety, obsessional thinking, compulsive behaviors, stress-related physiological symptoms such as high blood pressure, interpersonal friction, and so on. Overvigilant processes tend to produce rigid, stereotyped responses while they stifle creativity by preventing access to new information. The individual becomes locked in a highly reactive stance vis à vis others and the world. Ironically, the individual whose perceptual processes become narrowly organized around certain stimuli associated with danger runs the risk of being "blind-sided," victimized by other factors in the environment that escape scrutiny.

Signal Sensitivity: Overvigilance Operating on the Perceptual Level

We all know of visually impaired individuals who have honed their skills of hearing and touch far beyond the levels normally attained by their sighted peers. Some of our clients also have developed exquisitely tuned perceptual abilities in response to traumatic or chronically threatening family environments in childhood or adolescence. They now automatically scan the perceptual field (which includes both internal and external stimuli) constantly for signs of danger or threat. They learn to see certain forms of danger coming from a long way off, although they may generate many "false positives," and much unnecessary anxiety, in the process. Moreover, as we shall discuss in a subsequent section, the same individuals may also fail to recognize other even more serious threats closer at hand.

Once acquired, habits of overvigilance may persist more or less unchanged into adulthood, often without the explicit awareness of the individual. In fact, the individual may be tense in certain situations, or may be unable to ignore certain stimuli, without knowing exactly why. The following examples illustrate the development of signal sensitivity and its manifestations in adult life:

Joseph was a bright, articulate 9-year-old whose father, a successful lawyer, had physically abused both his wife and his children on a number of occasions. The father himself recalled having been beaten as a boy on a regular basis by his mother. Joseph's father was rigid and authoritarian in his approach to parenting. Since his academic expectations were enormously high, he insisted on personally reviewing his son's homework each evening, despite the fact that the wife was home with the children all day long. It was during the homework sessions that the bulk of his angry episodes with Joseph had occurred. In terms surprisingly articulate for a little boy his age, Joseph described the threatening interactions that began each night as his father returned from work. He told the therapist that he could tell what kind of mood his father was in "by the way he walks up the stairs." Not surprisingly, he reported becoming quite nervous during the nightly review of his schoolwork, scared to the point of not being able to answer questions from his father. According to Joseph, the more difficulty he had responding to questions, the angrier his father became. The therapist asked Joseph if he knew in the past when he was going to be hit. Joseph replied that he could always tell "by the look on Daddy's face." When the father did hit him, the boy said he would try as hard as he could not to cry, because if he wept, the father would grow even angrier and hit him again.

It seems clear that Joseph's stressful experiences with his father had already begun to exert a profound influence on his basic attentional mechanisms. How many typical children of his age who have not been abused would report attending so carefully to the way a parent walks up the stairs? By 9 years of age, Joseph had already learned to gear his moment-to-moment awareness in the home to anticipating the threat of being hit by his father.

Maria grew up in a household dominated by an authoritarian father who physically abused her mother and her older brother on many occasions. The father tended to be moody and unpredictable, capable of lashing out in a violent manner at any time. As a child, Maria learned to monitor all ongoing interactions between members of her family. No matter where she was in the house, she always remained fully aware of where everyone else was and what they were doing. During stressful family interactions, she generally withdrew to the comparative safety of her room, where she kept herself occupied with art work and a wide range of other intellectual pursuits. In adulthood, Maria always found family gatherings, which now included her siblings' spouses and children, to be inordinately stressful. On such occasions, she invariably experienced a profound sense of relief as soon as she returned home. In the course of treatment, she recognized that she felt compelled to follow every conversation and monitor every interaction going on around her at these family functions. No wonder she found herself exhausted after a few hours!

Both of Ernie's parents were extremely rigid about cleanliness and tidiness in the house. As he described it, they "went nuts" when the kids spilled something or failed to pick up after themselves. He remembered having been spanked regularly for very minor infractions, such as leaving the lights on in a room after he left it. He also described beatings with sticks and other objects that left bruises and lacerations, necessitating medical treatment on a few occasions. His parents habitually used terms such as "asshole" and "shithead" to address their children. Ernie was determined to treat his own children, who were still preschoolers, in a less abusive manner. However, at times he found himself extremely tense around the house, particularly toward the end of the day, when toys and clothes were strewn about. Having little things out of place in the house really bothered him. Try as he might, he found it impossible to ignore it when his wife left the lights on or the kids tracked dirt into the house. Although he generally avoided persecuting the children, he did become enraged quite frequently with his wife over minor infractions. Ernie entered treatment because his angry outbursts had prompted his wife to initiate a separation.

Obsessive Thinking: Overvigilance Operating on the Conceptual Level

Themes of physical and/or psychological threat often dominate the thought processes of our clients. Sensitized on a sensory/perceptual level to threatening stimuli, they often find themselves unable to stop thinking about the implications of such stimuli. According to the cognitive model, sustained rumination on a particular theme produces sustained arousal of the relevant affective states. For example, continued reflection on one's mistakes and imperfections will perpetuate feelings of self-loathing and shame. Similarly, obsessive thoughts about potential calamities in one's life will produce continuing feelings of apprehension and anxiety. As we discussed previously, obsessive thinking and dysphoric affect can begin to resonate together to produce a vicious cycle for the individual. Continued rumination produces continued unpleasant emotions, which in turn constrict and channel thought further, so that the individual's ability to embrace alternative perspectives progressively dwindles. The individual's thinking may become so rigidly patterned that he or she can no longer process additional information that might relieve, or at least reduce, unpleasant feelings. In many instances, the client will also report a complete inability to turn off obsessive thoughts even when he or she has recognized that further reflection on a particular topic will be unproductive.

As our clinical examples illustrate, obsessive thinking is a coping strategy gone awry. In one's family of origin, continually anticipating and rehearsing for threatening interactions may have been a very sound survival tactic, either because it helped the individual to learn new coping skills or reduced anxiety by creating the illusion of control over future events. Unfortunately such strategies may remain central in the individual's survival repertoire even when they are no longer necessary and/or effective. Although the ostensible goal of obsessive thinking is to reduce anxiety, it ultimately produces the reverse effect, raising discomfort in the long run, for reasons explained in the preceding paragraph.

Below are three case examples that depict patterns of obsessive thinking that we observed in our clients:

Joey, a muscular, athletic-looking college student, had been sexually abused by an older man in his neighborhood for a period of over 2 years, between ages 10 and 12 years. Since early adolescence, Joey had been obsessed with issues of masculinity and sexual identity. He was desperately afraid that he would appear effeminate to others, particularly his male peers. He carefully monitored his posture, his physical gestures, and his vocal inflections in order to insure that he appeared as "masculine" as possible. Likewise, he often obsessively reviewed his conversations with other males after the fact, in order to determine whether he had come across as virile or effeminate. Not surprisingly, Joey exercised compulsively, and at times, self-destructively. He often pondered taking steroids so he could "bulk up" even further. On the other hand, Joey found himself longing for an intimate relationship with another man and developed a series of intense but unrequited crushes on his weightlifting partners.

Fritz's father was a stockbroker who worked long hours and often returned home intoxicated. The father's behavior when drinking was highly unpredictable, ranging from abusive to affectionate. Fritz felt responsible for protecting his mother and younger sister from his father's abuse, often blaming himself when violent altercations took place. Shortly after college, he married Joanne, who had also grown up with an abusive alcoholic father. Over the 20 years of their marriage, Joanne experienced a wide range of physical and psychological symptoms which frequently interfered with her day-to-day functioning. During periods of distress, she was prone to make frantic calls to Fritz at work, sometimes summoning him home so that he could take care of her. Like other individuals locked into "codependent" relationships, Fritz worried about Joanne's emotional state almost constantly. If he didn't hear from his wife during the day, he often found himself wondering whether she was all right. While driving home after work, he usually tried to visualize how Joanne would behave on his return, so that he could rehearse his responses to her. He planned all his activities, particularly those he engaged in independently, according to how much they might upset his wife. Because of his wife's escalating objections, he had greatly curtailed visits with his mother and his sister, so that he now saw them for little more than a few hours each year. Whenever his therapist opened a session by asking him how things were going, Fritz invariably replied with a description of Joanne's emotional state and a list of her current concerns.

Carol was the second oldest child in a highly enmeshed Lebanese-American family, which was characterized by overprotective parenting. When Carol was 10, her older brother found their father dead, the victim of a heart attack while still in his 30s. Thereafter, Carol began to take a strong caretaking role toward her mother, her maternal grandmother, and her two brothers. After Carol's father died, her mother's brother Anton served as a surrogate parent in the family. He remained very involved with Carol and her siblings even after they had each married and left home. When Carol was in her 20s, Anton began to experience a series of severe depressive episodes marked by delusional thinking, aggressive behaviors, and chronic suicidal ideation. True to her caretaking role, Carol spent a great deal of time "babysitting" for her uncle when he was depressed, despite the fact that many other family members could have become involved. When he ultimately shot himself, not only did she hold herself responsible, she was also blamed by a number of other family members.

Not surprisingly, given the sudden deaths of both her father and her uncle, Carol spent an inordinate amount of time worrying about some form of harm coming to the members of her family. Wherever she was, if she heard a siren, she immediately assumed that something had happened to her mother or grandmother. Likewise, she often expected to hear bad news about someone when the phone rang. She regularly found herself calling her mother and her brothers several times a day with no specific agenda in mind other than to relieve nagging fears for their well-being. Carol seldom traveled out of town overnight, but she could not recall ever having done so without daily phone contact with the family members back home. If another member of the family was home with a cold or the flu, she usually would feel too anxious to enjoy herself if she went out for an evening with her husband.

We believe that basic schemas set the stage for the themes that are reflected in the person's obsessive thoughts despite fluctuations in content that may occur across situations and developmental stages. An individual who believes that he or she is worthless, for example, may obsess about physical appearance during adolescence, educational attainments in young adulthood, and financial security in middle age, all the while expressing the same underlying belief about the self. As we shall illustrate in subsequent chapters, a cognitive orientation to treatment does not oblige the therapist to pursue every manifestation of distorted content in the client's thinking. The therapist may choose to pursue recurring themes or underlying schemas more fruitfully in another area of the client's life rather than attempt to address the specific content of obsessive thoughts, particularly if these are associated with a high degree of belief and intense emotional arousal. Moreover, as we discuss later in this chapter, the content of obsessive thoughts may be quite peripheral to the real sources of threat in the client's life, especially when substantial areas of denial coexist with the patterns of over-vigilance.

Compulsive Behaviors

In our discussion of Solomon's dogs, we emphasized that although compulsive behaviors often lead to self-defeating consequences for the individual, they generally reflect an attempt to cope with perceived physical or psychological threat. It should be noted that any action an individual feels compelled to perform, regardless of its social desirability, can be considered a compulsion. As the following case examples illustrate, signal sensitivity and obsessive thinking serve as the foundation for compulsive coping strategies of all sorts:

Lori had grown up with a much younger sister and a brother just 2 years her junior. Her father had experienced recurring episodes of severe depression during her formative years, necessitating innumerable hospitalizations, as well as many rounds of electroshock therapy. Episodic alcohol abuse further impaired the father's ability to function. Lori remembered her father as cold, critical, and rejecting, completely uninvolved with everyone else in the family, except her younger brother. Somehow the father would rouse himself sufficiently to attend the boy's athletic events on a regular basis, whereas he had not even shown up at Lori's high school graduation. Likewise, although the parents had made it clear early on that Lori would have to finance her own education, they had found a way to pay for her brother's tuition when he attended college. Moreover, despite the fact that the brother had become more and more physically and verbally abusive to Lori throughout his adolescence, neither parent had intervened on her behalf. In fact, the mother had frequently accused Lori of deliberately provoking her brother to violence! As an adult, Lori found herself desperately afraid of showing favoritism or preferential treatment to either of her two preschool-aged sons. If she said, "I love you," to one of her sons, she would feel uncomfortable until she spoke the same words to the other. She kept careful track of the one-to-one time she spent each day with the children so that each would receive equal amounts of attention. In similar fashion she took care to spend identical amounts on Christmas gifts for each boy, despite the fact that, like most toddlers, her sons had little or no concept of money! At one point Lori became quite enraged with her husband when he questioned her approach to purchasing Christmas presents for their sons.

Raised in a family with a history of physical and sexual abuse that spanned several generations, April described a series of productive, but highly driven behaviors beginning when she was 9 or 10 years old. Like some of our other clients, she became a compulsive house cleaner in late childhood, apparently as a means of creating a greater sense of safety for herself in the household. As an adolescent, she became so involved in gymnastics that she did little else except eat, sleep, and attend school. Having married just after her high school graduation, April had two children by the time she was 21 years old. Discouraged by the weight she had gained during her two closely spaced pregnancies, she became a chronic abuser of laxatives for several years during her early 20s. A few years later, April turned to running as a means of weight control. She quickly progressed to the point where she was entering marathons on a regular basis, and her menstrual periods stopped completely. When injuries forced her to stop running, she decided to go to law school, where she pursued her studies with almost maniacal determination. Despite her many other time-consuming responsibilities, April usually became restless and uncomfortable during school vacations. Shortly before her graduation, she seriously considered abandoning law and applying to medical school!

Having been rejected by her father and sexually abused by her step-brother, Audrey drew a sense of self-worth in her family of origin from being a confidante to her mother and a surrogate parent to her younger sister; in fact she felt responsible for the functioning of the entire family. On the other hand, Audrey prided herself on her stoicism and imperviousness to physical pain. She asked for nothing in the way of support from anyone in the family, and of course, she received none.

In her late teens, Audrey married a passive but decent man 10 years older than she was. Within 5 years, she had borne three children despite the fact that her physician had suggested she limit herself to just two pregnancies because of some chronic health problems. Audrey also took a strong interest in her husband's son by a previous marriage. At Audrey's urging, the couple eventually assumed custody of the boy. After her second child was born, at a time when many mothers might feel justifiably overwhelmed, Audrey began taking in foster children. She bristled at the therapist's suggestion that such behavior might represent a self-defeating coping strategy, stating rather uncharacteristically at one point that God Himself had commanded her to become a foster mother. Audrey cared for as many as five foster children at one time and ultimately undertook legal adoption of three of her charges. She also concurrently ran a small business in her home—a day-care center of course! Audrey indicated again and again, in a number of ways, that any critical examination of her caretaking activities was off-limits for the therapist.

We suspect that compulsive behaviors generally lead to progressively more negative consequences over the life span of the individual, perhaps because they inevitably collide with the escalating demands of work, marriage, and family. Compulsive behaviors seem to produce a widening range of ripples in the real world, resulting in legal, financial, and career problems, and perhaps worst of all, impairment in the individual's ability to function as a spouse and a parent. Moreover, such behaviors also reinforce a sense of worthlessness on the part of the individual, particularly if he or she repeatedly engages in futile attempts to change. On the other hand, as Solomon's dogs, clients may well experience considerable discomfort if and when they do stop their compulsive behaviors. They are unlikely to tolerate such discomfort for any significant period of time unless they are truly convinced that the behaviors in question are destructive or unacceptable. In the meantime, they will react defensively, perhaps in an extremely hostile manner, if they think they are being pressured to change by their therapists or any of the other important people in their lives.

Perseverative Interactional Patterns: Overvigilance Operating on the Systemic Level

Just as an individual becomes obsessed with particular concerns, so do marital and family systems become organized around repetitive themes. Spouses and other family members may perseverate on the same issues, year in, year out, with no sense of closure or resolution.

Moreover, denial and overvigilance can coexist within a family system, just as they coexist with an individual. As other writers have pointed out (Black, 1981; Brown, 1988), persisting cycles of conflict between various family members may serve to obscure other serious problems in the household, such as alcoholism.

Over a period of 4 or 5 years, Tim and Irene brought three of their children to the therapist, all for adjustment difficulties in adolescence. During each treatment contact, the symptoms were acute and quite serious. The first identified patient, Scott, had been thrown out of high school for assaulting a gym teacher. A year or two later, Angela became severely bulimic, to the point of requiring a brief hospitalization to stabilize her symptoms. Finally, Tim Jr., then 14 years old, took the family car for a test drive while drunk and stoned on Quaaludes, getting himself arrested in the process. During each treatment contact, the family rallied around the identified patient generally in a constructive, if somewhat overblown, fashion. Both mother and father obsessed constantly about the welfare of the children, particularly whichever one was experiencing adjustment problems at the time. At times they seemed to function in a permanent state of panic. Calls to the therapist between sessions from both parents were an ongoing problem whenever the family was in treatment. The fourth and final time the parents sought treatment, they sought help for Tim Sr.'s drinking, a problem the therapist had long seen as the real source of all the uproar in the family.

Fritz and Joanne, a couple we discussed in the previous section, engaged in the same repetitive, stereotyped interactions for many years. Their relationship was organized around Joanne's physical and psychological complaints. She needed a great deal of verbal support from her husband, whose substantial efforts always seemed to fall short of her expectations. The couple would spend literally hours discussing Joanne's problems, particularly her recurring complaints about the marriage. Despite the fact that Fritz was generally obsessed with the subject of his wife's well-being, both spouses seemed to assume that he was too "emotionally tuned-out" to respond properly to his wife's needs without frequent criticisms and admonishments from her. Meanwhile, Fritz's reactions and expectations concerning the marriage never came up for discussion. Likewise, although Joanne's thoughts and feelings were the central focus of most of the dialogue between the spouses, her behavior, and its impact on Fritz, seldom if ever received any attention during their interminable conversations.

We assume that just as boundaries, roles, and other systems parameters tend to rigidify, cognitive distortions and information-processing styles often also remain frozen in place in distressed families. In our view, effective marital or family treatment often involves redirecting attentional processes within the system so that new beliefs and behaviors can emerge.

HOW DENIAL AND OVERVIGILANCE COEXIST WITHIN THE SAME INDIVIDUAL

The authors find that the typical client from a dysfunctional family of origin will present maladaptive patterns of *both* denial and overvigilance. In fact, clients will often focus obsessively on an issue that may be peripheral, mundane, or incapable of immediate resolution at the same time they utilize denial mechanisms to cope with a problem or situation that should be of much more significant and immediate concern. Presenting complaints, such as anxiety symptoms, may occupy most of the client's attention, whereas other problems, such as a spouse's drinking, remain embedded in the perceptual background. The client may be quite comfortable talking at length about his or her symptoms but may be unwilling or unable to acknowledge certain other difficulties, particularly those that could threaten the survival of intimate relationships.

Lena, a woman in her 40s, provides a vivid illustration of how denial and overvigilance patterns can coexist in the same individual. Lena was married for the second time to Mario, whom she not affectionately dubbed, "Mister Wonderful." The spouses, both now sober, had met when they were still drinking. Both of them had left their respective spouses and families in order to be together. Mario's children, all daughters, were younger than Lena's, and perhaps as a consequence, they required more in the way of time, energy, and money from him.

Lena often found herself obsessed with the topic of Mario's relationship with his daughters to the point of scrutinizing his every interaction with them. She often resented the time he would spend with them and complained bitterly about the way he showered them with expensive gifts. She continually second-guessed his parenting style and was quick to blame him for any of his daughters' difficulties. Her frequent attacks on the subject of Mario's children seemed to accomplish little other than to drive her husband deeper and deeper into his own bind of conflicting loyalties.

Eventually, Lena disclosed to the therapist that "Mister Wonderful" had physically abused her over two dozen times in the 10-year history of the relationship. Periods of reconciliation had followed each episode of battering, although neither spouse would explicitly discuss the violence afterwards. Just thinking about the physical abuse would

cause Lena to be flooded with self-recrimination and shame. Consequently she had never spoken of the battering to anyone else, nor did
she even reflect on it privately to any substantial degree. However, she
was able to acknowledge that she was always aware of her husband's
potential for abuse whenever she had to interact with him. Her reactions
to Mario, particularly during periods of conflict, were often based on
her fear of his becoming violent again.

Even after she had disclosed the marital violence to her therapist,
it was still difficult to move Lena off the subject of Mario's daughters.
She would usually begin each session with a vignette that illustrated
Mario's deficiencies as a parent, and unless the therapist interrupted
her, she would appear quite content to spend the entire session on the
matter. As treatment progressed however, Lena began to recognize that
her main issue was with Mario, not with his daughters. She confronted
her husband about the battering on a number of occasions making it
clear to him that she would no longer tolerate physical abuse in the
marriage. With her physical safety no longer at risk in the marriage,
Lena turned her attention to other matters including Mario's frequent
verbal abuse and the impact her own lack of self-esteem had on the
marriage.

Most of the treatment cases we discuss in this volume required the
therapist to attack *both* overvigilance and denial in order to achieve a
satisfactory long-term outcome. It was nearly always necessary to direct
the client's attention *away* from certain stimuli through a variety of
interventions (e.g., by discouraging discussion of selected topics, by
exposing cognitive distortions through the use of Socratic dialogue, by
identifying certain obsessive patterns of thinking as symptomatic responses to stress, and so on). On the other hand, it was also vital to keep
the client oriented *toward* certain stimuli, again through a variety of
strategies (e.g., repetitive discussions of painful or threatening topics,
extensive reviews of stressful or victimizing relationships, and so on).
As we illustrate in later chapters, we look for opportunities to underscore the nature and effects of information-processing styles, particularly denial mechanisms, more or less continually throughout the treatment process. If our clients can internalize our model just as we have
presented here to the reader, so much the better. To our delight, we have
found that many of them are fully capable of doing so.

HOMEOSTATIC RELATIONSHIP BETWEEN SCHEMAS AND INFORMATION-PROCESSING STYLES

The individual's basic schemas and information-processing styles resonate with one another, so that the result is a sort of homeostatic balance

in the person's attitudes and behavior. The individual attends to a relatively narrow set of stimuli that have high personal valence, while he or she ignores or blocks other potentially relevant information. Likewise, the person tends to assimilate only data that are consistent with his or her beliefs, while he or she discounts or otherwise minimizes the significance of information that might be discrepant with basic schemas. Consequently, without assistance, the individual may never have the opportunity to process new data that could challenge the validity of a schema or facilitate the development of competing belief systems. As the following case vignettes illustrate, one dysfunctional schema can block the person from addressing and correcting other distorted belief systems.

Audrey grew up with an abusive alcoholic father who made no attempt to hide a long series of extramarital affairs from his wife and his children. Audrey's mother was far more concerned with her husband's sexual escapades than she was with his binge drinking and his maltreatment of the children. She solicited her daughter's aid, as a confidante and as a surrogate mother for the younger children, beginning when the girl was still in elementary school. From age 10 to 13, Audrey had been involved in an incestuous relationship with a stepbrother who was 4 years her senior. Although she recognized some of the degrading components of the relationship, she held herself primarily responsible for the sexual abuse. Her reasoning went as follows:

No force was involved. I could have said no. I was a willing participant. I always knew it was wrong. I went back for more because sometimes it made me feel good. Therefore, there is something basically wrong with me.

Like most victims of childhood sexual abuse, Audrey believed that the incestuous relationship reflected her essentially sinful nature. Not surprisingly, her sense of worthlessness affected many aspects of her adult life. She told the therapist that it was best for her to avoid thinking or talking about the incest, since it only made her feel worse about herself. Moreover, she was convinced that any examination of the sexual abuse would erase any doubts she might have had regarding her culpability, thereby only confirming her most terrible thoughts about herself. Ironically, Audrey's inability to process the implications of the incestuous relationship kept her a prisoner of the shame it had originally stimulated. Unless she was willing to take the risk of processing the sexual abuse with the therapist, she might never be able to absolve herself of blame. As long as she held herself responsible for the incest, Audrey would probably continue to experience the sense of underlying worthlessness that served as the foundation of many of her current patterns of thinking and behavior.

Like Audrey, Maria also found it difficult to assimilate new information about herself and her family background but for a different set of reasons. As we mentioned earlier, Maria grew up with an extremely frightening, physically abusive father. Having been identified somehow as her father's "favorite," Maria was largely spared from the direct impact of his wrath during her formative years. She idealized her mother and wanted to protect her from the father. Having assumed that her mother preferred her three sisters to her, Maria grew up believing that her siblings were warmer, more personable, more feminine, and more "normal" than she was. Despite her attractive looks and her wide range of talents, Maria struggled with poor self-esteem and depression throughout her adult life. Constantly fearing that others would see the deficiencies she perceived in herself, she tended to obsess over her failures and shortcomings.

As her treatment progressed, Maria began to describe current difficulties with her now elderly mother. The therapist was struck by the critical, competitive, and ultimately rejecting quality of the mother's behaviors toward her daughter. He began to suspect that Maria's lifelong struggles with worthlessness stemmed from chronic rejection by the mother. Maria struggled with tremendous guilt whenever she felt the least bit irritated or annoyed with her mother. Likewise, she became visibly uncomfortable whenever the therapist commented on the mother's rejecting, critical behaviors, or otherwise tried to validate her angry reactions to such treatment. Maria told the therapist she was afraid that sustained examination of the relationship with her mother would lead to uncontrollable feelings of anger, which in turn would stimulate destructive confrontations with her elderly parent. After all, she had always been told by the mother that she had her father's temper.

The preceding case examples suggest that the therapist needs to attend to the *sequence* in which he or she addresses issues with certain clients. For example, the therapist believed that it was vital for Maria to recognize the connection between her obsessive thoughts about her own flaws and deficiencies and the critical, rejecting attitude of her mother. He believed that she would ultimately feel more worthwhile if she could perceive her own deprivation and victimization during childhood more accurately. However, Maria was unable to acknowledge fully the negative impact of her mother's behavior until she could feel more confident that increased insight into conditions in her childhood would not lead to angry, destructive actions on her part. In later chapters, we discuss Maria's treatment in greater detail and describe our work with other clients whose issues also demanded a sequential therapeutic approach.

COPING STRATEGIES AND PATHWAYS INTO THERAPY: WHY NOW?

We assume that family of origin issues such as physical abuse or neglect, incest, or parental substance abuse will produce effects that reverberate throughout the life span of the individual. An understanding of individual and family development often provides the therapist with hypotheses as to why the presenting symptoms have appeared or intensified at a particular time. In our view, life transitions such as marriage or parenthood will challenge the individual's belief systems in new and unexpected ways, often revealing unresolved family of origin material as a result. Each developmental stage taxes existing schemas and coping strategies, demanding cognitive and behavioral accommodations to new roles and responsibilities. Individuals with rigid cognitive styles and fear-driven, stereotyped coping strategies may find themselves unable to make the necessary accommodations. Symptoms of psychological distress in the cognitive, affective, behavioral, and/or interpersonal realms will then appear. The following cases illustrate how the changing demands associated with the family life cycle create "natural" crises that expose the presence of underlying individual and/or systems issues:

Prudence was the youngest child of a prominent judge and the last one to leave the home. While the judge drank himself into a stupor each night, Prudence and her mother would draw the draperies, screen his telephone calls, intercept unexpected visitors, and otherwise conceal his intoxication from the public eye. Prudence acted as a confidante and an advisor to her mother, who was more concerned about her husband's pretty young secretary, than about his late-stage alcoholism. After graduation from high school, Prudence matriculated at a prestigious university about a half hour's drive from her home. She had difficulty adjusting to dormitory life and became embroiled in petty conflicts with her female neighbors in the residence hall. Meanwhile, the friction between her parents seemed to have increased in her absence and, with it, her father's drinking. Late in her freshman year, Prudence began to experience agoraphobic symptoms and panic attacks, which eventually caused her to withdraw from school. She returned to her parents' home, where she remained for the next 2 years, rarely venturing past the mailbox at the end of the driveway.

Victor's mother had been addicted to prescription drugs. Throughout his childhood and adolescence, she showed a steady physical and psychological deterioration. When Victor was a sophomore in college, he withdrew from school in order to take care of his mother, whose health was failing rapidly at that point. Six months later she was dead.

When he was in his mid-30s, Victor moved in with Stephanie, a bright, attractive woman who was completing her law degree. The couple planned to be married within a year or two. Still "engaged" 3 years later, Victor and Stephanie began couples therapy. Although he could not bear the thought of losing Stephanie, Victor was terrified by the prospect of making a commitment to her. During his most distressed moments, he would ask, "Why would any rational person want to get married and have children?" Stephanie clearly wanted to marry Victor but was distressed about his indecisiveness and his constant attempts to control her behavior. He monitored her diet and would chide her if she ate junk foods or sweets, as his mother had done during her last years. He would become particularly annoyed if Stephanie curled up on the sofa with a paperback book. Later in treatment, he remembered his mother languishing in bed for hours on end, reading "cheap dime novels." At times, Victor expressed his fear that instead of finding a job after graduation. Stephanie would simply give up her own aspirations and allow him to support her for the rest of her life.

Daisy's father had abandoned the family when she was just entering kindergarten. Her mother, who could best be described as an "ambulatory schizophrenic," was often unable to provide even minimal care for Daisy and her younger sister. From grade school on, Daisy pretty much came and went as she pleased, without any supervision. Even in the poor neighborhood where she grew up, Daisy's shabby clothes set her apart from her peers. From an early age, she realized that her home environment deprived her of many things other children seemed to take for granted. Daisy sought treatment because of escalating conflicts with her oldest daughter, who was 4 years old at the time. She described her little girl as verbal and opinionated, particularly about the clothing she wore. Instead of selecting the pretty outfits that filled her closet, the daughter demanded to wear wildly mismatched combinations of her own creation, frequently throwing tantrums if she was prevented from doing so. Daisy would feel anxious and embarrassed if her daughter left the house in clothes of her own choosing, thinking that the little girl "looked as if no one took care of her."

As we illustrate in the case vignettes above, the ways in which family of origin issues manifest themselves will depend on the developmental stage of the client and his or her current family. The developmental tasks of young adulthood, which call for the establishment of independence from the family of origin, vocational mastery, and the beginnings of intimate relationships, often force the individual to confront issues of worthlessness, especially if they experience rejection or failure. By their late teens or early 20s, many clients already will have established a pattern of unsatisfying, abusive, or otherwise dysfunctional relationships with the opposite sex. On the other hand, many of our clients report having achieved apparent mastery over the vocational challenges of young adulthood through a combination of hard work, incredible persistence, and the ability to "fake it." Although they may emerge from this developmental stage with all the trappings of success, they may report that they never experienced the gains in self-esteem commensurate with such progress.

We find that the experiences associated with parenthood, including infertility problems, abortions, and miscarriages as well as actual child-drearing, often lead to powerful symptoms of anxiety and depression in individuals who have hitherto appeared quite adequate and successful, at least to the outside world. *For most of us, whether we are psychologists, educators, or garbage collectors, the primary data base for parenting, particularly in the early stages of family formation, remains our own childhood experiences.* Clients may find themselves behaving in the same unacceptable ways their parents did or parenting in an overcompensated, extreme manner so as to avoid duplicating conditions in the family of origin. In some instances, the caretaking of children forces individuals to confront intrusive memories of their own victimization, as was the case with our client, Audrey, described above. Young parents are faced with the greatest responsibility of their lives, yet they must learn to tolerate a lack of control and an abundance of anxiety over many aspects of their child's health, temperament, and behaviors. Mothers or fathers of young children may become obsessed with irrational fears for the health or safety of their offspring. Some clients simply report diffuse, unaccountable feelings of anxiety or discouragement associated with family life, despite an apparent lack of objective difficulties in the home.

For a variety of reasons, marital distress will occur in families with young children, particularly if one or both of the spouses come from a dysfunctional family of origin. The hormonal changes triggered by childbirth, as well as the sleep deprivation, fatigue, tedium, and tension associated with parenting infants, naturally create a breach in the spouse subsystem that may be slow to repair even in the best of marriages. Moreover, fussy infants may grow into intrusive, unreasonable toddlers with short attention spans. Individuals who are primed by traumas or other historical issues to be overvigilant and overly responsible in their parenting, may become too anxious about their children to devote any substantial attention to their marriages. Some parents may find it hard to keep children out of the marital bed. Survivors of sexual abuse may be terrified of leaving young children with babysitters, so that the couple may end up spending little or no one-to-one time together. In some cases, they may even become obsessed with the thought of a spouse perpetrating incest. Parents who drive themselves relentlessly to actualize unrealistic visions of a perfect family may alienate their spouses by becoming compulsive and controlling about earning or saving money, about cleaning or housekeeping, about establishing family rituals, about exposing their children to just the right kind of stimulating activities, and so on.

The desire to nurture and protect children may also give rise to issues in the marriage that are far from irrational. The attitudes and behaviors of one spouse, which hitherto had been tolerated by the other partner, may begin to appear in a new, more unflattering light now that children are involved. The wife who has been battered by her spouse may now begin to worry about the safety of her children, and quite justifiably so. The husband who always turned a deaf ear to his wife's verbal abuse may now become quite distressed to find her speaking to the children in the same way. A wife who has always worked at a good job and maintained her own finances, may feel the direct economic consequences of her husband's compulsive gambling now that she has resigned her position to become a full-time mother. Individuals who had perhaps blamed themselves for their spouses' dysfunctional be-haviors in the past may now begin to see their children as helpless victims. Although they may never have stood up to their victimizers in the past, they may now begin to defend their children, perhaps with very destructive consequences for themselves.

Many of our clients have no life experiences indicate that there is even the most remote chance of correcting difficulties in intimate rela-tionships. Although they may feel adequate in many of the roles they assume in life, when it comes to intimate relationships, they see them-selves as helpless children. In typical all-or-nothing fashion, they believe that they must either tolerate a destructive relationship exactly as it is, or they must end it. At the same time that dissatisfaction with the marriage may be at its highest level, the potential ramifications of divorce also become the most serious, particularly for women and chil-dren. Finding the consequences of divorce too destructive to ponder but lacking any sense of what else they could possibly do to improve their marriages, many individuals with young children feel increasingly trapped and hopeless.

On the other hand, new strains can begin to emerge in a marriage as the tasks of parenting are beginning to wind down. When children start to leave the home, the parents may lose a sense of common pur-pose as well as a source of distraction from other frustrations in their lives. At a time when many couples finally have the leisure to enjoy one another's company again, problems in the relationship may begin to stand out in increasingly bold relief. With fewer responsibilities, de-creased accountability, and less structured schedules, the behavior of substance abusers and other impaired individuals may begin to deteriorate. In the meantime, disgruntled spouses, who are no longer saddled with the responsibility of children to raise, may find it hard to justify remaining in troubled marriages indefinitely, particularly if they have the potential to be financially independent.

PRESENTING COMPLAINTS AND THE THERAPEUTIC CONTRACT

It can be a difficult task, particularly early in the treatment process, for the therapist to combine interventions directed at the presenting complaints with strategies intended to modify the underlying mechanisms responsible for the symptoms. Jay Haley (1976) outlines a model of therapy that assumes that presenting complaints about children and adolescents often reflect underlying flaws in family structure and communication, particularly in the spouse subsystem. He advocates that therapists begin to address the broader difficulties in the family by working within the metaphor of the presenting complaints. Once the therapist joins the family system, over time he or she may find opportunities to move the focus beyond the problems as perceived by the family, perhaps toward issues in the parents' marriage or problems the adults have in separating from their own families of origin. Treadway (1989) offers a similar model for working with families with underlying alcohol problems who seek treatment for other issues. The approaches advocated by authors such as Haley and Treadway demand great patience and subtlety on the part of the therapist, who may understandably want to address the "real problems" instead of dawdling around with the presenting complaints.

In our experience, a relatively small percentage of our clients actually initiate treatment with the explicit goal of working on family of origin issues. Indeed, as we discuss in Chapters 6 and 9, many clients may not even be able to identify traumatic or otherwise dysfunctional elements in their early lives when the therapist first takes a history at the start of treatment. Clients who are seeking treatment for anxiety, depression, marital friction, or problems with their children have a legitimate desire for the therapist to attend to the presenting complaints. If possible, they deserve immediate access to any behavioral techniques or other relatively short-term interventions that have the potential to produce symptom relief. It is our belief that whenever possible, the therapist should attempt to respond to the client's treatment agenda as presented at the initial office visit.

If family of origin issues lie at the heart of the presenting problems, there are many pathways that the therapist can follow in order to redirect the client's attention to the relevant material. The therapist can label attempts to change presenting complaints as *behavioral experiments* suggesting, for example, that failures in symptom control will indicate a need for a different therapeutic direction. Symptom-based interventions that are successful, although they may lead to termination, increase the client's respect for the therapist and the treatment process. As discussed in Chapter 14, on termination the therapist may sow the seeds for more of a family of origin focus during subsequent treatment contacts. Often it takes a series of therapeutic contacts before a client is truly ready and/or motivated to identify and confront family of origin issues. On the other hand, if the therapist structures the client's expectations carefully from the outset, symptom-based interventions that are unsuccessful or only temporarily successful can help to provide the client with an eventual justification for working explicitly on family of origin material. The therapist's skill at interweaving historical material with current manifestations, particularly the presenting complaints, will often be a crucial factor in moving treatment away from a symptom focus. Therapists who refuse to be flexible in the kinds of interventions they offer, or who communicate a cavalier attitude about presenting symptoms, will alienate clients long before they can build a data base convincing enough to shift the focus of treatment to the examination of basic belief systems and coping strategies.

4

The Goals of Recovery and Treatment

THE GOALS OF RECOVERY

As we emphasize again and again, recovery will follow a unique path for each client. We believe that for individuals from particularly traumatic backgrounds, certain vulnerabilities may be present throughout the life span, and may retain the power to stimulate symptoms over a period of many decades. Such clients may be involved in long-term treatment experiences, or they may engage in a large number of serial therapeutic contacts, perhaps spanning many life stages. Similarly, some of our clients may also opt for long-term participation in Twelve Step Programs as a way of preventing symptom relapse and promoting continued personal growth. We find that individuals *can* sustain such long-term involvements in treatment or self-help programs without sacrificing a sense of competence.

The following items reflect potential recovery goals for the typical client:

Symptom reduction.
A coherent, comprehensive understanding of the basis of symptoms.
Mastery of symptom control strategies.
Improvements in self-esteem and self-efficacy.
Quicker recognition and modification of cognitive distortions as they occur in daily life.
Greater freedom from irrational self-blame and feelings of worthlessness.
Increased tolerance for self-examination, and an increased ability to utilize legitimate critical feedback from others.

Recognition of dysfunctional conditions in the family of origin, including impaired parenting, parentification of children, boundary violations, traumatic experiences, chronic rejection, distorted cognitions, and/or distorted communications.

A coherent, comprehensive understanding of the impact of family of origin experiences on past development and current functioning, with particular emphasis on basic schemas, information-processing styles, coping strategies, and recurring relationship patterns.

Recognition of victimization in past relationships and, if relevant, of one's own role in perpetuating such treatment in the past.

Recognition and prevention of victimization in current relationships.

Increased assertiveness, along with decreased inappropriate expressions of anger or rage.

A reduction in the frequency, intensity, and scope of irrational anxiety.

Quicker recognition of *irrational* threats to one's safety and self-esteem.

Greater control over self-defeating patterns of obsessive thinking.

Elimination or marked reduction in self-defeating compulsive or addictive behaviors.

Greater resistance to participation in perseverative interactional patterns with significant others.

A higher degree of accountability for, and control over, one's own actions, along with decreased externalization of blame.

Increased sense of clarity regarding the limits of one's responsibility for the thoughts, feelings, and behaviors of *others*.

Increased ability to recognize and tolerate *appropriate* emotions, in oneself and in others.

Greater sense of choice and/or control over unpleasant thoughts and feelings.

Reduction in self-defeating use of denial strategies, including signal blocking, positive distortions, avoidance behaviors, and collusion.

A greater capacity to respond in an assertive or self-protective manner to legitimate areas of concern, threat, or anxiety in one's life.

Establishment and maintenance of more appropriate personal and familial boundaries.

Development of more adaptive and realistic beliefs about others and relationships.

An increase in the ability to establish and sustain intimacy.

Improved parenting resulting in the prevention of dysfunctional family patterns being repeated in succeeding generations.

A Personal Recovery Program, based on an awareness of personal issues, information-processing biases, and behavioral tendencies that require ongoing monitoring, for the foreseeable future.

It should be emphasized that the above items represent a "wish list." The authors do not expect that each client will leave treatment having accomplished all of the goals enumerated above.

We emphasize again that working on family of origin issues in treatment is not a matter of shifting responsibility away from the client. The bulk of our clients are individuals who have precious little trouble shouldering responsibility (indeed, often they bear too much responsibility), for events that never were under their control. Understanding the familial roots of one's difficulties ultimately may absolve the individual of irrational blame, but such understanding should also lead him or her to assume an even greater degree of responsibility and control over current behaviors, coping strategies, and communicational patterns. It goes without saying that the therapist must avoid colluding with the client to excuse current choices on the basis of his or her having had a dysfunctional family background.

Some clients seem to be in a hurry to confront family members with a litany of past sins long before they have developed a thorough understanding of their own issues. To our dismay, some authors of self-help literature seem to insist that such confrontations are essential to the recovery process for individuals with dysfunctional family backgrounds. Our treatment model does not emphasize the intrinsic healing power of such confrontations. In fact, in many instances, we find that the net effect of these intense confrontations on all concerned, including our clients, is decidedly negative. The aftershocks often distract clients from working on their own issues. Indeed, as case examples in later chapters illustrate, we often attempt to restrain our clients from moving prematurely to restructure significant relationships.

In the authors' experience, clients who readily use popularized expressions such as "codependent," "ACOA," or "shame-based" to describe themselves are not necessarily fully aware of the personal implications of such labels. The therapist may need to use alternative descriptive language with such clients that steers them away from the hackneyed or popularized terms back toward the powerful original experiences themselves. Statements such as "I've resolved those issues," "I've come to terms with my husband's alcoholism," or "I've already worked on my sexual abuse in therapy" should alert the therapist to the presence of denial in the client's repertoire of coping strategies.

SIGNIFICANT FEATURES OF OUR
TREATMENT APPROACH

Below we have attempted to summarize a number of the key elements of our approach to the treatment of family of origin issues. In doing so, our intention is to provide the reader with a introduction of sorts to many of the themes which we will cover at length in the remainder of the volume. The treatment model described in this book includes the following features:

> Multidimensional utilization of the therapeutic relationship, for example as a source of data on the client's recurring interactional patterns, as a vehicle for affirming the individual's worth, as a model for more constructive relationships, and so on.
>
> The use of a consciously formulated therapeutic *posture,* aimed at achieving a variety of treatment goals, for example maintaining secure boundaries, preventing resistance, and so on.
>
> Ongoing, continuous, and deliberate use of embedded messages to facilitate various treatment goals.
>
> Ongoing, continuous attempts to affirm and promote the client's basic sense of self-worth through the use of direct interventions and embedded messages.
>
> Ongoing attempts to identify, underscore, and preempt the barriers (e.g., family loyalty, fear of affect, and so on) that prevent contemplation of significant issues by the client.
>
> Use of the therapist's affect and other reactions on the part of the clinician, as a source of data for developing and altering the treatment plan.
>
> Extensive *educational* focus, using the client's learning experiences in treatment as a primary data base.
>
> Use of varied techniques to promote awareness of family of origin experiences and their impact on the client's psychological development and current functioning.
>
> Use of highly structured treatment sessions with agenda items typically selected in a collaborative manner by the therapist and the client.
>
> Active, ongoing efforts during each treatment session to orient, to focus, and to sustain the client's attention on significant themes.
>
> Continuous attempts to help the client organize content and integrate historical information with current difficulties.
>
> Persistent efforts to maintain a sense of continuity in treatment through the use of frequent capsule summaries and repetitive presentation of formulations.

Emphasis on teaching the client various strategies (e.g., containment techniques) to control a range of symptoms.

Persistent attempts to highlight and facilitate remediation of boundary problems in the client's current life.

Emphasis on helping the client learn how to identify and resist current victimization, particularly in intimate relationships.

Frequent attempts to intensify affect by raising the client's distress regarding areas of legitimate threat or concern.

Emphasis on exploration and remediation of affective *deficits* (e.g., instances when expected or appropriate emotional responses fail to occur) as well as affective excesses.

Emphasis on normalizing appropriate affective reactions on the part of the client and/or significant others.

Ongoing efforts to help clients reprioritize their concerns, so that legitimate threats to self and/or significant others move to the foreground, whereas obsessions and irrational fears move to the background.

Direct, persistent confrontation of addictive, acting out, and/or compulsive behaviors on the part of the client.

Explicit emphasis on repetition and practice as long-term growth strategies.

Regular assignment of homework, including bibliotherapy and cognitive self-monitoring.

Opportunistic use by the therapist of attitudinal and behavioral shifts on the part of the client, such as those that occur during instances of successful coping to promote a variety of treatment goals.

Emphasis on stress-inoculation, most typically involving anticipation of cognitive distortions.

Frequent use of multiple treatment modalities and self-help groups.

Emphasis on *family recovery* in addition to individual recovery, as demonstrated by frequent inclusion of family and/or marital therapy as part of the treatment process.

Extensive use of serial therapeutic contacts.

Use of the termination process to seed subsequent therapeutic contacts.

5

Diagnostic Considerations

We assume that in each case, a unique configuration of biochemical, psychological, and interpersonal factors have united to produce and maintain the client's presenting complaints. In attempting to account for the presenting symptoms, the skilled diagnostician must consider the *full range* of *organismic* and *contextual* influences that operate in the client's life. Organismic influences include biochemical factors, cognitive mechanisms, and behavioral excesses and deficits. Contextual variables include severe life stresses, relationship problems with significant others, socioeconomic factors, conditions in the work place, and so on. Despite the fact that it may be useful at times to focus on either organismic or contextual influences separately for descriptive or therapeutic purposes, we assume that the two factors never operate independently of one another. Since every individual participates in an ongoing, continuous process of reciprocal influence with the environment, it is important for the clinician to view the causal processes in the client's life as circular, as opposed to unidirectional.

The therapist cannot assume a cavalier attitude regarding diagnostic considerations, even when it seems obvious that the client's current distress is directly connected to cognitive mechanisms rooted in family of origin dysfunction or other childhood trauma. The therapist has the obligation to inform the client about the various types of treatments available for his or her difficulties. We also would argue that the therapist has a responsibility either to provide the client with any known techniques for relief of presenting complaints (e.g., systematic desensitization for specific phobias) or to facilitate referral to another professional who is more familiar with such methods. Moreover, we believe that the client should receive any treatments available for symptom relief before, or at least concurrent with, engaging in therapeutic work on broader psychological issues. Likewise, we assume that for certain clients, marital or family therapy may be more appropriate than individual treatment, or at least should be combined from the outset with one-to-one sessions.

MEDICAL DISORDERS

The therapist must always leave open the possibility that the presenting symptoms of the client, such as anxiety, depression, fatigue, and so on, may be secondary manifestations of a nonpsychiatric medical problem. It is unreasonable to expect that the typical mental health professional will have a working knowledge of the incredible range of medical disorders that could give rise to psychological symptoms. The nonmedical therapist has no right to express (or, some may contend even *to hold*), any opinion on the presence or nature of physical problems on the part of the client. The therapist does have an ethical obligation to facilitate referral for the appropriate medical evaluation, however. In such instances, the therapist and the client must rely on the wisdom of physicians in order to rule out a medical cause for the presenting symptoms. However, there is no guarantee that the client's doctor will be thorough or competent. Although the therapist cannot necessarily comment directly on the quality of medical diagnosis and treatment, he or she can encourage the client to be a well-informed consumer, not a passive victim.

Many clients we encounter present a complex set of symptoms, including significant physical complaints. Our impression is that medical practitioners vary widely in their responses to complaints of fatigue, pain, sleep difficulties, mood swings, and the like. Perhaps physicians increasingly lack the time and the financial backing of health insurers to conduct extensive investigations of chronic, but semitolerable physical complaints. They may become impatient with the client because of their own feelings of frustration over not being able to solve the presenting problems. Moreover, some physicians may lack the training or the temperament to deal with an emotionally distressed client who refuses to be "brave" (and perhaps most important of all, *quiet*) about his or her symptoms. The medical practitioner may offer the client a referral for psychotherapy, perhaps with the not-so-subtle message that the medical complaints are not legitimate. If the client is already in treatment, the physician may begin to scapegoat the therapist for the client's ongoing medical complaints. In our experience, all the relationship difficulties discussed in this paragraph seem to be strongly influenced by sexual politics, in that they are most likely to occur between male physicians and female patients. We suspect that men's physical complaints generally are treated differently by male doctors. We also suspect that male patients are much less likely to hear intimations that their complaints of pain or other physical distress are exaggerated, illusory, or psychogenic in origin.

In our experience, clients with known psychiatric histories may find it very difficult to have their physical complaints taken seriously by the medical profession unless they can produce lesions or other concrete, demonstrable pathology. The failure to be taken seriously by a powerful authority figure throws many of our clients (and at times their therapists) into a severe inner conflict that resonates strongly with feelings of worthlessness, fear of rejection, and other family of origin issues. Incest survivors, for example, may already have difficulty monitoring and correctly labeling bodily sensations. "Is it pain or is it me?" they may ask. Flooded with shame for having made a mistake, or besieged by anxiety over the threat of being rejected, they may try to accommodate to the physician's views. Clients may then blame themselves for the physical complaints and may attempt to deal with symptoms of pain or illness by suppressing awareness of them.

As we have observed, many victims of childhood trauma, particularly incest survivors, may become inordinately skilled at screening out sensations of pain and other symptoms of illness. Unfortunately, such a highly advanced ability to deny pain, coupled with severe problems of self-worth can lead to potentially disastrous consequences for certain clients.

Betsy, a single woman in her mid-30s, regularly consulted an internist who was aware of her history of psychiatric hospitalizations. A survivor of extensive physical and sexual abuse, she experienced overwhelming anxiety over being rejected by others, which led to a lifelong pattern of avoiding close relationships. Predictably, visits to a physician elicited terror in her, particularly when a physical examination was involved. Compounding Betsy's lack of assertiveness with authority figures was the brief but powerful sense of relief she experienced whenever her doctor dismissed a physical complaint as due to "nerves" and declined to investigate it further. Moreover, she was well accustomed to seeing problems in her life as all her fault anyway. For several months, Betsy had complained to her therapist about recurrent abdominal pains severe enough to cause her to double over in distress. Having worked with Betsy for several years, the therapist knew her psychological symptom picture well enough to recognize the woman had never before complained of abdominal pains even during periods of extreme stress. Time and again, he encouraged Betsy to return to the physician with the gastrointestinal complaints. Although she was unable to assert herself with the internist, who persisted in labeling the pain as psychogenic in origin, Betsy found the therapist's suggestion that she seek a second opinion far too threatening to even consider. One weekend the searing pain finally drove Betsy to an emergency room, where her symptoms were evaluated on their own merit, and not in light of her psychiatric history. The resident on duty at the emergency service ordered a series of gastrointestinal tests immediately. Within hours, Betsy underwent emergency surgery in order to remove a badly diseased gall bladder.

PSYCHOSIS AND BIOLOGICALLY BASED PSYCHIATRIC DISORDERS

We believe in the concept of mental illness, at least as it refers to biologically based and/or genetically transmitted disturbances in thinking, emotions, and behavior. Schizophrenia and manic–depressive illness are the best examples of disorders that fit in such a category. The history of psychiatry is replete with concepts such as "schizophrenogenic mother," which have emphasized psychological causes (and ultimately parental culpability) for essentially biological disorders. In our opinion, the burden of proof must rest heavily on the shoulders of any clinician who claims that a particular client's psychotic or manic symptoms originally stem from nonbiological causes.

Individuals who show evidence of mania or psychotic thought processes will not benefit from psychotherapy unless appropriate medical interventions occur first. They should receive an evaluation as soon as possible from a competent, biologically oriented psychiatrist. If the mania or the psychotic symptoms respond to medical treatment, then the individual may well be a good candidate for the therapeutic interventions described in this volume. There is every reason to believe that medication and psychotherapy should operate in concert on the client's behalf, particularly if the psychiatrist and the nonmedical therapist have a good working relationship. In fact, with the possible exception of the use of minor tranquilizers for anxiety symptoms, it is difficult to imagine instances where appropriate utilization of medication would interfere with the goals of psychotherapy.

MULTIPLE PERSONALITY DISORDERS

Since we do not consider ourselves sufficiently experienced with the multiple personality disorder (MPD) population to offer anything in the way of treatment recommendations at this time, we urge interested readers to consult recent volumes on the treatment of MPD (e.g., Putnam, 1989; Ross, 1989). At one time, clinical lore held that multiple personality disorders were exceedingly rare. Like many of our colleagues, however, we now suspect that over the years we treated certain individuals who, in retrospect, appear to have been "multiples." We look forward to learning from other therapists, particularly those with a cognitive orientation, who have achieved success in treating patients with multiple personality disorders.

"GARDEN VARIETY" DEPRESSION

As Beck (1976) has described, depression involves the "cognitive triad," a negative view of the self, the world, and the future. It is easy to see how the basic beliefs developed in a dysfunctional family of origin would render an individual vulnerable to recurring feelings of worthlessness, helplessness, and hopelessness later in life. We encourage our readers to assess the presence of depressive symptomatology carefully, particularly with reference to vegetative symptoms, and of course, suicidal wishes. Clients who are experiencing insomnia, appetite loss, concentration difficulties, and related symptoms may not be able to benefit from psychotherapy until they can eat and, most importantly, sleep properly. As we indicated in a previous section, there should be no inherent incompatibility between the use of antidepressant medication and involvement in psychotherapy.

There are many straightforward cognitive and behavioral interventions available for use with moderately and severely depressed individuals (Beck et al., 1979; Bedrosian & Beck, 1980; Hollon & Beck, 1979). These treatment techniques enable clients to become more active and productive and assist them in modifying current distortions in thinking. Early in the treatment process, we typically combine such interventions (aimed at securing immediate symptom relief for the client), with our efforts to link pertinent family of origin material with the current distress. If the "traditional" cognitive therapy techniques help a client to become mobilized, even to the point of terminating before addressing broader issues, so be it. However, our model of psychopathology would predict that clients who come from dysfunctional family backgrounds will continue to experience recurring symptoms unless they begin to change basic schemas and coping strategies. We assume that the individual who declines to work on family of origin issues will want to resume treatment at a later date, particularly if he or she had a positive experience the first time around. As we discuss in Chapter 14, the therapist should reframe any termination as a behavioral experiment, carefully sowing the seeds for a non-stigmatizing return to treatment if the client experiences difficulties in the future.

Any clinician who works with depressed clients must become skilled in the assessment and treatment of suicidal wishes. Although a detailed exploration of the topic is beyond the scope of the current volume, we refer the reader to a number of publications which approach the assessment and modification of suicidal ideation from a cognitive perspective (Beck, Kovacs, & Weissman, 1975, 1979; Beck, Rush, et al., 1979; Bedrosian, 1986, 1988; Bedrosian & Beck, 1979; Bedrosian & Epstein, 1984). Like other cognitions, suicidal wishes may fluctuate considerably in response to contextual influences, such as marital or family relationships. As discussed in greater detail elsewhere, involvement of spouses and/or other family members in some form of treatment is usually essential when a client is suicidal (Bedrosian, 1986, 1988).

Nearly all of the chronically suicidal clients we have seen were raised in highly dysfunctional families. In addition, nearly all of them were victims of childhood sexual abuse. In many instances, they reported obsessive suicidal ideation dating as far back as late childhood or early adolescence. Often there were multiple instances of suicide attempts and/or completed suicides in the family tree, a pattern that served to reinforce the client's view of such behavior as an acceptable coping strategy.

Patricia, a woman in her early 40s who suffered from chronic depression remembered having her first suicidal thoughts when she was in sixth grade. Each night as she tried to sleep, she would soothe herself with the image of warm blood flowing from her slit wrists down the length of her forearms. As an adult, Patricia consistently experienced similar imagery *automatically* in a wide range of stressful situations, particularly those that involved interpersonal conflict. A maiden aunt, who had always identified Patricia as her favorite, had a long history of suicide attempts, using a variety of methods. When the client was 14, the aunt hanged herself in the family's garage. During the course of treatment, Patricia recognized that at the same time her own suicidal images began, she was the victim of ongoing sexual abuse at the hands of two perpetrators, a great-uncle, and a male cousin. Over the course of several years of treatment, Patricia's therapist illustrated to her again and again how the suicidal ideation served as a coping strategy for her, dating back to a time when she was helpless to affect the circumstances in her life in any other way. She began to see the connection between the suicidal imagery and the current stressors in her life, especially those that stimulated feelings of worthlessness on her part. The more she viewed her suicidal thinking as a *symptom* of something else occurring in her life, the less she wanted kill herself. Instead of nurturing the suicidal imagery, she eventually began to disregard it as "noise" and found other means of coping with uncomfortable situations.

The therapist who works extensively with incest survivors and other victims of severe childhood trauma must also learn to discriminate between self-mutilative wishes and behavior and more explicitly suicidal thoughts and actions. Clearly not every client who cuts, or who thinks about cutting, wishes to die. On the other hand, clients who have no wish at all to die, as well as those who are ambivalent about living and dying, are still capable of tragic miscalculations. The therapist may still need to be concerned for the safety of self-mutilative clients even in the absence of explicit suicidal wishes. Likewise, we urge clinicians to reflect carefully before dismissing any self-destructive act as a "suicidal gesture." *All* suicidal acts (and indeed, all suicidal ideation) should be taken seriously until conclusively proven otherwise. In order to gauge the seriousness of a suicide attempt, it is necessary to investigate thoroughly the individual's cognitions *at the time of the act*. Interested readers should consult the references listed earlier in this section for ideas on conducting such assessments. Since young victims of incest and other sexual abuse are prone to engage in acts of self-mutilation, we encourage clinicians to rule out the presence of such traumatic circumstances in the environment *first*—before considering more complex and potentially stigmatizing explanations (e.g., personality disorders) for the client's difficulties.

Treating chronically suicidal and/or self-mutilative clients can be a stressful experience for even the most experienced of therapists. Clinicians must be careful not to overwhelm themselves by accepting too many cases with self-destructive symptoms. Likewise, through experiences in supervision and in their own treatment, therapists need to confront personal issues that might sabotage their interventions with suicidal clients.

ANXIETY AND PANIC DISORDERS

Therapists with cognitive and/or behavioral training have much to offer in the way of symptom control to the client who suffers from anxiety or panic. We believe that particularly in cases of acute onset, the therapist has a responsibility to offer the client symptom-relief techniques, such as relaxation and imagery procedures *first* before progressing to more lengthy and complex treatment options. We urge interested readers to consult both professional texts (Barlow, 1988; Beck & Emery, 1985) and the self-help literature (Goldman & Babior, 1991; Bourne, 1990; Weekes, 1968, 1972, 1976; Wilson, 1986) for an overview of cognitive and behavioral strategies for coping with anxiety.

As we have indicated in previous sections, we are strong advocates of the use of medication for a variety of psychiatric disorders. We are more ambivalent about the use of medication with anxiety and panic disorders, however, than with other psychiatric conditions. We find that medication seems most helpful as a *time-limited strategy*, particularly in anxiety cases that involve acute onset of symptoms and/or severe impairment in day-to-day functioning. As we discuss below, long-term use of antianxiety medication, or "anxiolytics," can directly interfere with certain cognitive and behavioral treatment goals. Clients who benefit from medication seem to do so quickly, often reaching a plateau beyond which they will not progress without fundamental changes in the way they *perceive* anxiety and its potential effects. We want our clients to accept the biological fact that every person has the capacity to experience anxiety at any given time. Further, we want our clients to learn that if they have to, they can tolerate very high levels of anxiety without going crazy or being damaged in any way. Unfortunately, the use of medication does not necessarily help our clients develop a greater *tolerance* for anxiety. Indeed, in the absence of overt symptoms, clients may not have the opportunity to acquire and practice new strategies for coping with anxiety. Although they may show less behavioral impairment, they might still be "afraid of fear." As long as they attribute clinical improvements solely to medication, they will continue to be overly intimidated by their symptoms. Consequently, they may be reluctant to challenge themselves to the fullest by reapproaching fearful situations. As a result, they will continue to show pockets of avoidant behavior, some of which may be quite significant, despite clinical improvements in many areas.

As our readers know, some of the most commonly prescribed minor tranquilizers are highly addictive. Unfortunately, we are aware of a number of physicians who think nothing of keeping our clients on such medications for years without adequate monitoring or follow-up. Since many clients are not even aware that the medications they are taking are addictive, they obviously cannot identify the signs of withdrawal, which, ironically enough, often resemble the symptoms of anxiety they sought treatment for in the first place. Some individuals may be prone to experience withdrawal symptoms in a matter of a few *hours* if they do not take their accustomed dosages of medication. Not surprisingly then, some clients erroneously label drug withdrawal as a recurrence of their symptoms, mistakenly concluding that they need to continue taking medication when what they really require is medically supervised detoxification.

Needless to say, we become concerned when clients with known family histories of alcoholism and/or drug addiction take minor tranquilizers for more than a few days or weeks. Although we do our best to discourage clients with substance abuse problems of their own from using such medications except on an emergency basis, there are definite limits on our ability to influence them. Unfortunately, as nonmedical therapists, we do not make medication decisions. In fact, the physician writing the prescriptions, who in many anxiety cases is more likely to be an internist or a family practitioner than a psychiatrist, may not even be interested in our input on the client in question! Moreover, since we have an ethical obligation to keep our recommendations confined to areas of true professional competence, we must be careful about second guessing medical decisions.

Clinicians who treat substantial numbers of clients with anxiety or panic disorders need to keep a number of differential diagnostic issues in mind, some of which are beyond the scope of the current presentation. We have seen very few legitimate "simple phobias" in our clinical practice. Likewise, except for those instances involving acute, first-time onset of symptoms, most of the anxiety cases we treat involve more pervasive and complicated life difficulties. When clients fail to respond to reasonable symptom control strategies for anxiety or panic disorders or experience frequent relapses, the therapist may need to explore and address other important diagnostic factors. These include:

1. *Substance abuse or other compulsive behaviors, possibly hidden from the therapist.* In our experience, it is not unusual to find that clients who request treatment for anxiety have unacknowledged substance abuse problems, which sometimes do not surface until a variety of treatment options have proven to be unsuccessful. Other addictive or compulsive behavior, such as bulimia or sexual behaviors of a degrading nature, may also bear a direct relationship to the presenting complaints of anxiety or panic.

2. *Ongoing life stressors, which the client cannot confront or perhaps even recognize.* For many of our clients, anxiety symptoms may reflect the fact that there is something in their lives of extreme importance that requires their attention. Clients who seek treatment for panic attacks and other anxiety problems often manifest mixed patterns of overvigilance and denial. At the foreground of the client's awareness, of course, are the anxiety symptoms and the related cognitions. Sensitized to signs of autonomic arousal, the individual habitually scans for the physical sensations of anxiety. He or she becomes preoccupied with identifying and avoiding stimuli or situations associated with fear. Likewise, the individual obsesses about the potential consequences of experiencing anxiety (e.g., insanity) perhaps to the point of *inducing* panic. In the meantime, the client who is so preoccupied with symptoms may not recognize the connections between the anxiety and other ongoing prob-

lems of a serious nature, particularly those involving relationships with significant others. By continually diverting the individual's attention away from these other difficulties, the anxiety symptoms actually facilitate denial. Further, the symptoms may also play a role in the family system keeping the client in a dependent, relatively incompetent position that undermines his or her ability to confront difficulties with significant others. Finally, the anxiety symptoms themselves may escalate every time the client attempts to address the marital or family problems in a more direct manner. The client may be unable or unwilling at first to acknowledge the presence of such additional life difficulties to the therapist. Symptom reduction, an increased level of trust in the therapeutic relationship, and changes in information processing may make it possible for such a client to acknowledge broader areas of distress as treatment progresses. In many instances, the client may become involved in family or marital therapy at some point in the treatment process.

3. *Secondary gains.* Unlike depressed individuals, who may feel quite badly no matter where they are and what they are doing, clients with anxiety problems can structure their lives so that they are comparatively symptom-free while enjoying the benefits of various secondary gains in the process. Indeed, some secondary gains, such as disability payments, certainly encourage continued avoidance of anxiety-provoking situations, if not outright malingering. As we discussed above, the client's marital or family system may be organized in such a way as to discourage improvements in his or her functioning. The client may lack sufficient motivation to confront fear-provoking situations as long as significant others continue to reinforce avoidant and dependent behaviors. The presence of such relationship patterns in the client's life would argue for the inclusion of family or marital sessions in addition to individual therapy, as part of the treatment plan.

4. *Family of origin issues, including historical material of a traumatic nature.* Many years ago, an esteemed colleague of ours, Patricia Waldeck, observed that family of origin issues are usually implicated whenever a client with an anxiety disorder fails to respond to symptom-oriented interventions. Our subsequent clinical experiences seem to have borne out her prediction. We have difficulty recalling a single case of chronic anxiety or panic that did *not* involve demonstrable family of origin pathology. Obviously, many of the schemas that develop in response to destructive childhood experiences insure that a tense, fearful undercurrent will accompany daily living in adulthood, thereby increasing the likelihood that the individual will experience autonomic arousal at inappropriate times. Moreover, clients who have been abused or otherwise traumatized in childhood, may show clear symptoms of

(PTSD), *even if they are unable to acknowledge the existence of the precipitating events themselves.* They may not understand the true significance of their symptoms, and the fears underlying them, until they undergo a process of trauma revelation, as we describe in Chapter 11. Many of our clients may require a *series* of therapeutic contacts, along with several cycles of improvement and relapse, before they begin to recognize that family of origin issues, as reflected in basic schemas, information-processing styles, and other coping strategies, have created a *predisposition* to experience anxiety or panic.

SUBSTANCE ABUSE AND "ADDICTION-LIKE" COMPULSIVE BEHAVIORS

Ongoing substance abuse clearly limits the potential benefits of psychotherapy for any client, no matter how motivated or insightful he or she may be. Many of our clients have engaged in high levels of substance abuse beginning in early adolescence and have continued literally for decades thereafter. Until such individuals attain sobriety, they are likely to experience continuing difficulties in most, if not all, major areas of life functioning. *We emphasize that clients do not have to be physically addicted or dependent to be significantly impaired by their use of substances.* In our experience, even clients who experience only infrequent or episodic substance abuse also may not realize appreciable gains in treatment until they achieve sobriety.

Despite our remarks on the limitations imposed on treatment by ongoing addictions, we do not advocate the summary dismissal of clients who are not yet ready to acknowledge such difficulties. Along with other writers (e.g., Treadway, 1989), we believe that it is possible for a therapist to be helpful to clients and their families during periods of active substance abuse, as well as in the early stages of sobriety. The therapist may decide to continue working with the individual who is in the throes of an addiction, with hopes of either stimulating a crisis directly, or of developing a trusted role in the client's life, so as to be helpful in arranging appropriate treatment when the addicted person finally "bottoms out." The therapist may be aware that a spouse or another significant person in the client's life is working hard in his or her own treatment and/or in a Twelve-Step Program. Soon there may be powerful new relationship currents in the client's life that will facilitate confrontation of the addiction. In the meantime, the therapist may choose to build a relationship with the substance abuser, all the while scanning the horizon for signs of an imminent crisis.

We assume that the symptoms or relationship problems that stimulated the client's involvement in treatment in the first place will continue, and perhaps even intensify, until the chemically dependent individual confronts the addiction in question. This period in the treatment process can be quite frustrating for the therapist and perhaps even frightening, depending on the extent of the client's impairment. The therapist may struggle with feelings of excessive responsibility when, for example, he or she knows that the client is regularly drinking and driving. Referral sources or significant others, particularly those who are locked into "codependent" or enabling roles vis à vis the client, may have extremely inappropriate expectations of treatment, believing, in effect, that the therapist will be able to control the client's behavior. Such inflated expectations of the therapist and of treatment merely reflect an inability to acknowledge powerlessness over the addicted individual.

Unwilling and/or unable to take appropriate responsibility for their actions, chemically dependent clients often try to recruit therapists in their efforts to blame their difficulties on significant others. The addicted individual may wish to devote the entire treatment hour to complaints about spouses and other family members, while resisting any of the therapist's attempts to shift the focus back onto the self. He or she may habitually twist the therapist's words in order to gain advantage during arguments in the home, thereby encouraging significant others to focus blame on the practitioner and the treatment process.

While addicted clients continue to escalate their irresponsible, destructive behaviors, they also may scapegoat the therapist. The addicted client may resent the therapist for not helping to silence critics in the family or may blame the therapist because the presenting complaints, such as anxiety attacks, marital friction, or problems with an adolescent, have not improved. Their blaming attitudes and behaviors can make life even more stressful for the therapist, especially if he or she is already struggling with a sense of blurred boundaries and responsibilities. Despite the therapist's involvement and input, the client may ultimately suffer tragic, or even fatal, consequences as a result of his or her addiction. The therapist will need support in order to remain in such a powerless position without taking unnecessary responsibility for the client or experiencing inappropriate guilt over negative outcomes. Consultation with colleagues or supervisors can be extremely helpful in reducing the pressure on the therapist in such instances.

The therapist who continues to work with an addicted individual in hopes of facilitating recovery efforts at the appropriate time must be wary of sending dangerously mixed messages to the identified patient, the family, and in some cases, referral sources as well. Although on some level, the therapist cannot control the distorted expectations and perceptions others may hold about treatment, he or she does have a responsibility to be clear with the client and other interested parties about what therapy can realistically accomplish as long as the addictive behaviors continue. On the one hand, the therapist must take pains to avoid knowingly colluding with the identified patient's denial while he or she attempts to sustain some sort of constructive bond with the client. On the other hand, the therapist needs to find a way to indicate to the family and/or the referral source that continuing to see the addicted individual in treatment in no way implies that he or she has even an *infinitesimal* level of control over the client's attitudes and behaviors.

Individuals whose substance abuse remains hidden may receive extensive psychiatric treatment, including psychotropic drugs, with no discernible success. For years, they may consult therapists and/or physicians complaining of recurrent or unremitting symptoms of anxiety or depression. When assessing a client's ability to benefit from treatment, the clinician should take failed psychotherapy experiences that occurred prior to sobriety with the proverbial grain of salt.

Active substance abusers readily behave in a manner that makes them appear "characterological" or "personality disordered" to the clinicians who come into contact with them. However, therapists need to remember that alcohol and drugs produce neurological deficits, labile moods, and symptomatic patterns of thinking and behavior that may not reflect the individual's basic values or psychological structure. We find it quite difficult, if not impossible, to predict what a chronic substance abuser will look like after 1 or 2 years of sobriety. It may take the therapist a comparable length of time to develop a reasonably accurate assessment of the client's potential for change. The clinician may find that the individual still retains many of the presobriety attitudes and behaviors, albeit without the earmarks of intoxication, despite a lengthy period of successful abstinence. In some instances, new compulsive behaviors, including eating problems, sexual acting out, or workaholism may come to occupy the central role in the individual's life once played by substance abuse. Some individuals seem to resume their lives at about the same developmental point where the substance abuse first began. Those clients who began habitual use of drugs and alcohol in late childhood or early adolescence will clearly have a lot of catching up to do. As they move from the sobriety phase to more of the recovery phase of treatment, they will need to remediate many deficits in their social, intellectual, and moral development.

We concur with what appears to be the conventional wisdom offered by the Twelve-Step Programs, namely that sobriety, as opposed to recovery, ought to be the primary focus for the recovering individual during the first 1 to 2 years of abstinence. We prefer to undertake therapeutic work on family of origin issues with formerly addicted clients only after they have achieved a reasonably stable period of sobriety. We generally do not feel comfortable delving into family of origin material, especially if we have reason to suspect that there is considerable traumatic content, until the individual has been sober or abstinent for at least 1 year. Major aspects of the client's lifestyle, including friends, leisure time, and even the job, having been inextricably linked with the addiction, may need to be completely restructured—this time around sobriety. Such restructuring may require severe changes and losses in the client's daily life resulting initially in boredom, social isolation, and/or a sense of disorientation.

We realize that there is justifiable controversy over whether compulsive behaviors such as gambling, overeating, bulimia, and sexual acting out should be classified and treated as true addictions. We do find however, that there are some legitimate parallels between individuals who engage in such compulsive behaviors and those who victimize themselves with substance abuse. Both types of clients are apt to rely heavily on denial mechanisms, particularly with respect to the adverse, and in some cases life-threatening, consequences of addictions or compulsive behaviors. Like the conventionally recognized addictions, these other compulsive behaviors can retard progress in any treatment targeted at larger issues. Compulsive behaviors and the associated negative consequences distract clients and keep them trapped in a narrow, self-perpetuating frame of reference. Like addictions then, compulsive behaviors need to be under control before the individual can benefit from examination of basic schemas or other family of origin material. In addition to providing social support and an established framework for recovery, client involvement in a Twelve-Step Program targeted at compulsive behavior can free the therapist from having to play the role of a parent or watchdog.

LEARNING DIFFICULTIES AND RESIDUAL ADHD EFFECTS

We are struck by the number of our clients who suffer from learning disabilities, attention deficit disorders, and related difficulties. Perhaps we should not be surprised, however, since attention deficit hyperactive disorder (ADHD), for example, is the most common childhood psychiatric disorder, accounting for over half of all referrals to child mental health clinics (Ingersoll, 1988). Moreover, the majority of ADHD children suffer recognizable symptoms in adult life as well (Barkley, 1990). Current research now indicates that many ADHD adults will demonstrate impairments in social, educational, and occupational functioning, and as many as 25% will show serious levels of antisocial behavior (Barkley, 1990). Often such problems were not detected in childhood or adolescence, so that the individual had to endure being labeled as lazy, stupid, or willful by parents and teachers. Some of our clients who had always seen themselves in similarly negative terms eventually sought out psychological testing at our urging, only to discover that they suffered from legitimate impairments. In other cases, the parents may have known about the difficulties but because of their own deficiencies were unable to respond constructively to the child's problems. Consequently, the child's self-esteem, as well as his or her academic foundation, may have been severely compromised in the course of development.

We urge therapists to be alert to any signs of learning problems on the part of their clients, including some of the following:

- Chronic school or vocational underachievement
- Undue difficulty performing less demanding aspects of current job
- Difficulty prioritizing tasks
- Poor organizational skills, at home as well as at work
- Recurring problems with deadlines and time limits
- Compulsive avoidance of tasks involving reading, writing, basic computation, or other academic skills
- Recurring difficulties with concentration or memory, not attributable to other factors such as anxiety or depression

Although it may include a substantial family of origin component, psychological treatment of individuals with learning and/or attentional difficulties may often focus on repairing self-esteem deficits directly tied to the disabilities. The therapist must conduct treatment in a way that capitalizes on the client's unique learning style, otherwise the individual may find it unreasonably difficult to utilize or even retain material from the sessions. Unfortunately, some of our clients have spent a lifetime "fakin' it," pretending to follow or understand a discussion when they really do not. Consequently, the therapist needs to monitor the client's ability to absorb material from treatment. Needless to say, it may be extremely inadvisable to assign readings, written exercises, or other types of homework assignments to clients with certain learning problems. Apart from work on issue-related content, therapists and/or educational specialists also may need to help the client acquire new attentional or organizational strategies.

PERSONALITY DISORDERS

We remain stubbornly ambivalent on the subject of personality disorders. On the one hand, as we mentioned earlier, we know that we have worked quite successfully with some clients whom other clinicians might label as personality disordered. We avoid using terms such as "borderline" or "narcissistic" in a casual manner, since in our opinion they often unfairly stigmatize the individuals involved and provoke unreasonable feelings of hopelessness on the part of clinicians. We do not want to feel intimidated just because a client has many types of symptoms, pervasive relationship difficulties, or even a history of treatment failures. Moreover, any given client may have areas of substantial competency that are not readily apparent early in treatment. Consequently we tend to be extremely conservative about diagnosing personality disorders.

In addition to avoiding the obvious pitfalls of basing our interventions solely on Axis II labels, we try to bear in mind the infinite number of "moderator variables" that might render an apparent nightmare of a case quite workable. A number of these variables have research support. For example, in a summary of the literature relating client variables to treatment outcome, Prochaska and DiClemente (1984) found that lower levels of defensiveness, less externalization of blame, the presence of felt emotional pain such as anxiety or depression, and positive expectations for therapy all bore positive relationships to treatment outcome. These data converge with our clinical experiences. We consistently find that clients who present to therapy in obvious pain, who have the capacity for self-examination, and who are willing to acknowledge at least some responsibility for the problems in their lives, have an excellent chance of benefiting from treatment irrespective of their presenting diagnoses.

On the other hand, we do not see how it is possible to work with certain personality-disordered clients, for example, those who truly lack empathy for others, fail to experience remorse over legitimate wrongdoing, and/or habitually externalize all responsibility for their actions. We assume that at least some measure of dissatisfaction with oneself is a necessary precondition for psychotherapy. Unfortunately in our clinical experiences we have never observed any exceptions to such an assumption. Clients who externalize all blame and responsibility for their difficulties will not sit still for the kind of self-analysis demanded in active forms of psychotherapy. These individuals would prefer to rail ad nauseum against people and situations that are unfavorable to them. When it becomes clear to them that they will be expected to examine their own attitudes and behaviors, they tend to drop out of treatment.

Consequently, accounts of purportedly successful cognitive therapy with *true* paranoid or antisocial personality disorders would appear to lack credibility in our eyes.

When dealing with a client who externalizes blame to such an extreme degree, the therapist should not work too hard trying to fashion an area of self-dissatisfaction out of whole cloth. Let the client define a problem within himself or herself on which to work. If the client cannot sustain even a minimal focus on the self, he or she probably should be dissuaded from wasting time and money on treatment. Clients certainly cannot benefit from the specialized skills of a therapist unless they are ready for a modicum of self-examination.

LIMERANCE

The symbolism contained in many popular songs illustrates how the images of erotic love and those of the addictions become intertwined in the human experience. Songwriters as diverse as the urbane sophisticate Cole Porter and the gritty blues man Willie Dixon have alluded to the similarities between being in love and being high on drugs. We prefer to use the term "limerance" coined by Tennov (1980) to describe the transient, but powerful, experience associated with falling in love. Individuals who are experiencing limerance are in the grip of the strongest drug known to humanity. They will wrestle with a constant, seemingly insatiable desire to be with their new partners. In the presence of their lovers, they may report feeling more secure, more accepted, more optimistic, and more worthwhile than ever before. Other interests and relationships may cease to exist for them for a time. Although they may appear to be reasonable and receptive in treatment, at least on a superficial level, they will resist any rational analysis of the romantic relationship. Until the negative features of the relationship begin to escalate, or the infatuation subsides, these clients will be unwilling to process information that could lead to alienation or separation from the adored partner. Often they will react to the therapist's attempts to examine the relationship by defending the individual reflexively, just as a defiant teenage girl might defend her boyfriend to her parents.

By pushing too hard on the limerant relationship, the therapist may unwittingly force the client to give up treatment. The therapist may drift into such a triangulating mode with the client out of an ill-advised desire to rescue him or her from yet another hurtful or otherwise inappropriate relationship. In such situations, the therapist must recognize once more his or her essential helplessness over the choices the client makes and retreat to a more detached treatment posture. It may be painful for the therapist to have to watch the client make decisions that could produce negative consequences for years to come. However, the therapist must remember that the client will begin to choose more suitable partners only when his or her underlying belief systems change. Unfortunately, the beliefs which accompany a limerant experience can best be described as "quasidelusional," that is, so strongly held as to be impervious to new data. To facilitate future changes, the therapist must be willing to wait until the client is more receptive to self-examination. If the therapist's assessment of the client's limerant relationship is correct, then there will be ample opportunity for relevant issues to surface in treatment. Soon enough, the limerant aspects of the relationship will fade away, as they always do, forcing the client to confront a more painful, distressing reality. At that point, the client may be more ready to work with the therapist, provided he or she has not been alienated in the meantime.

Rather than confront the client in a heavy-handed manner, we recommend that the therapist step back and let the limerant experience unfold even if it means allowing the client to withdraw from treatment. All the therapist's efforts should go toward seeding the subsequent treatment interactions that will occur when the strains in the limerant relationship begin to appear. The therapist should maintain a posture that allows the client the opportunity to acknowledge such strains when they occur without having to lose face. The therapist's message to the client, which may be conveyed either implicitly or explicitly, should be: "Although I've explored with you some of the potential difficulties that might occur in your relationship, I'm going to defer to your judgment. I hope it continues to be a source of happiness for you. You deserve to have a good relationship in your life. I want to remind you, however, that I'm still here to support you if any problems occur."

Clients who are participating in ongoing affairs may pose a number of additional complications for therapists. Limerant relationships appear to thrive when the partners lack accessibility to one another. If there had not been a blood feud between the Montagues and Capulets, Romeo and Juliet might have wound up singing "The Thrill is Gone" instead of committing suicide together. In an affair, the relative lack of contact and daily involvement seems to keep the limerant experience going for longer periods of time than would typically be the case for partners who have ready access to one another. As a consequence, the client's reality testing is impaired for a longer period of time. Moreover, he or she may habitually compare an attractive, exciting lover who has few, if any, discernible flaws, with a spouse whose deficiencies are all too apparent. Clients who are purportedly in the process of deciding between two lovers, or a lover and a spouse, can be extremely boring to treat. Unless they can remain focused on their own issues, as opposed to the characteristics of their partners, they may lead the therapist down the same unproductive pathways again and again, all the while juggling two relationships in a precarious manner. The therapist may have to watch and wait somewhat helplessly as these clients remain bogged down in a cycle of obsessive thoughts and compulsive behaviors centered on the competing relationships in their lives. Until they begin to detach from the all-consuming limerant experience itself, it will be difficult for them to devote sufficient attention to the more central issues that have helped to stimulate their affairs. Likewise, as the clients become less stimulated by the new partner, it should be easier for them to recognize some of the cognitive distortions that have accompanied both the marriage and the extramarital relationship.

It is important to note the relationship between *denial* and infidelity. Probably the majority of our clients who participate in ongoing extramarital relationships do experience discomfort of some sort regarding their actions. Only through engaging in various levels of denial, are they able to sustain the affairs without feeling overpowered by dysphoric emotions, such as anxiety and guilt. Telling themselves that their extramarital affairs are not affecting their families, they may block out thoughts of the other person while spending time with their spouses. On the other hand, they also may find it necessary to screen out cognitions that involve their spouses or families in order to enjoy time with their paramours. They may minimize the significance of the outside relationship (e.g., "It's only a sexual thing"; "Neither one of us intends to get seriously involved.") They are likely to idealize their extramarital partner while ignoring rather obvious character defects in the process and may be particularly forgiving of his or her participation in the acts of betrayal and deception that are necessary to maintain the affair.

They typically assume that their lovers would have been their lifetime partners had they met them sooner, yet we find that relatively few affairs actually culminate in marriage or long-term commitment once both participants are free of their former spouses. If the partner in the affair is married, the client may dismiss the relationship (e.g., "Their marriage is essentially over") or bitterly scapegoat the spouse for all the difficulties in the relationship. Likewise, the client who is engaged in an affair may present a seemingly airtight case (at least in the client's eyes) against being able to produce any constructive changes in his or her marriage. Clients may prefer to see themselves as having "outgrown" their spouses, thereby rationalizing their own avoidance of intimacy in their marriages. In many instances, it turns out that the client's spouse had recognized significant indications of infidelity on the part of his or her spouse but had ignored or minimized the information. Some spouses of unfaithful partners find themselves unable to call the issue of an affair to question with their mates for fear of the answers they might receive. In fact, both partners may collude to avoid the topic for some time, even when the facts point quite obviously to an affair.

Lastly, most of our clients who conduct affairs fail to recognize how they lose self-esteem in the process. The ongoing rewards of an extramarital relationship may be so compelling that they fail to process the subtle, but often mounting loss of self-respect that occurs as a consequence of deception and disloyalty. Parenting in particular may suffer as a result of such an insidious loss of self-esteem. Needless to say, a therapist who rationalizes his or her own participation in extramarital affairs may be quick to support the denial processes of clients who find themselves in similar circumstances.

As the previous paragraph suggests, one of the therapist's major strategies with a client who is conducting an ongoing affair involves the repetitive identification of denial processes. In a supportive, collaborative manner, the therapist must help the client to become fully aware of all the personal psychological issues and potential "real-world" consequences associated with infidelity. While avoiding a judgmental posture, the therapist must identify and highlight data that challenge the client's beliefs about the character of the extramarital partner, the quality of the affair and its likely outcome, the impact on ongoing relationships with significant others, the long-term efficacy of deception, the potential effects of discovery, the consequences of separation and divorce, and so on. A more accurate appraisal of such topics should produce a legitimate rise in the client's emotional discomfort and sense of dissatisfaction with the self, thereby facilitating constructive involvement in treatment. The therapist also needs to reframe the client's compulsive and indecisive behaviors as *choices* (e.g., "So although you are uncertain about the future, right now you have *chosen* to stay with your husband and continue on in the affair"; or "What made you *decide* to start seeing her again?"), thereby maintaining the posture that the individual has the capability to resolve his or her situation, without being controlled by dark, unseen forces. Above all, the therapist wants to direct the client's attention back toward basic personal issues that continue to affect his or her behavior regardless of whichever relationship happens to prevail at any given time.

Although cases involving ongoing infidelity can turn out to be boring in a clinical sense, they may be quite stimulating for the therapist on a personal level, particularly in the early stages of treatment. As the publishers of supermarket tabloids and the programmers of prime-time television know all too well, affairs make people pay attention. Our clients' amorous adventures may well resonate with our own marital frustrations, escapist fantasies, sexual insecurities, parental loyalties, and a variety of other very hot issues. The therapist must be careful about over-identifying with *any* character in the romantic triangle created by an extramarital affair, so that he or she can continue to address the client's actions as *symptomatic of other underlying issues* without adopting a judgmental tone or applying unreasonable pressure for behavior change on the one hand, or colluding with various forms of denial on the other. Therapists should monitor their own reactions carefully when they treat cases involving infidelity. Some clinicians may conclude from their responses to such cases that they need to address their own problems with intimacy, perhaps in individual or couples therapy.

6

Generating Hypotheses about Family of Origin Issues

ASSESSMENT AS A DYNAMIC PROCESS

In our clinical work, the assessment process is inextricably woven into the treatment process. The purpose of our assessment is not only to determine the kind (e.g., panic disorder, depression) and degree of pathology presented but also to generate and test hypotheses about family of origin issues. As treatment begins, a personal and family history provides the basis for the therapist's initial hypotheses regarding the probable impact of early life experiences on the client's current functioning. As treatment progresses, client and therapist remain engaged in a process of gathering and sorting data relative to core beliefs, information-processing styles, and coping strategies.

Throughout the early stages of treatment, the therapist develops speculative hypotheses as important guides for subsequent exploration. In fact, it is useful for the therapist to be as fluid and creative as possible in his or her initial attempts to understand the client. Over time, however, the therapist's initial speculation should serve as a springboard to a more scientific, data-based process in which hypotheses about the client are evaluated and modified *continuously*, as new information about the individual comes to light.

PARSIMONY

As clinical psychologists, the authors were trained in the "scientist–practitioner" model. The scientific training we received has influenced our clinical work in a number of important ways. First of all, as we mentioned earlier, we regard all our assertions about human behavior in general, and about specific clients, as *hypotheses* that are subject to disconfirmation. Consequently,we assume an obligation to question our assumptions and to revise them constantly in the light of new experiences. Second, although we do not adhere to a strictly behavioral orientation by any means, we do aim whenever possible to tie our basic psychological assumptions to observable phenomena. Third, we have respect for the research tradition. Although we conduct no empirical studies ourselves, we do at least make an effort to integrate some relevant research results into the complexities of our clinical work. Moreover, we must always attempt to evaluate the effectiveness of our therapeutic interventions, and to face up to treatment strategies which simply do not work. Maintaining a clinical practice in one location for more than a decade has forced us to confront the distinction between short- and long-term treatment outcomes. In many instances, follow-up contact with clients has indicated that therapeutic strategies, sometimes based on sound research studies, which may have produced quite dramatic reductions in presenting symptoms, were not effective in preventing long-term, recurring difficulties in our client's lives. As we discuss Chapter 14 on termination, such clinical experiences lead us to question both the ethics and the efficacy of certain approaches to managed care.

One of the cornerstones of a scientific orientation is the concept of parsimony. The doctrine of parsimony requires us to avoid a more complex explanation when a simpler one will do. If two theories can explain a particular phenomenon, the one that uses the fewest assumptions in doing so is preferable. Practitioners of psychotherapy must also exercise parsimony in their formulations about their clients. Before they move to more complex explanations of an individual's psychological symptoms, therapists have an obligation to rule out simpler, more straightforward formulations first. Clinicians must remain aware that readily discernible factors such as ongoing medical problems, situational stressors, and so on, may be sufficient to account for the client's presenting complaints. We concur with Prochaska and DiClemente (1984), who argue that case conceptualizations that contain the least complexity will lead to less client defensiveness, fewer therapy dropouts, and less overall treatment time. Later, we shall describe how we encourage clients themselves to utilize more parsimonious explanations for their own behaviors as well as other occurrences in their lives.

It is the therapist's responsibility to meet the client where he or she happens to be at the start of therapy, and to build a case gradually for the relationship between current difficulties and suspected problems in the family of origin, if the data support it . The therapist has an ethical obligation to let the *data about the client*, not his or her preexisting assumptions about human behavior, ultimately decide whether historical material needs to be an integral part of the treatment of a particular case. Clearly not all of our clients' problems have historical antecedents. As therapists, we need to retain enough humility to allow us to acknowledge information that runs counter to our hypotheses. Nonetheless, in our experience, therapists who do observe some of the typical signs of childhood abuse or trauma in their adult clients will often find that their initial hypotheses were on target if they remain patient and continue to sustain a collaborative atmosphere in treatment.

USING ANOMALOUS DATA

In work with certain clients, the therapist may encounter attitudes, behaviors, and/or emotional reactions that simply do not fit with prior formulations. We have often found that such anomalous data reveal aspects of the client that must be integrated into the case conceptualization in order for the treatment plan to be successful. Like any good scientist, the therapist has an obligation to keep a mental file of anomalous data and to evaluate his or her hypotheses on an ongoing basis in light of such information. The therapist needs to be able to tolerate ambiguity and uncertainty and must be willing to scrap prior formulations that no longer account for the data. Persistent investigation of anomalous data by the therapist may result in a profound change in the subsequent course of treatment.

Peter and Sherry had concealed from the therapist the fact that they had slept apart for over a decade. When the information surfaced during a couples session, they maintained that Peter's snoring had necessitated the separation, while they discounted the therapist's conjecture that such an arrangement might reflect a need to maintain distance in the relationship. The therapist knew that Peter had suffered from episodic erectile dysfunction a few years previously, which had elicited a demeaning, angry response from Sherry. The couple assured the therapist, however, that Peter had not experienced problems with sexual performance for some time, and no longer worried about it occurring. The therapist still believed that the separate sleeping arrangements *together* with the failure to disclose the information to him indicated that one or both partners found it necessary to maintain distance in the relationship and to prevent any mechanisms that promoted such a goal from being addressed in treatment. He continued to look for data that would help him achieve a more complete understanding of the couple's behavior.

About a year later, Sherry began to experience intrusive imagery of a sexual nature. In an individual session, she tearfully acknowledged long-standing aversions to a number of very normal sexual behaviors. She admitted that she avoided any opportunities for lovemaking with her husband, participating in amorous activities only to keep him from becoming overly distraught about the lack of sexual activity in the marriage. She had been secretly relieved when Peter announced that, because he could not stand to be rejected by her so consistently, he would no longer make sexual overtures in the relationship. Through a series of recollections over the next several months it became clear to Sherry that she had been the victim of childhood sexual abuse perpetuated by a close friend of her parents. Thereafter, her individual treatment focused intensively on the effects of the childhood sexual abuse.

HISTORY TAKING

In our treatment model, the therapist should have a number of essential goals in mind when initially obtaining a history from the client:

1. Establishing the presence of factors typically associated with family of origin dysfunction (as we described in Chapter 1), impaired parenting, parentification of children, boundary violations, chronic rejection, traumatic experiences, distorted cognitions, and distorted communications.
2. Outlining the client's course of development from childhood onward, highlighting any significant gaps or delays.
3. Identifying the client's basic beliefs, preferred coping strategies, information processing styles, and recurring relationship patterns, as they have manifested themselves from childhood onward.
4. Generating preliminary hypotheses as to how family of origin dynamics might account for the client's current difficulties.

History taking, like other aspects of the treatment process, will be facilitated by the therapist's sensitivity to issues of race, ethnicity, religion, and socioeconomic class. There is unfortunately no substitute for direct knowledge and experience with a particular culture. A white therapist is never going to know what it is like to be black. Nonetheless, a good therapist from any background should be willing to learn from his or her clients. Presuming more knowledge than one truly possesses is ultimately patronizing and disrespectful of the client. On the other hand, confessing one's cultural ignorance and asking to be taught by the client can be a powerful joining maneuver. We urge interested readers to consult excellent volumes by a number of authors (McGoldrick, Pearce, & Giordano, 1982; Propst, 1988; Sue, 1981) that address the impact of race, ethnicity, and religion on the therapeutic endeavor.

In our opinion, a good therapist should be curious about various ethnic groups, races, cultures, and religions, particularly those which are significantly represented in the area where he or she practices. A broad knowledge of history and geography can also be vital in providing the therapist with a framework for investigating the client's background. For example, a client in his early 20s mentioned that his father had emigrated to the United States in the late 1950s from Hungary. The therapist had acquired some knowledge of the bloody Hungarian Uprising of 1956, in which Russian tanks roared into Budapest itself to crush the revolt. As a result of asking whether the events of 1956 had played a role in the history of the client's family, the therapist found out that the man's father had participated directly in guerrilla warfare and political assassination, while still a young teenager. The client's experiences growing up made much more sense to the therapist when viewed in light of the father's shattering, traumatic experiences during the Hungarian Uprising.

We recommend that the therapist fill out a basic genogram (Guerin & Pendagast, 1976) for each client. In our opinion, a multigenerational emphasis enables the therapist to obtain a clearer picture of the individual's family of origin, particularly if the client's parents themselves had experienced trauma or victimization of any sort during their formative years. Below, we have summarized various classes of information the therapist should attempt to obtain from the client, if possible, at intake. As we emphasize repeatedly, however, we expect that the therapist will continue to probe and highlight various aspects of the client's history throughout the treatment process.

Structure and Characteristics of Family of Origin

Ethnic identification of parents
Religious identification and involvement of parents and family
Circumstances around parents' meeting and marriage
Parents' relationships with in-laws or extended family
Nature and extent of client's involvement with extended family during childhood and adolescence

Occupational and economic status of parents
Career progression of parents
Parents' social adjustment
Demographic characteristics of neighborhood or community
Nature and extent of impairment on the part of parents, relatives, and other caretakers
Nature and extent of alcohol and drug use in the family
Unusual stressors (e.g., genocide) experienced by parents or grandparents
Birth order and gender of siblings
Occurrences of miscarriages, stillbirths, or other losses of children
Medical problems, handicaps, or other forms of impairment on the part of siblings
Perceived roles and characteristics of siblings
Perceived role of self in the family
Perceived attitudes of parents and siblings toward self
Authority structure of family
Coalitions in family, especially cross-generational ones
Disciplinary practices of parents
Extent of parental involvement in day-to-day life of children
Values or issues parents emphasized in childrearing practices
Manner of expressing anger or conflict in the family, between spouses, between parents and children, and between siblings
Boundary violations in family (see examples in earlier section)
Nature and extent of sex education in the family
Reactions of parents to victimization of children outside the home
Current level of functioning of family members
Current or recent stressors experienced by family members
Status of current relationships between client and family members

Social and Academic Functioning in Childhood and Adolescence

Physical health and body image in childhood and adolescence
Developmental delays or learning difficulties
Academic skills, interests, and achievements
Nature of client's attributions for academic success or failure
Nature and extent of extracurricular interests and achievements
Parental reactions to achievements
Nature and extent of involvement in institutions outside of school and family (e.g., church)
Quality of relationships with authority figures outside the family
Quality of peer relationships
Age of and experiences associated with onset of puberty

Dating history
Extent and nature of sexual activity in childhood and adolescence

History of Medical and/or Psychological Complaints

Nature and extent of previous medical or psychiatric symptoms
Presence of untreated or unrecognized psychological symptoms, particularly in childhood or adolescence
Parents' reactions to childhood medical or psychiatric symptoms
Nature of previous psychiatric treatment and client's perception of its effectiveness
History of miscarriages or abortions in female clients
Prior occurrences of substance abuse, impulsive behaviors, or antisocial actions

Adult Career History

Nature and extent of career progression, including job stability
Circumstances surrounding prior job losses or job changes
Degree and sources of satisfaction in career
Areas of interest and/or competency in current job
Nature of relationships with supervisors or other authority figures at work
Quality of interactions with peers at work
Areas of regret over past vocational decisions
Nature and extent of achievement-oriented activities not directly connected with employment (e.g., triathlon competition, church choir)

History of Current Family Configuration

History of long-term intimate relationships in adulthood
History of sexual behavior in adulthood
Circumstances of bonding with current spouse or partner
Reactions of families of origin to marriage
Family background and current level of functioning of spouse or partner
History of relationships with children from previous marriages
Current status of marital or intimate relationship

As we shall discuss in Chapter 9 on building awareness of family of origin issues, the simple act of asking historical questions also serves an important *orienting intervention*. That is, regardless of the immediate yield, the questions themselves begin to draw clients attention to various topics which the therapist wants them to begin thinking about. In the meantime, the therapist will begin to formulate tentative hypotheses regarding the client's core beliefs, information-processing styles, coping strategies, and recurring relationship patterns.

The therapist may have difficulty obtaining a vivid picture of the client's history if he or she simply uses a blunt, telegraphic style of questioning. In order to conduct a good historical interview, the therapist must accommodate to the client's vocabulary and speaking style, carefully noting and reusing words and phrases that stimulate elaboration on important topics. Moreover, the therapist may need to be creative in fashioning questions, particularly with clients who find it hard to provide details or who otherwise fail to bring the past to life in their responses to more straightforward inquiries. Below are some examples of questions that, when posed during the initial historical interview(s), might help the client elaborate a bit further on specific areas of childhood or adolescence experience that have particular relevance for treatment. In Chapter 9 we discuss more elaborate strategies for increasing the client's awareness of family of origin data.

Beliefs about the Self

How would you have described yourself when you were a child or teenager?

What did you like about yourself as a child? What didn't you like?

How do you imagine your parents/teachers/siblings/friends would have described you as a child?

What were you good at as a child? What were you not so good at?

What would you have liked to change about yourself as a child or teenager?

Beliefs about Others

When you were growing up, how would you have described your parents?

Could you give me three adjectives to describe how you saw each of your parents/brothers/sisters when you were growing up?

As a child, how might you have finished the statement: "In general, I think other people are...(or, "I think adults/teachers/ kids/parents are ...")"?

Beliefs about the World

> As a child, how might you have finished the statement: "In general, I think the world is. . . ."? or "When I think about the future, I see . . .?", or "What I like best/least about this world we live in is . . .?"

Beliefs about Relationships

> What was your parents' relationship like growing up?
> How would you have described your own relationship with your mother/father?
> What were your relationships like with your brothers/sisters/friends/teachers/grandparents?
> Are there ways in which current relationships of yours resemble those you were part of or observed when you were growing up?

Roles

> Children in families often take on certain roles. For example, one child in a family might sometimes act like another parent in the home and take on the role of "the caretaker" or "the responsible one." Other children sometimes have roles such as "the smart one," "the pretty one," "the sick one," "the troublemaker," or "the social worker." Can you think of any roles that you played in your family? Did you tend to play any particular roles with your friends? What roles did your siblings take?
> What roles or jobs did your mother/father handle? Which ones were shared?
> What do you think you learned from your family about the role(s) you were expected to play in future relationships?

Communication

> What did you observe in your family about how people dealt with conflicts?
> What was your parents' style of solving problems together? How were big decisions made?
> What did you like about how people communicated in your family?
> What do you wish had been different about the ways family members communicated?

How did family members express their concern for one another?
How did family members express their displeasure with one another?
Are there ways you communicate in relationships now that you see
as having roots in your family experiences?

Areas of Denial and Overvigilance in the Family

In your family, if you had really stepped back and thought about
certain things, might you have said: "Hmmm. How come we
never or rarely talk about that?" If so, what were those things?
Families also often have some topics that seem to be discussed all
the time. For example, some families seem to be obsessed with
topics such as school performance or money problems or health
problems. Other families might focus a lot on a particular child's
accomplishments or a particular child's behavior problems.
Were there any topics that your family seemed especially focused on?

Coping Strategies

When you were upset as a child/teenager, what did you tend to do
to help yourself feel better?
If you saw something going on in your family that upset you, such
as your parents fighting or one of your parents having had too
much to drink, what did you tend to do in those situations?
In general, people tend to cope with conflict or problem situations
either by directly confronting the situation in some way or by
avoiding the situation. Which of these styles would have best
characterized you growing up? Can you give me some examples?

REVISIONIST HISTORY

Even when the therapist has obtained a fairly detailed history from a
client, he or she should view it as tentative and provisional. Individuals, like nations, indulge in historical revisionism through the operation of denial mechanisms. The narrative of the past may well include
significant omissions and distortions, that will only come to light as a
result of subsequent therapeutic work with the individual. In some

cases, it has taken months or even years in treatment before clients have been able to recall traumatic childhood experiences in sufficient detail to understand the impact on their current functioning. Without specific images or recollections, neither the therapist nor the client can achieve a full understanding of the client's current difficulties. We discuss the trauma revelation process in greater detail in a subsequent Chapter 11.

In other instances, the client's perspective on the past will change radically during the course of treatment, not through recollections of traumatic material, but because of the recognition of more subtle, but powerful historical forces.

For example, from the very start of treatment, Teresa was able to give a clear account of the way in which her irresponsible alcoholic father had affected her and the rest of the family during her formative years. She experienced considerable anger at both her father and other incompetent males in the extended family. As Teresa portrayed childhood, she became a surrogate parent to her younger sibling because she was moved by the plight of her tired, overwhelmed mother. The mother, meanwhile, always took on a somewhat saintly air when Teresa described her. Teresa also habitually referred to herself as her mother's "favorite," suggesting that she had received preferential treatment over her siblings as a consequence. During the course of treatment, a more complex picture of the mother began to emerge, perhaps as a result of the client's increasing ability to challenge her own denial processes. Teresa began to describe more and more interactions, both past and present, in which the mother had behaved in a highly critical, rejecting manner toward her. A packet of letters written to her by her mother when she was away from home briefly as a young adolescent was particularly instructive for both Teresa and the therapist. In the correspondence, the mother came across as embittered, demanding, and guilt-inducing. One note, written after Teresa's last response had arrived a few days late, particularly epitomized the mother's hostile-dependent style. Consisting largely of punitive remarks, the letter was signed, "Your mother (I think)." As it turned out, the issues involved in Teresa's relationship with her mother probably played a more significant role in her current symptoms, and in her recovery, than any other aspect of her family background.

Family loyalty is often closely linked with historical revisionism. By acknowledging dysfunction in the family of origin, some individuals believe that they will dishonor the memory of a deceased parent or ruin an ongoing relationship with a living one. Since many of our clients tend to think in all-or-nothing, black and white terms, they fear that recognition of victimization or other stressors in childhood will destroy any positive feelings they currently have toward their parents or other family members. Another aspect of loyalty involves strictures against disclosing family secrets to outsiders. For some clients, acknowledgment of childhood stressors to a therapist constitutes an unacceptable betrayal of family trust, a moral transgression for which they fully expect to be punished somehow.

Issues of worthlessness also retard the acknowledgment of family of origin pathology. Many of our clients wonder if they played a role in causing the problems in their families, whereas others who were mistreated, in various ways believe that they somehow deserved the ill-treatment. In Chapter 3, we described the case of Audrey, who resisted discussion of an incestuous relationship with an older step-brother because she feared that such conversations would only place the blame for what had occurred even more securely on her shoulders. Some clients have achieved a relative sense of worth in their lives by putting their families of origin out of their thoughts as much as possible while they created positive identities for themselves in the extrafamilial world. Looking back to recognize the chaos or abuse associated with childhood presents a significant threat to self-esteem. As one client put it, "If my family was abusive, that means I was an abused child. What kind of problems does that mean I have?"

Generally clients cannot identify the belief systems that support historical revisionism during the early stages of treatment. As far as some of our clients are concerned, the family history is a cut and dried matter that does not need to be revisited. For many individuals, recognition of painful and/or threatening historical realities will come only if they acquire a compelling data base in the course of the treatment process. As we discuss at length in Chapters 7, 8, and 9, the client must have a trusting relationship with the therapist in order to begin to build such a data base.

The authors are unaware of any normative data on the degree to which the average adult can recall events experienced prior to the onset of puberty. We suspect that it is comparatively rare to find individuals in the general population who, like some of our clients, report that they remember little or nothing before the age of 13 or 14. Consequently, we would typically assume that powerful denial mechanisms of various types, probably stimulated by traumatic experiences, are involved when a client reports such a complete paucity of childhood recollections. Further, we would also expect that the client who has difficulty remembering childhood experiences will also manifest problematic use of denial strategies in his or her current life.

"READING" THE HISTORY PRIOR TO TREATMENT

Most clinicians tend to anticipate a more negative prognosis when the client has experienced multiple symptomatic episodes of a similar nature in the past, particularly if there has been a history of failed psychotherapy experiences as well. Even the most self-confident therapist cannot be so grandiose as to expect automatically to achieve success where other clinicians have failed. On the other hand, we mental health professionals are perhaps all too painfully aware of the distressing number of colleagues to whom we would *not* refer a friend or family member. Unless we know the particular therapists involved, it is difficult to make any assumptions about either the quality or the focus of the client's previous treatment experiences. Moreover, even good therapists can falter with cases that others end up treating successfully as a result of limitations in training or expertise, unresolved personal issues, poor "chemistry" with the client, and so on.

It is vital for the therapist to question the client rather explicitly about his or her previous treatment experiences. What was the relationship like with the therapist? How were the sessions structured? Was homework ever a part of the treatment? What did the client learn about him or herself as a result of treatment? Did the client acquire an understanding about how family of origin issues might have been related to the presenting complaints? Did the therapist offer much feedback or interpretation? Was there an explicit focus on the therapeutic relationship? How did the client feel about the therapist? What were the client's expectations? Were they fulfilled? How did the client think the therapist felt about him or her? What did the client think the therapist's expectations were? How and why did the client terminate? Why didn't the client return to the previous therapist when the current difficulties occurred?

Unfortunately, we find ourselves outraged all too often by stories of clients who have been victimized financially, sexually, or psychologically by other therapists. The disastrous consequences of therapist–client sexual contact have been well documented in the research literature. For example, Pope (1988) found that clients who had been sexually involved with their therapists suffered long-term consequences similar to those of incest victims. Common aftereffects included guilt, severe depression, feelings of emptiness and isolation, sexual confusion, impaired trust, and increased suicidality. Although many victims of sexual exploitation do not seek out further treatment (Bouhoutsos Holroyd, Lerman, Forer, & Greenberg, 1983), those who do often find their subsequent therapeutic experiences to be severely hampered by the negative effects of the prior, abusive relationship.

We find that therapists abuse the enormous power inherent in their positions in a number of ways, not just by taking sexual liberties with their clients. Many of our clients have undergone prior treatment experiences that may not have provided sufficient grounds for malpractice suits or complaints to licensing boards but were clearly psychologically harmful. We hear too many stories of therapists who routinely tolerate or enter into various types of dual relationships with their clients, for example, or who impose rigid beliefs and idiosyncratic values on their clients. Not surprisingly, in a number of instances, these destructive therapeutic relationships directly replicated difficulties the clients had experienced in their families of origin. We expect that many individuals who were raised in abusive families will continue to be ripe targets for exploitation by authority figures they encounter later in life. In the hands of a predatory therapist, who has been privy to all their secrets and frailties, such clients would be absurdly overmatched—indeed, to the point of being defenseless.

There are other factors aside from outright victimization that may have rendered the client's past treatment experiences ineffective. There may have been some basic incompatibility with the previous therapist, perhaps the result of actual differences in temperament, style, or personality, or the *attributions* the client makes about the therapist's race, age, gender, marital status, and so forth. Working in a closely knit private practice, with the same group of mental health professionals for many years, the authors have grown to appreciate the unique skills—and blind spots—of each therapist with certain types of clients and clinical situations. Naturally, we assume that all therapists see a certain number of clients whom some of their colleagues could probably treat in a more powerful, effective manner.

We find it distressing to note how many clients are unable to offer substantive details about what they learned in their previous therapy experiences. Clients often seem to have completed past treatment with reductions in symptoms, improvements in well-being, and the sense of having been listened to and cared for by the therapist but without explicit concepts or coping strategies to bring to bear on future difficulties. Evidently many therapists do not set up treatment as an explicit investigatory or learning experience for their clients, nor do they typically use strategies, such as homework, to facilitate retention of therapeutic insights. As we stress repeatedly throughout this volume, we strive to send our clients out the door at termination armed with a clear understanding of their past difficulties and a framework for preventing similar problems in the future.

EXAMINING CURRENT FUNCTIONING

Areas of Greatest Competence

Although we must often examine our clients' psychological deficits in minute detail, we also need to remain attuned to their areas of strength and competency. Assessment of competence is crucial in order to prevent treatment from becoming exclusively centered on pathology. Since many of our clients tend be absorbed with their failures and defects, they often inadvertently conceal significant areas of talent and achievement from us. It would be natural for them to minimize or even ignore key areas of competent functioning. Consequently, the therapist needs to be continually vigilant for information about the client's skills and interests. Often such data come to light quite serendipitously in the course of discussions on other matters. We have also found that by asking clients to record their activities for a week or two, we can obtain considerable information about their habits, interests, and interpersonal contacts that might never have been elicited through direct questioning. The reader who is interested in a detailed description of the use of activity schedules should consult volumes by Beck (Beck, Rush, et al., 1979) and Burns (1980).

Knowledge of the client's areas of competence enables the therapist to couch subsequent discussions in metaphors that are familiar and palpable to the individual. Clients who have learned a foreign language, competed in gymnastics, or played the violin will be able to draw on past experiences in order to appreciate the therapist's remarks on the role of practice and repetition in the recovery process. Likewise, such clients are likely to remember, when reminded by the therapist, that the acquisition of new skills can be a frustrating and unpredictable enterprise at times during which periods of growth alternate with periods of stagnation and even apparent regression.

Whether the client recognizes it or not, every area of competence contains cognitive and behavioral components that could be profitably utilized in other areas of life. The therapist needs to identify the mechanisms that support competence and bring them to the attention of the client, particularly when such components have potential relevance for current situations of a stressful nature. Moreover, it is always useful to understand why the client's characteristic difficulties *don't* occur in a particular situation. For example, the therapist might ask a long distance runner who is experiencing difficulties with procrastination the following questions: "I suspect most people would agree that it takes quite a bit of self-discipline to train for a marathon. How do you get yourself out there to run day after day? How do you fight fatigue and discouragement?" As we describe at length in Chapter 12, the therapist must also analyze carefully any instances, both past and present, in which the client copes more successfully with problematic situations. When conducted on a regular basis in the course of treatment, such reviews of successful coping will facilitate generalization and transfer of the client's skills.

An awareness of the client's areas of competence provides the therapist with additional opportunities to affirm the individual's worth in various ways. By asking the individual questions about special interests or experiences, the therapist allows the client to act as an expert on subjects about which the clinician may be totally ignorant. Clearly, many clients will downplay or reject direct compliments from their therapists on their special skills or talents. However, the client does not have to acknowledge an area of competence in order for the therapist to utilize it as a metaphor or as a vehicle for validating the individual's worth. The therapist can send the client embedded messages that affirm competence but in an indirect way, which preempts direct refutation by the client, for example, "I'm sure that being an artist you can see so much more in a painting than the average person. As a lay person though, I had a powerful reaction to El Greco's work," or "I'll bet that it really upset you to hear how that teacher spoke to your daughter, especially since you do such a good job of bolstering the self-esteem of your children." We shall discuss the use of embedded messages to amplify competence in greater detail in Chapter 7.

Special skills and interests also provide a useful vehicle through which a client might communicate more comfortably with the therapist. Clients may want to share samples of their poetry, music, or art work with their therapists. The therapist should emphasize, however, that he or she will not be able to offer a critical appraisal of the client's creative work but will examine it only in light of what it discloses about the individual who produced it.

The therapist needs to examine the motivational sources of the client's competence as well as the actual manner in which the individual pursues his or her goals. The client's academic, vocational, and/or interpersonal successes may only tell a portion of the story. Is the hard work and perseverance motivated simply by a love of achievement for its own sake, or by the individual's chronic feelings of worthlessness? Do the client's accomplishments obscure a pattern of superficial, impoverished, or conflictual relationships? Does the individual's achievement-oriented activity operate as a *compulsion*, resulting in self-defeating consequences, such as exhaustion, ill-health, and interpersonal friction? Is the client pursuing highly unrealistic goals, such as a career in show business or professional athletics, without formulating alternative plans?

Many of our clients appeared to have been "depressions waiting to happen" for many years before they actually became symptomatic or entered treatment. As long as the rewards, the recognition, and the promotions kept coming, our clients were able to continue functioning at a fairly high level. If, either through performance problems or external circumstances, they were unable to continue forward movement in their careers, they were apt to become severely depressed and consumed with self-loathing. Later, clients may report that they actually never had felt particularly good about themselves, despite their outward successes. As they look back they see that they were dogged by a powerful fear of failure and often felt uncomfortable when they were not working toward some defined goal. They may recognize that they had become overly reliant on *one* source (e.g., career advancement, accumulation of wealth, success in an intimate relationship and so on) as a means of affirming self-worth. As they begin to feel more secure in the therapeutic relationship, some clients may reveal pockets of compulsive, self-defeating behaviors such as addictions, affairs, degrading sexual practices, and so on, that co-existed with the more adaptive career behaviors.

Distortions in Current Self-Image

As discussed previously, negative beliefs about the self can stimulate lifelong habits of overvigilance. The vast majority of our clients are obsessed with their defects and failures. They may be able to cite voluminous data, both current and historical in nature, that support their negative self-perceptions. Some clients constantly scan for any signs of criticism or rejection from individuals in the environment, perhaps acting defensively or absorbing blaming messages from others in the process. The client's concerns about his or her inadequacies may reach a truly monomaniacal level, as in the eating disorders or other conditions that involve a distortion of body image. Likewise, many compulsive behaviors also may reflect the individual's attempt to compensate for perceived deficiencies in the self.

In each case, the therapist needs to map out the characteristic pattern of reciprocal influence that occurs between contextual or systems factors, particularly involving close relationships and themes of worthlessness on the part of the client. The better the clinician understands this area, the better he or she will be able to identify and even anticipate threats to self-esteem as they crop up in the client's life. Armed with such knowledge, the therapist should find it easier to prioritize the content to be covered during treatment sessions and to assist the client to recognize how seemingly minor or even innocuous events in the environment may trigger powerful emotions or defensive behaviors. Likewise, a detailed map of trigger points that stimulate a sense of worthlessness on the part of the client also should enable the clinician to anticipate, discuss, and avoid distorted perceptions of the therapeutic relationship.

However, not all distortions in self-image involve issues of worthlessness or self-blame. In fact, the client may express certain beliefs about the self which, although *positive* in nature, may also be *inaccurate* or *distorted*. Such positive distortions in self-image typically reflect the operation of denial strategies on the individual's part. For example, the client may state, "I don't get upset about things the way others do," "I'm pretty even-tempered", "Those things don't bother me anymore," or "I can continue my affair without affecting the way I act with my wife and kids", while much of the available evidence, including accounts of his or her behavior from significant others, suggests otherwise. Even although some of our clients view themselves as attentive, considerate spouses, or nurturant, reasonable parents, it may become all too apparent to the therapist that their performances in such crucial roles are, at best, inconsistent and, at worst, severely flawed. The therapist must take note of such distorted self-perceptions and look for opportunities to address them in a constructive manner with the client during the course of treatment.

Clients who consistently see themselves as small, weak, vulnerable, and/or inadequate often have no idea what kind of a powerful emotional impact they may have on others. When threatened, they may lash out at those around them in an extremely destructive manner. Ignorant of the interpersonal consequences of their behavior, such individuals may persist in seeing themselves as meek or ineffectual, whereas, ironically, significant others may find them to be overpowering, or even abusive. Unless these clients truly understand the impact of their actions on others, they will continue to experience high levels of rejection and interpersonal conflict without knowing why. During the course of the treatment process, they can become increasingly aware of their victimizing behaviors, particularly if they can achieve a strong relationship with a therapist who is skilled in confronting such behavior patterns.

Areas of Denial

As described in Chapter 3, denial processes manifest themselves in the sensory, conceptual, and behavioral/interpersonal domains. In some instances, the therapist will be able to identify denial mechanisms at work with a particular client almost at the outset of treatment. In other cases, the denial processes may be much more subtle and insidious, so that a large body of pertinent information about the client remains concealed from the therapist. Since we assume that denial mechanisms enable the individual to avoid threatening information and the emotional responses associated with it, it is likely that the missing information will often involve some of the most significant areas of the client's life. As most readers surely know from their own experiences, the distorted picture presented by the client may even mislead the therapist into making the wrong diagnosis and/or offering the wrong treatment.

Let us review some of the typical signs that should alert the therapist to the presence of significant (and dysfunctional) denial processes on the part of the client:

Hazy, impoverished, or missing recollections of childhood or adolescence.

Sketchy or chronologically confusing rendering of significant portions of adult life, such as career or history of intimate relationships.

Poor recall of prior therapy sessions (in the absence of learning disabilities, neurological problems, or biologically based mental illness).

Resistance to or a dread of recounting details of potentially painful or upsetting life events.

Use of the phrase, "It wasn't that bad" to describe childhood in a dysfunctional family of origin, or other clearly stressful life experiences.

High threshold for physical pain.

Inappropriate laughter or joking with the therapist.

Willingness to indulge in excessive small talk with the therapist.

Inability to formulate a clearly-defined contract with the therapist.

Flat affective response in recounting events with significant content.

Affective responses of therapists and/or significant others far exceed those of the client in response to important events or relationships in his or her life.

Minimal usage of "feeling words" in description of life events.

The frequent need to substitute less affectively charged words or phrases for those which the therapist has offered (e.g., When the therapist says, "Boy, you must have been furious about that!" the client responds by saying, "I wasn't furious. I was irritated").

Inability to recognize disturbed behavior on the part of spouse or significant other.

Recurring complaints from significant others that the client is withdrawn or "emotionally unavailable."

Recurring intense anger from a spouse or significant other without a complementary emotional response of similar intensity from the client.

Frequent usage of explanations for behavior of self and particularly others, that favor external causes over the assignment of responsibility to the individual.

Recurrent and generally convoluted explanations for why it would not be a good time to raise a pertinent issue with a significant other.

The presence of affairs and other important secrets in the client's life.

Chronic inaction in response to ongoing life difficulties, particularly involving children or adolescents in the family.

Chronic procrastination or avoidance behavior.

Areas of Overvigilance

For the most part, it is not a difficult task to obtain a fairly detailed picture of the issues that habitually capture the client's attention. The most common presenting psychological problems, such as depression and anxiety, seem consistently to involve multiple levels of overvigilance, including signal sensitivity, obsessive thinking, compulsive behavior, and perseverative interpersonal interactions. For example, a 45-year-old depressed woman seems constantly on the alert for signs of rejection or disapproval from others. Once she perceives such a sign in a relationship, she obsesses about her interactions with the other person, carefully reviewing who said what to whom, preparing justifications for her actions in case she has to defend herself, rehearsing for later encounters with the individual in question, enumerating past failures and other evidence of her deficiencies, and so on. Suicidal or self-mutilative thoughts may also be part of her obsessive "loop." The woman may also report that, while obsessed and upset about these matters, she overeats, makes unnecessary purchases on her credit cards, or finds herself engaging in some serious and threatening flirtation with the husband of a close friend. Lastly, the therapist may observe that many of the woman's relationships have become organized around her fear of disapproval and rejection. She seems to fall over herself to please others, yet it seems as if her spouse and children continually give her negative feedback, frequently blaming her for their difficulties.

Clients will generally lead with their sensitivities and their obsessions, *except for cases in which there are secret compulsive or addictive behaviors*. Clients who engage in such behaviors may feel so worthless that they cannot disclose the information to the therapist, perhaps despite frequent and repeated resolutions to do so. Given their negative attitude toward themselves, and their prior disappointments in relationships, they cannot conceive of the possibility of continued acceptance and support from the therapist after such a disclosure. Moreover, the client will probably also be struggling with severely conflicting beliefs regarding the addictive or compulsive behaviors themselves. The desire to continue the self-defeating behaviors at all costs may be strong enough to keep the individual from making disclosures that might hinder his or her freedom to act out in the future. Consequently, the therapist may proceed on the basis of an incomplete picture of the client.

Distortions in Perceptions of Others and the World

Clients who have grown up with neglectful or abusive parents may show the effects of their childhood experiences in a rather straightforward manner, by expecting such victimization to continue on in their current lives. They may be afraid of being assaulted when others are angry with them, even when the likelihood of such attacks occurring is nonexistent. They may experience significant others, who are ordinarily supportive of them, as rejecting, physically threatening, or sexually coercive. They may also become fearful about the therapist's attitudes or intentions toward them. Individuals who have experienced childhood abuse may also express a strong sense of mistrust in a more subtle way, through fault-finding and blaming directed at others. They may react as if normal and entirely understandable lapses in attention, judgment, or sensitivity on the part of others consistently reflect intentions of a more hostile or manipulative nature. Consequently they may often behave in an angry and/or defensive manner with others. They may also find it hard to believe that someone in an authority position, such as a therapist, could be either concerned or competent enough to help them with their difficulties.

On the other hand, because of the operation of denial mechanisms, victims of childhood abuse or neglect may fail to recognize when they really are being victimized. Clients who find themselves stuck in enabling or "codependent" patterns with significant others will often present perceptions of their partners that are distorted in a positive direction. They may prefer to attribute the other person's misbehavior either to situational causes (e.g., Vinnie is drinking more because he's under so much pressure at work") or worse, to their own behavior (e.g., She wouldn't have gone out that night if I had chosen my words more carefully".). Similarly, they may consistently focus on the other's *motivations* or *intentions*, which might appear to be quite honorable, as opposed to his or her *actions* and the negative consequences thereof. Such

clients may attempt to short-circuit prolonged contemplation of a partner's difficulties by insisting that he or she is "really a good person
underneath it all." They might derive an unwarranted sense of optimism from minute or chance fluctuations in the other person's attitude
or behavior, while ignoring clear signs that past problems in the relationship are likely to recur.

A number of our clients assume that they must constantly orchestrate or manipulate events behind the scenes in order to accomplish
certain objectives in their relationships. For example, a wife who wants
her husband to spend more time with their two young sons might
simply leave him alone more often with them rather than ask him
directly to be more active with the children. At the heart of such behind-
the-scenes orchestration lies a problematic assumption, namely, that the
spouse is incompetent or irresponsible on some level and needs to be
"handled" much as one might cope with an unruly child. Indeed many
"helpful," ostensibly benign, relationship behaviors are predicated on a
rather negative assessment of the other person's capabilities.

Many clients will readily express the belief that a significant other
is *dangerously* vulnerable or incompetent. If factors such as substance
abuse or mental illness are involved, many of the client's perceptions
may be valid. Their enabling behaviors may be based on an assumption
that could be quite accurate in many instances—namely, that if left to
his or her own devices, the impaired individual will commit suicide or
fall victim to foul play of some sort. The therapist cannot afford to be
cavalier about the client's legitimate fears for the safety of the impaired
individual. On the other hand, being a suicidal risk does not give the
person license to abuse or exploit others or to live a life free from
responsibilities. As one of the authors is fond of pointing out to clients
who are prone to assume enabling roles,even state hospital patients
must conform to certain rules and limits. That is, despite their obvious
organic problems, *psychotic individuals are not allowed to mistreat others
with impunity.*

Perceptions of others and the world may harmonize with perceptions of the self in a variety of ways. As mentioned above, many of our
clients see themselves as weak, vulnerable, powerless, and/or incompetent. Not surprisingly, they may see other key figures in their lives in
complementary terms as strong, confident, proactive, and/or competent. They may habitually compare themselves to a particular friend or
sibling only to come up on the losing end every time. In such situations,
the client usually overestimates the positive attributes of the individual
in question or fails to take into account other aspects of the person that
may not be admirable at all. Clients who cannot recognize the vulnerabilities of their intimate associates not only feel alienated for irrational
reasons but also run the risk of being needlessly hurtful to others dur-

ing periods of conflict simply because they underestimate their own power.

Processes that our psychoanalytic colleagues would label as "projection" or "projective identification" also exemplify the close connection between perceptions of the self and perceptions of others. The client with a strong sense of worthlessness will expect to be criticized and/or rejected on some level, in any relationship. For such individuals, the closer the relationship, the greater the danger of being hurt. Consequently, they will look carefully for—and invariably find—signs of dissatisfaction or disapproval on the part of significant others. These individuals may well appear tense, defensive, and ironically enough, critical or rejecting in their interactions with significant others. As a result, they may find themselves driving away partners who might otherwise be supportive of them. Needless to say, they may also respond in a similar manner in the therapeutic relationship by assuming that the therapist will also find them objectionable or unacceptable. In the course of treatment, however, they can begin to recognize that what they perceive as rejection coming from their partners is often actually a reflection of the self.

If the client is a parent, the therapist should investigate the individual's perceptions of his or her offspring. Some clients identify so strongly with one or more of their children that the differences between the individuals in question begin to disappear. Parenting functions cannot help but suffer when such an extreme process of identification occurs. For example, a strongly self-loathing incest survivor may be at risk of being overly rejecting, punitive, or outright abusive when his or her most objectionable characteristics or behaviors appear to show up in an offspring. On the other hand, she may also perceive others as being destructive or abusive toward the child when they make appropriate efforts to set limits.

Individuals who view their children as carbon copies of spouses, parents, or other members of the family of origin are also likely to experience difficulties executing their parenting duties. Our clients seldom describe positive inheritances in their children from the family tree (e.g., "Junior is such a good singer and dancer, just like my wife's uncle"). Instead, we find that our clients often see qualities or behaviors in their children that reflect the most upsetting attributes of the family member who is the object of the comparison. In our experience, a child of divorce who has been labeled by the custodial parent as identical to a former spouse may be at risk for behavioral difficulties, particularly in adolescence. The custodial parent may be unable to respond effectively to the adolescent's challenges to authority, just as he or she had no way to cope with the former spouse's angry or oppositional behaviors.

A number of our clients grew up in families that were marked by extensive superstitions and unreasoning fears of divine retribution for past misdeeds. Not surprisingly, as adults they may also hold beliefs of a religious or cosmological nature that lead to similar irrational fears and superstitious rituals. Such beliefs usually reflect themes of worthlessness and victimization that originated in the family of origin. The client's early experiences in organized religion, particularly in faiths that tend to portray an angry, vengeful Deity, may have resonated with his or her experiences at the hands of abusive or rejecting parental figures. Consequently, the individual may expect God to behave in an arbitrary or vindictive manner, just as his or her parent did. Not surprisingly, a number of our clients with such beliefs have fallen prey to religious cults, coercive fundamentalist religious movements, or abusive clergy from mainstream denominations.

We do not share the reflexive disdain expressed by some well-known cognitive therapists toward beliefs of a spiritual or religious nature. In fact, we do encourage our clients to seek active connections with the *positive* spiritual forces they experience in their lives in whatever manner feels comfortable to them. Many of our clients who participate in the various Twelve-Step recovery programs, often begin to derive more spiritual comfort from the general concept of a "Higher Power," put forth by the self-help groups than from the more doctrinaire messages of organized religion. Since ideas of a religious or cosmological nature tend to be associated with very high degrees of belief, they must be approached with great caution by the therapist. Fortunately, as other long-standing cognitions begin to change, some clients begin to question their religious beliefs on their own, so that the therapist can become involved in the reevaluation process without eliciting a defensive reaction. Although we tend to avoid direct confrontation of religious beliefs unless they are actively impeding recovery, there are times when we must address such cognitions head-on relatively early in the treatment process. We refer the reader to an outstanding volume by another cognitive therapist, Rebecca Propst (1988), who offers a number of constructive treatment strategies for use with religiously committed individuals.

Recurring Relationship Patterns

Ongoing stressful relationships often prevent the individual from being able to examine, let alone change, cognitive distortions or information-processing mechanisms of a problematic nature. Even when the primary complaint is an identifiable organismic problem (such as a biological depression), the therapist may still need to combine individual treatment with marital or family systems interventions designed to block abusive or otherwise destructive interactions (Bedrosian, 1986; 1988). In the meantime, the clinician also will attempt to provide a cognitive foundation for the establishment and maintenance of new relationship patterns in the client's life. Without such a foundation to support more healthy patterns of interactions, we predict that positive changes in the client's marriage or family relationship, if they occur at all, will tend to be transient or superficial in nature. If significant others in the client's life are willing to examine ongoing relationship issues and their own material as well, so much the better, since then the therapist can design a very powerful treatment plan that combines the cognitive and systems elements.

Whether or not the therapist chooses to work with the family system, there is no substitute for first-hand information regarding the client's significant relationships. Even when occasional conjoint sessions with spouses or partners are geared solely toward facilitating individual treatment, the therapist will gain considerable insight into the client's style of relating from such meetings. Moreover, having had direct contact with the individuals in question, the therapist will be in a better position to help the client identify distorted perceptions of the significant other. Otherwise, the clinician may have to rely only on the client's descriptions of the individual, which, as discussed in the previous section, are likely to contain distorted elements.

Every therapist, regardless of his or her orientation, ought to be able to describe the client's relationships in systems-oriented terms, taking into account variables such as reciprocal influence, circular causation, boundaries (see next section), coalitions, triangulation, family hierarchy, and so on. Further, the therapist should be capable of articulating how interactional sequences resonate with individual issues triggering cognitive distortions, information-processing errors, and self-defeating coping strategies. The clinician should also be able to identify how relationship dynamics keep the participants locked into dysfunctional patterns of thinking and behavior, thereby perpetuating the limitations of each individual. The therapist must remember that, despite outward appearances, partners in intimate relationships often function at comparable levels of maturity. In fact, the overt impairment or symptomatic behavior of one spouse may merely serve to obscure the psychological limitations of the other. Such limitations may become much more apparent when the impaired individual becomes less symptomatic. Likewise, overtly disturbed or destructive behavior on the part of one spouse may divert attention away from victimizing or rejecting behaviors of a more subtle nature coming from the other partner. The therapist needs to keep in mind that in a distressed marital or family system, *everyone* may be victimized in some manner.

Peter and Sherry, a couple discussed in the previous chapter, exemplify a typical interlocking relationship pattern, one involving
blurred boundaries, as well as multiple manifestations of denial and
overvigilance.

Peter's mother was a prescription drug addict from the time he was
in elementary school. From an early age, he played a caretaking role for
her in a variety of ways. Peter even remembered being instructed to
make the rounds of local pharmacies in order to obtain narcotics for his
mother. He often found himself extremely anxious while at school
during the day, worrying about what kind of situation he might encounter when he returned home. Rather than socialize with his peers or
participate in extracurricular activities after school, Peter would feel
compelled to rush home, in order to make sure that his mother was safe.
As an adult, Peter was compulsive, anxiety-ridden, and responsible to
a fault.

Sherry's parents were rigid, moralistic, and physically abusive. She
recalled that even minor breaches in table manners might be rewarded
with a backhand slap in her household. As a preschooler, Sherry was
diagnosed with juvenile diabetes. Thereafter, her parents kept tight
reins over her schedule, her activities, and of course, her diet. Sherry
learned to be overtly compliant and dutiful, while she engaged in covert
acts of rebellion, primarily involving eating. Starting in elementary
school, Sherry would bribe other children into obtaining candy for her.
Thus began a lifelong pattern of hoarding and binging on sweets. Because of her diabetes, Sherry's binging produced wild swings in her
moods and her metabolism, sometimes driving her to the brink of losing
consciousness.

Neither Peter nor Sherry entered the marriage with a strong sense
of self-esteem. From the early days of their courtship, Peter established
himself as his wife's protector, projecting a false sense of self-confidence
to her in the process. With the advent of children, he grew increasingly
anxious about his responsibilities, so that his behavior toward Sherry
became more intrusive and controlling rather than nurturant. Peter
often found himself calling home several times a day, just to determine
if Sherry and the children were all right. By acting in such a parental
manner toward his wife, Peter constantly reinforced her sense of helplessness and incompetence.

Although Sherry expressed resentment about her husband's controlling behaviors, she often drew him into her decision making, only to
blame him later for unsatisfactory results. She used her health problems,
which were certainly a legitimate source of concern, to elicit sympathy
from her husband and to avoid difficult or uncomfortable situations.
Sherry's blaming and abdication of responsibility tended to reinforce

Peter's sense of inadequacy and self-reproach and kept him in a paren-tified role. Because she viewed herself as weak and vulnerable, Sherry tended to become uncharacteristically vindictive if Peter showed any signs of inadequacy. She ridiculed Peter for having panic attacks and derided his manhood when he experienced a brief period of sexual dysfunction. Such behaviors hardly encouraged her husband to show his vulnerability or otherwise relinquish the comparative safety of his controlling, parental role in the relationship.

On the other hand, although Peter would accuse his wife of using her health problems to evade responsibilities, he never confronted or even openly acknowledged her binge eating, which regularly interfered with her ability to function as a wife and a mother. During the early stages of treatment, the couple colluded to conceal Sherry's eating dis-order and her phobic avoidance of sexual relations. Had Peter's self-esteem been stronger, he might well have confronted his wife earlier regarding the lack of physical intimacy in their marriage. In the absence of external pressure from her husband, it was comparatively easy for Sherry to continue to avoid confronting her problems with eating and sexuality. In the meantime, her chronic problems with self-worth per-sisted.

Many clients come to treatment for the first time as a result of a crisis that has occurred in an intimate relationship. If possible, the therapist should determine whether the current crisis is largely a one-shot occurrence or simply the latest in a chain of similar events, perhaps spanning many years of the client's life. The presence of the kinds of cognitive distortions described in the previous section or demonstrable family of origin pathology would suggest that the client's relationship difficulties are of a recurring nature. After obtaining an initial history, the therapist may be able to identify specific interaction patterns in the family of origin that seem to be repeating themselves in the client's relationships. At times, it may also be clear to the therapist from the initial history (although probably not to the client) how circumstances in the family of origin have primed the client to assume a certain role in relationships again and again.

For a variety of reasons, however, it may take the therapist con-siderable time to develop a full picture of the client's relationship diffi-culties, particularly the underlying cognitive components. Denial mechanisms may prevent the client from even recognizing certain re-lationship dynamics, let alone communicating such data to the thera-pist. Family loyalty certainly makes it difficult for many clients to depict their relationships in a realistic manner, particularly if they are afraid of being told to leave the individual in question. As we discussed in the previous chapter, denial processes are apt to be particularly virulent during the limerant phase of a relationship. Under such circumstances, the client will resist any efforts by the therapist to analyze the relationship, or the partner, in objective terms. Rather than pressure the client, the therapist simply may have to wait patiently for difficulties in the relationship to unfold.

Many of our clients automatically assume responsibility for anything that happens in their important relationships. If their significant others habitually *externalize* blame, these individuals can easily remain stuck in an endless cycle of conflict and self-recrimination. Although such clients may view themselves as responsible for their relationship problems, they may paradoxically fear being blamed by the therapist. Consequently, efforts on the therapist's part to explore the client's relationships may yield distorted information and/or defensive reactions from the individual. In Chapters 7 and 13, we describe various ways in which the therapist can make discussions of ongoing relationships less threatening for clients.

Some of our clients with the most severe relationship difficulties spend the least amount of productive time attempting to analyze the inner experiences that accompany such problems. On the other hand, they may expend great time and effort obsessing about their partners' inner workings. These clients may find themselves automatically monitoring and/or anticipating the other individual's every mood and reaction. Such individuals may find it much easier to discuss their views on what the *partner* thinks and feels, rather than articulate their *own* thoughts and feelings. The tendency to center the conversation with the therapist on the other party is a direct reflection of the client's obsessive inner dialogue, which likewise tends to concern itself primarily with the partner. Over the course of treatment, the therapist should strive to make the client keenly aware of the tendency to focus obsessively on the other party and the personal costs that accrue as a result. We sometimes ask our clients to chart periods of rumination about their partners in order to underscore the amount of time and energy actually consumed. The client will also need to identify the underlying fears that help to maintain such rumination. The major thrust of the treatment process, in many cases, may involve stimulating a greater degree of psychological separation between the client and his or her partner. In the meantime, it may require continuous redirecting by the therapist to enable such clients to sustain even minimal discussions of their own reactions to a relationship. The therapist may need to make statements such as, "You're telling me about him. I want to know how *you* reacted to this situation" repeatedly, almost to the point of rudeness in order to begin to obtain a picture of the client's inner experience of the relationship. By forewarning the client that such efforts to redirect attention will be a regular part of treatment sessions, the clinician can avoid creating unnecessary disruptions in the therapeutic relationship. The therapist may say, "I think we both agree that we can use our time most productively if we focus on you, rather than on others. I want you to remember that I'm going to keep redirecting your conversation back to yourself, so that you won't think I'm being impolite when I do it."

Encouraging the client to pay attention to the manner in which he or she experiences a relationship is not only a device to facilitate assessment, but it is also an important therapeutic intervention aimed at changing a basic attentional pattern. Many of our clients simply never even consider asking themselves what *they* thought, how *they* felt, or what *they* wanted in connection with a particular interaction. Only through persistent but supportive direction from the therapist can the client begin to move his or her attention back to the self. Even with the therapist's help, it may not be easy for the client to acquire the ability to report on inner reactions to events in a relationship, since it may run so contrary to his or her normal mode of operation, which involves an obsessive focus on the other individual.

Some clients take an enabling position in their close relationships, but they do so in a subtle, ostensibly benign framework, one which only becomes clearer to the therapist over time. They do not describe disturbed or impaired behavior on the part of the significant other, nor do they experience intense dissatisfaction with the relationship. In fact, they may believe that they idealize their partners. However, the significant others may begin to complain about certain aspects of the relationship, particularly involving controlling attitudes or behaviors on the part of the client. The therapist may observe that the client habitually withholds important bits of communication from the significant other while citing the partner's potential negative reaction as the rationale. Sometimes the information the client withholds is trivial or even laughable, although the relationship implications of such a withholding communicational style are more negative.

Leon failed to tell his wife that he had not enjoyed the meal she had cooked for him, because she was "having a tough time lately." Predictably, she served the same unpalatable concoction just a week later. If his wife was too psychologically fragile to tolerate negative feedback on her cooking, the therapist asked, then how was Leon ever going to address more serious issues with her as they arose? Further, how would he know when she was capable of handling greater candor on his part? Not surprisingly, the cooking vignette alerted the therapist to find many more instances in which Leon viewed his wife as helpless and incompetent and/or withheld significant reactions from her.

In the course of his treatment, Leon was able to recognize that regardless of his good intentions, many of his behaviors in the marriage communicated a lack of respect for his wife's competency, her emotional resiliency, and her freedom of choice. He began to understand the distinction between *manipulation* and *communication*, so that, for example, instead of attempting to orchestrate success experiences for his wife, he encouraged her to talk to him about her feelings of insecurity. Most importantly, Leon realized that his *own* sense of inadequacy had played a significant role in determining his behavior in the marriage. It was safer for him to relate to his wife from a distance, as a wise, competent parental figure, rather than risk making himself more vulnerable by disclosing his own fears and insecurities. Through self-monitoring assignments, Leon discovered that his compulsive, controlling behaviors at home were most likely to surface whenever he himself was entertaining doubts about his wife's feelings toward him. He was amazed at how threatening it was to share his innermost thoughts and feelings with his wife. Through considerable effort and practice, however, he was able to disclose more and more to her. As he began to experience a sense of true intimacy in his marriage, Leon also recognized just how withdrawn and distant his earlier role in the relationship had been.

Boundaries

As we discussed in Chapter 1, many of our clients were the victims of various types of boundary violations in their families of origin. We find that individuals who have experienced boundary violations as children often unknowingly replicate similar circumstances in adult life. Their lack of a "normal" frame of reference allows them to function in relationships in which infringements of personal, intergenerational, and/or hierarchical boundaries regularly take place. If the therapist can identify a clear pattern of boundary violations in the client's history, he or she must continue to assume that analogous difficulties exist in the individual's current relationships, even if these are not immediately apparent. These clients may report affairs or other exploitative relationships with authority figures such as professors, bosses, or therapists. The feelings of worthlessness and self-blame the individuals experience from these encounters keep them in a vicious cycle, so that they never achieve sufficient self-esteem to demand better relationships for themselves. Clients may create difficulties for themselves by sharing highly personal information indiscreetly or find themselves unable to keep intrusive family members or friends from interfering in their lives. They may become overinvolved with family members or friends to the point of submerging their own identities in the process. Accompanying such overinvolvement is a strong sense of responsibility and self-blame for the actions of the other party. In our view, so-called codependency patterns reflect the inability of the participants to remain intimately involved without invading one another's psychological space. If individuals with boundary issues choose careers in the helping fields, they may be unable to separate personal and professional roles clearly and may act out issues with clients as a consequence.

In our clinical experience, even clients with considerable insight will not be able to recognize the degree to which boundary difficulties have become woven into the fabric of their daily lives. Moreover, they may be handicapped by some of the very same factors that prevent abused children from protecting themselves: (1) ignorance as to what constitutes a normal, nonexploitative relationship; (2) a crippling sense of responsibility for the abusive or exploitative behavior of the other individual; (3) an attitude of loyalty and/or protectiveness toward the perpetrator that results in guilt over betraying secrets; (4) a belief that they have no power to prevent continuing mistreatment; and (5) a fear of losing the relationship with the victimizer and whatever positive elements have been associated with it. Just as in childhood, these factors will prevent the individual from even acknowledging current boundary violations in adult life—let alone acting to prevent them.

Let us review some strong indicators of boundary problems in the client's relationships:

Involvement in cross-generational coalitions in current family relationships

Separation problems in offspring, for example, school refusal.

Sexual relationships that cross hierarchichal lines, for example, with bosses, professors, students, therapists, and so on.

Recurrent involvement in promiscuous, degrading, painful, unpleasant or anxiety-provoking sexual experiences.

Involvement in sexual behavior for nonhedonistic reasons, for example, to placate an angry or demanding partner.

Continued voluntary contact with individuals who have manifested repeated sexual advances or sexual harassment toward the client.

Self-disclosure of intimate personal information in inappropriate contexts or to inappropriate individuals.

Obsessive focus on the thoughts, feelings, and behaviors of significant others.

Repeated involvement with highly dependent, overly demanding individuals, or development of similar dependent attachments to others.

Repeated unwanted intrusions on physical privacy by neighbors, friends, family members, or work associates.

Chronic, recurrent inability to shield personal time from work demands or interruptions.

Overinvolvement with clients in a human services or business context.

Recurrent intense involvement in the personal affairs of acquaintances, neighbors, and other somewhat peripheral figures.

Recurrent assumption of a go-between role with friends or family members who are experiencing conflict.

Overinvolvement with therapists, physicians, and other individuals who are engaged with the client in a professional capacity.

Recurrent efforts to learn more personal information about the therapist.

Persistent difficulties with time norms, insurance arrangements, payment of fees, and other limits imposed on the therapeutic relationship.

As we discuss in Chapter 8, clients with boundary difficulties necessitate ongoing adjustments in the therapist's posture. Likewise, in Chapters 10, 12, and 13 we describe various cases in which the client's boundary problems were a major focus in treatment.

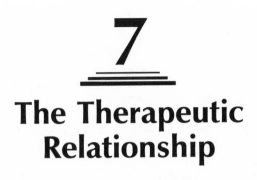

7

The Therapeutic Relationship

Whether its serves as a "corrective emotional experience" in itself, or as a rich source of data regarding the client's interpersonal functioning, the therapeutic relationship is the engine that drives the treatment process. When treatment involves a family of origin focus, we expect to find that some of the client's key issues will play themselves out in the therapeutic relationship. Over the next two chapters, we describe how we approach the therapeutic relationship, primarily from a cognitive perspective with an assist or two from a few other sources.

COLLABORATIVE EMPIRICISM

Carl Rogers (1951) proposed that treatment success was contingent on the therapist's ability to create an environment characterized by accurate empathy, nonpossessive warmth, congruence, and unconditional positive regard. Beck (1976) agreed that the Rogerian conditions were essential for effective treatment but added the notion of *collaborative empiricism*. Collaborative empiricism refers to a relationship in which the therapist and client work as *partners* at the task of identifying, examining, and modifying maladaptive cognitions. By maintaining a spirit of collaborative empiricism, the therapist helps to keep the client in a competent, empowered position while minimizing defensiveness and resistance. The collaborative spirit of therapy is enhanced when: (1) the roles and responsibilities of both the client and therapist are spelled out early in treatment; (2) the therapist and client jointly set and prioritize goals; (3) therapists provide information and feedback in a clear and straightforward fashion; and (4) therapists regularly request and encourage feedback from clients about both the content and process of therapy.

In our view, an emphasis on collaborative empiricism does not mean that the client is always right, nor does it demand that the therapist never utilize confrontation as a treatment strategy. In fact, other cognitively oriented therapists (e.g., Walen, DiGiuseppe, & Wessler, 1980) have discussed the appropriate use of confrontation as a highly effective strategy for enhancing rapport. Similarly, within the spirit of collaboration and empowerment of the consumer, the therapist still must function as an expert in many areas vis-à-vis the client. In the final analysis, it is the therapist who is responsible for maintaining a sense of direction and continuity in treatment. Similarly, the therapist must be the one to decide what kind of emphasis in treatment will result in reductions in the client's symptomatology. When family of origin of issues are involved, effective treatment may involve moving in directions that may seem counterintuitive to the client but that, in the therapist's experience, have been associated with remediation and long-term prevention of symptoms. The therapist may well move away from some of the client's most significant obsessions, preferring to concentrate, for example, on areas of the individual's life that have been hitherto obscured through the use of denial mechanisms. In the strictest sense, such efforts on the therapist's part could hardly be termed "collaborative" in nature. However, once the therapist sets a course, it is up to him or her to orchestrate learning experiences for the client that produce data that support the clinician's hypotheses. As we discuss at length in Chapter 8, it is also incumbent on the therapist to change direction when his or her interventions have proven to be destructive or ineffective.

Just as we want our clients to learn as much as they can about their difficulties, so do we also seek to have them understand the actual treatment process itself. We begin treatment by discussing the parameters of confidentiality and by obtaining written confirmation of clients' understanding of these issues. We then proceed to outline the typical structure of treatment for the first few sessions We tell clients that our initial aims are to understand presenting complaints, to gather relevant history, and to set goals. At the close of the first session, we leave time to discuss fees, billing practices, and procedures to be followed in the event of an emergency. By clearly defining the limits of confidentiality, by discussing fees and other practical considerations, and by structuring the early stages of treatment, we seek to provide clear expectations and secure boundaries in the therapeutic relationship.

We want our clients well informed as to where they are, where they have been, and where they are going in the treatment process. Consequently, we tend avoid the use of highly noncollaborative methods, such as paradoxical intention. However, we also assume that there are times when the therapist would be ill-advised to disclose all the motives for every one of his or her actions in treatment.

THE THERAPIST'S POSTURE

Successful treatment inevitably requires the therapist to find and sustain a posture, a workable position from which to confront the client's thinking and behavior. Our clinical experiences suggest to us that something more is involved in the concept of "posture" than the basic building blocks of the therapeutic relationship discussed in previous sections.

Human relationships contain both communication of content and metacommunication (Watzlawick et al., 1967). Loosely defined, metacommunication consists of all kinds of messages, whether implicit or explicit, verbal or nonverbal, that define a *relationship* between two or more persons. Metacommunicative messages articulate boundaries, distance, hierarchies, and other relationship variables between individuals. Often such messages are *embedded* in the social or familial context, without necessarily being acknowledged by the individuals involved. Family therapists such as Minuchin (1974) are skilled at both reading existing metacommunicative messages and at devising and sustaining new messages that stimulate the restructuring of relationships. Minuchin, Milton Erickson (Haley, 1967, 1971), and Jay Haley (1976) all excel at communicating with clients simultaneously on multiple levels in a variety of treatment situations, ranging from family sessions to hypnotic inductions. Messages are wrapped around one another, or embedded within other messages, so that clients can be supported and confronted at the same time, so they can acknowledge failings without losing face in front of their children, so that individual issues such as alcohol abuse can be disentangled from ongoing couples conflict, and so on.

Our emphasis on the therapist's posture reflects an attempt to integrate the work of the communication theorists, structural family therapists such as Minuchin, and other practitioners in the Erickson/Haley mold, while utilizing the highly collaborative treatment framework advocated by Beck. In our view, the term posture refers to the *totality* of the therapist's communications to the client, both content- and relationship-oriented, both explicit and implicit, both direct and embedded.

In this section, and throughout the following chapter, we attempt to describe some of the key considerations involved in formulating and sustaining a therapeutic posture with each client. A clear, consciously formulated posture enables the therapist to deal more effectively with traditionally uncomfortable issues such as collecting fees and setting limits on clients, and to be more circumspect about using such high-risk strategies as self-disclosure in working with a particular client. In our section on embedded messages, we show the reader how to confront a client with data while remaining in a strongly collaborative mode.

PSYCHOLOGICAL REACTANCE

Brehm (1966), a social psychologist who investigated the effects of interpersonal dynamics on attitudes, proposed a model of "psychological reactance" that has enormous relevance for the therapeutic situation. The model predicts that when an individual perceives that his or her *right* to hold a particular belief is being attacked, he or she will respond by clinging even more strongly to that belief. Anyone who has parented teenagers (or has acted as a surrogate parent to one in a treatment context) should understand perfectly how psychological reactance complicates the meaningful discussion of issues. If the parent continues to attack a hairdo, a style of clothing, a musical group, a girlfriend, or a boyfriend, the adolescent's beliefs grow stronger and more extreme. It is particularly frightening if an adolescent begins to argue with his or her parents about suicide. As some adult clients also do with their therapists, the teenager may end up arguing forcefully with the parents for the *right* to commit suicide, instead of examining the factors that may have caused the self-destructive wishes.

When psychological reactance occurs during a treatment session, the client stops processing new information pertinent to the topic currently under discussion. The client may argue vociferously, sulk, withdraw, or may attempt to "go through the motions" for the remainder of the discussion. Regardless of outward appearances, however, the client has ceased to listen to the therapist. On some level, the relationship with the therapist has now become unacceptable to the client. The client may resume processing new information, most likely involving a different subject, only if the therapist can reestablish the collaboration. Perhaps the concept of psychological reactance should be expanded to refer to *any* interpersonal process that leads to an intensification or a rigidification of an individual's beliefs. There are a number of instances in which the client may respond in such a reactive fashion:

When the therapist is actually behaving in a belittling, condescending, argumentative, rigid, authoritarian, and/or hostile manner, and the client accurately senses it.

When the client perceives anger, disapproval, or rejection on the part of the therapist.

When the client is afraid of being manipulated, exploited, dominated, or otherwise victimized by the therapist.

When the therapist persists in confronting or analyzing ideas that are currently associated with very high degrees of belief.

When the client feels stupid, ashamed, or otherwise defective, as a result of discussing the material in question.

When the client fears that the current discussion will lead to verification of his or her blameworthiness or worthlessness.

When the client believes that the current discussion will lead to disloyalty toward a significant other.

When the client senses that the current discussion will lead to conclusions that might threaten the future of an intimate relationship, particularly if it contains strongly limerant or enabling components.

When the client senses that the current discussion will prevent him or her from engaging in compulsive behaviors, addictive behaviors, or other coping strategies associated with the avoidance of pain or threat.

When psychological reactance occurs, the therapist's first priority should be to reestablish a positive alliance with the client. Restoring a collaborative atmosphere in the session often requires moving away from the specific content that initially stimulated the defensive reaction from the client. The therapist needs to learn how to "beat a hasty retreat" smoothly and gracefully when psychological reactance begins to prevent the client from working constructively on a particular topic. As we discuss in greater detail below in a section on therapist flexibility, it may also be vital in many cases for therapists to acknowledge openly when their comments or interventions have been ill-timed, poorly conceived, or hurtful in some way to their clients.

The therapist needs to determine why each particular episode of psychological reactance has occurred before returning to the topic in question. The therapist may then incorporate the dynamics involved into the therapeutic posture he or she takes with the client in the future. As we discuss in subsequent sections, the therapist can attempt to *preempt* attentional shifts that will move the client into a reactive position by using various embedded messages, changing tone, explicitly disavowing certain agendas the client fears, and so on. At the appropriate time, perhaps when a change in belief or mood has occurred, the therapist may also wish to highlight the issues that have predisposed the client to assume a reactive stance. The client can then begin to have an appreciation for the manner in which concerns such as blame, worth-lessness, family loyalty, and so on, interfere with the consideration of other equally compelling matters.

For example, Stan refused to acknowledge that his mother's recur-ring depressive episodes had any impact upon him during childhood and adolescence. Likewise, he seemed to become tense and irritated when the therapist attempted to explore how the client, as a young adolescent, had been recruited by the father to act as the mother's caretaker. Stan was unable to consider the possibility that his intense perfectionism and his overblown sense of responsibility in adulthood might be related to the parental role he had been forced to assume earlier in his life. Instead, he would deflect discussion by making state-ments such as, "My parents gave me so much, it's only natural to want to give back," or "It's just what you do when you're part of a family."

The therapist realized that he had to find a way to explore historical issues without threatening the client's strong sense of family loyalty. Consequently, he began to preface any discussions of Stan's parents by acknowledging the devastating impact of severe depression on indi-vidual clients and their families. The therapist emphasized that no one he had ever treated actually *chose* to be depressed. He said that he empathized particularly with anyone who, like Stan's mother, suffered from manic–depressive illness before lithium and antidepressant me-dications were extensively available. In a similar manner, the therapist portrayed Stan's father as an innocent, helpless victim, who struggled mightily on his own to cope as best he could with his wife's debilitating illness. The therapist described how vital it was in his own clinical practice to meet with the family members of depressed clients in order to provide significant others with realistic guidelines for dealing with the disorder. It was not uncommon in his experience, he said, to find that otherwise intelligent, well-educated individuals held a variety of mistaken assumptions about depression. He reminded Stan that marital or family treatment with depressed clients was hardly standard practice 20 years ago. Consequently, it was unlikely that Stan's father had re-ceived much professional advice on how to deal with his wife's depres-sion or how to help the rest of the family cope with her recurring impairment.

The therapist took care to include the statements described in the preceding paragraph in any discussion of Stan's family background. Although the therapist still had to be the one to bring family of origin material into the foreground, he allowed the client to stay pretty much in control of the conversations about his parents. Stan seemed to become increasingly comfortable with such discussions, probably because he began to recognize that the therapist had no intention of scapegoating the parents. Each time the topic of his childhood came up, Stan was able to volunteer more information regarding the impact of his mother's depressive episodes on the functioning of the family. He acknowledged that, as a child and as an adolescent, he had often been quite fearful for his mother's safety. He was able to recognize that at times he had blamed himself for his mother's depressive episodes. He also remembered having vowed to become a perfect son so as to avoid creating additional problems for his parents. Whenever possible, the therapist continued to underscore the connections between the family of origin dynamics and Stan's current difficulties but was able to avoid additional defensive reactions from the client. Later in treatment, the therapist used Stan's responses to the initial discussions about his parents as illustrations of the power of denial and the strength of the client's family loyalty.

THE USE OF EMBEDDED MESSAGES TO COMMUNICATE ON MULTIPLE LEVELS

With any given client, the therapist's posture will consist of multiple messages, addressing multiple issues, and delivered through multiple channels of communication. The therapist orchestrates and harmonizes these messages in the service of unfolding treatment goals. As illustrated again and again in subsequent case examples both in this chapter and in Chapters 8 and 9, the therapist seeks to promote treatment goals through indirect or implicit messages as well as through more explicit interventions. Moreover, the therapist must take care to ensure that he or she does not sabotage explicit treatment interventions by sending contradictory messages on an implicit or metacommunicative level. For example, let us suppose a therapist is working hard to help a client achieve an increased sense of competency, self-worth, and independence. Let us suppose further that the therapist persists in offering the client specific *advice* on how to handle various stressful life situations instead of identifying the *barriers* that prevent the client from resolving such problems in an independent way. Even if the client implements the therapist's solutions successfully (which seldom happens in our experience), the individual has not gained a greater sense of self-efficacy in the process. In fact, the client is likely to give the credit to the therapist. The client may also feel as if he or she did not *decide* to do anything different but merely followed instructions. In the meantime, if the client chooses *not* to follow the therapist's advice, he or she may begin to feel incompetent or disloyal in the process.

The therapist must look for opportunities to insert constructive embedded messages into the stream of communication with each client. When skillfully inserted into ongoing dialogue, embedded messages do not permit direct refutation by the client. Consequently, they can provide a forceful implicit challenge to established belief systems, particularly when they are combined with more explicit interventions by the therapist.

For example, suppose the therapist is treating a client who was raised in a household with two physically abusive parents. Now the mother of a 4-year-old and a 6-year-old, the client often feels overwhelmed by anxiety regarding the adequacy of her parenting. She finds it difficult to set limits on her children without becoming fearful that she has traumatized them in some way. Although she has never spanked her children and seldom even yells at them, she becomes frightened whenever she finds herself irritated with them, worrying that such feelings will inevitably lead to abusive behavior on her part. The therapist will of course want to help the client discriminate more effectively between her own childrearing methods and those to which she was exposed in her family of origin. Similarly, the therapist will also utilize various methods to enable the client to question out the belief that her angry feelings can lead to a loss of self-control and, ultimately, abuse of her children. Moreover, the therapist will want to provide the client with an awareness that negative emotions such as anger are a normal part of parenting.

At some point during a session, for example, the client may indicate that she will need to reschedule her next appointment, since it will conflict with a birthday party she is giving for her oldest child and his friends. While rescheduling the appointment, the therapist may remark casually that he always found birthday parties very stressful when his children were the same age as the client's son. He might recall how difficult it was to interact with an active, overly excited 6-year-old before the party without losing one's cool, let alone to keep a roomful of kids under some sort of control during the actual event itself. He may add with a chuckle that the one saving grace of birthday parties for young children was that they were mercifully brief, usually only an hour or so in length. Wishing the client well in her enterprise, the therapist might then turn the session over to other relevant topics, without necessarily eliciting a direct response from her.

The therapist's remarks above detail some of the difficulties inherent in managing young children, who are prone to become excited, impulsive, and/or unreasonable on special occasions such as birthdays and holidays, just when their parents are most invested in orchestrating loving, memorable experiences for them. The therapist has normalized the behavior of young children on such occasions and has also human-ized the affective responses of parents under such potentially stressful conditions. The clinician's remarks gain in credibility and power, however, from the fact that they were issued "spontaneously," that is, without reference to material the client had raised specifically for therapeutic consideration. Since the therapist's statements were "side comments" or "unofficial" in nature, the client is unlikely to dismiss them as attempts at reassurance or otherwise discount the messages he conveyed.

A good cognitive therapist must become adept at capturing the client's attention and directing it toward new data. Unless the therapist performs such an active *orienting function*, the client is liable to remain stuck in the same old cognitive grooves, habitually obsessing on famil-iar themes, while ignoring or discarding potentially important data. As we discuss in greater detail in Chapter 9, the therapist needs to analyze any instances in which he or she cannot successfully orient the client to new information. As the therapist becomes familiar with the client's thinking patterns, he or she can then begin to anticipate some of the individual's characteristic "attentional pathways." Armed with such knowledge, the clinician may then use various types of embedded messages to preempt certain attentional shifts in order to help the client to process new data. Below we describe several types of situations in which the therapist uses embedded messages to sustain a more effective posture with a client:

1. Whether they are in individual, marital, or family treatment, most of our clients find it hard to tolerate interactions with the therapist when they believe that the clinician is siding with another person against them. However, in many instances, unless the therapist can find a tactful way to keep the client focused on the self, the individual will engage in endless, unproductive discussions that center on the thoughts, feelings, and behavior of *others*. As the following example indicates, the therapist will often need to use multiple embedded mes-sages to redirect the client's attention in a successful manner.

During an individual treatment session, a client centers his remarks almost exclusively on his wife's behavior. The client, who is extra-ordinarily sensitized to blaming messages, has reacted defensively to any attempts to shift the focus back on to him during such discussions in the past. The therapist may listen empathically to the client's com-ments about his wife for a few minutes. During an opening in the conversation, the therapist may initiate a change in direction, by hold-ing eye contact with the client and speaking lines such as the following, in emphatic tones:

"It really sounds to me as if your wife's behavior hurt you a great deal. It's also clear that these interactions between the two of you happen much too often. I don't blame you for being unhappy. This kind of friction can't go on indefinitely in a relationship. We're going to have to talk a lot more about the relationship, that's for sure. We'll get back to that subject a little bit later. Right now, I need to understand what went on inside you just as you were returning home on Friday night. Can you think back, and tell me what you were thinking as you walked into the house?"

Note that the therapist does not change subjects until he or she has joined strongly with the client, validating the individual's sense of anger and discouragement. Pandering somewhat to the client's obsession with blame and wrongdoing, the therapist also suggests that he *does* see the wife's behavior as hurtful. (It should be noted, however, that the authors would be extremely cautious about utilizing such an approach with any client who is physically abusive to his or her partner.) Before leaving the topic of the wife, the clinician makes it clear to the client that the problems in the relationship will receive close attention in treatment, without of course specifying when or in what manner this will occur. The therapist may also attempt to minimize resistance during the subsequent discussion by saying: "I'm going to keep interrupting you if you begin to talk about your wife's behavior. You may start to feel like I'm blaming you for all the problems in the relationship, but I want you to remember that it's not true, as you clearly heard in what I just said a moment ago. All I'm trying to do is gain a better understanding of *your* inner experiences."

Although any extensive discussion of marital or family therapy is beyond the scope of this volume, the recovery process for most of the cases we see usually involves more than just individual treatment. The therapist's ability to shift alliances rapidly and smoothly is obviously crucial to the success of any conjoint treatment format. Therapists such as Minuchin and Haley are skillful at creating and maintaining serial alliances in a fluid manner during family treatment sessions. The use of embedded messages enables the clinician to join and confront an individual simultaneously in a conjoint session, just as the techniques above accomplished the same goal in an individual treatment context.

2. Many of our clients experience powerful feelings of disloyalty when discussing their families of origin. The therapist may precede conversations about family members with statements to acknowledge that family members had laudable characteristics or motivations, may have been victims themselves, and so on. The therapist may also insert

statements such as the following, *continuously* throughout such discussions:

- We know that your parents did the best they could.
- Your mother was impaired, not evil.
- We're not questioning the fact that your father loved you.
- We're only talking about your parents as they were then, not as they are now.
- Perhaps your father would be appalled if he truly realized the impact his behaviors had on you and your siblings.
- Naturally your mother was struggling with terrible problems of her own at the time.
- Of course I assume that it may not be necessary or appropriate for you to share any of these thoughts with anyone else in your family.
- Recognizing the impact of your childhood doesn't mean that you can't have a constructive relationship with your family members today.
- I know that you wouldn't want to do anything to jeopardize your current relationship with your parents.

The therapist may not want to discuss or elaborate on any of these messages when he or she inserts them into the stream of ongoing dialogue. Although each point mentioned above may legitimately deserve exploration in its own right, the insertion of messages aims only to acknowledge and steer past a side road, albeit one that may be quite tempting or compelling for the client. The *frequent* and *repeated* usage of such messages, particularly when they have been tailored to fit the individual's *specific* concerns, seems to give the therapist a much greater degree of control over the flow of the client's attentional processes during the session.

3. Many of our clients are afraid that acknowledging the negative components of a relationship will lead inevitably to its termination. It is also common for clients to fear that, as a result of information they disclose, the therapist will begin to advocate termination of a relationship. Unless the therapist addresses the individual's fears of loss, rejection, or abandonment, the client may not be able to sustain constructive discussion of a significant relationship. Again, the therapist will probably want to preface such discussions with relevant comments and to insert pertinent messages repeatedly into the stream of ongoing dialogue. Such messages may include the following:

- None of these problems means that the relationship has to end.
- Given your history, I can understand why you would think that acknowledging conflict would lead to the end of a relationship, but I'm not sure that it has to do that at all.
- I want you to try to stay focused on the nature of the relationship right now without worrying for the time being about what to do about it.
- Although you may believe differently at times, I truly have no opinion on whether this relationship should continue or not.
- Remember that I'm only interested in how *you* react in the most intimate relationship in your life. I'm focusing on *your* thoughts, feelings, and behaviors, not your partner's.
- I'm sure that like all of us, your husband has his good points and his bad points. I don't assume that just because a couple has problems, one of them has to be a bad person.

4. Many of our clients suffer from a decided lack of resolve when it comes to ending destructive or otherwise inappropriate relationships. They may enlist the aid of others somewhat inappropriately as they strive to implement their decisions by regaling them with stories of mistreatment or inventories of their partners' negative attributes. Our clients thereby induce others to side strongly with them against their partners. Alas, such support may not be sufficient for our clients, in that they may still find it extremely difficult to stick to their guns, particularly as the separation continues. Not surprisingly, if they resume their relationships, they may find themselves unable to face friends and family members without experiencing intense feelings of embarrassment. Since the client may undergo many such reversals in the course of his or her recovery, it is vital for the therapist to avoid becoming invested (or appearing to be invested) in temporary decisions the client makes. Consequently, the therapist must set the stage for the client's continued involvement in treatment, regardless of the outcome of decisions he or she makes. On the other hand, the therapist does not want to communicate that he or she does not take the client seriously, particularly when the individual feels fully committed to a decision. By inserting various phrases into the ongoing dialogue, the therapist can support the client while enhancing the likelihood that the individual can remain in treatment without losing face should he or she fail to execute the decision as planned. The therapist may use embedded phrases and statements such as:

- If you continue to believe that it's best for you to end the relationship. . . .

- If you continue on in the path that you seem to be choosing now. . . .
- Regardless of what you may decide to do in the future, it is clear that you've learned some important things, such as. . . .
- Even if you decide to go back to the relationship, it sounds as if your behavior will be quite different, in the following ways. . . .

As we discuss in greater detail in Chapter 13, the clinician should make every effort to communicate to the client that the therapeutic relationship is not contingent on his or her actions with significant others outside treatment. On the other hand, the therapist does need to maintain a posture that will encourage exploration of the conflicting attitudes that accompany difficult relationships. Consequently, the therapist may continue to acknowledge the ambivalent feelings of the client toward a relationship even when the individual claims to have made an irrevocable decision. The therapist may make comments such as "Even though you feel as if you've made up your mind, I'm sure you are going to miss the relationship at some point," "You will probably feel lonely in the future, just as you did in the past when you tried to end the relationship," or "It would be natural to miss him and to be concerned about him. After all, you did have a close bond."

In the remainder of this chapter, and in the Chapter 8 as well, we describe a variety of interventions that involve the deliberate use of embedded messages by the clinician. Indeed, to some extent, all of the cases described throughout the volume involved the use of embedded or implicit communications to facilitate changes in information-processing and belief systems on the part of our clients.

ANTICIPATING DISTORTIONS IN THE
THERAPEUTIC RELATIONSHIP

The therapist has an obligation at all times to look ahead and consider various potential developments in treatment, particularly those which might be difficult for clients to articulate to themselves, let alone to express directly to another person. Most of the clients discussed in this volume experienced significant cognitive distortions concerning the therapist and the therapeutic relationship, although given their family backgrounds, not without good reason. Although we do not attempt to stimulate such distortions by presenting an impassive and impersonal "blank screen" to the client, we seek to identify and utilize reactions to the therapeutic relationship as often as possible. As we have mentioned, some of the most significant periods in treatment begin with an examination of the client's experience of the therapeutic relationship.

As early as possible in the treatment process, the clinician should underline the importance of the client sharing his or her reactions to the therapist. The therapist should emphasize that the client's responses to the therapeutic relationship will serve as a significant data base, both for shaping the conduct of treatment and for establishing a better understanding of his or her attitudes and behaviors. If the therapist knows enough about the client's belief systems to make predictions from the outset about specific distortions that may occur, so much the better. For example, during the initial interview, the therapist may tell a chronically unassertive woman that she might find it hard to discuss areas of frustration or dissatisfaction with treatment while that therapist encourages her to share any such reactions. Likewise, the therapist might remind a client who has a history of rejecting or abusive relationships that he or she may see the therapist as angry or critical at times. The therapist may want to normalize the potential relationship distortions by briefly describing the reactions of another individual who had issues similar to the those of the client. With a client who might respond by minimizing the potential for distortions in the treatment relationship, the therapist might preface his or her remarks with phrases that anticipate denial, for example, "You may find this hard to believe, but . . .", or "Many people don't think this will apply to them when they hear it, but . . ." or "You may forget that I told you this, but. . . ." Should distortions in the relationship occur in the future, contrary to the individual's predictions, the therapist will have a wonderful opportunity to demonstrate the role of denial mechanisms in the client's life.

Victims of childhood sexual abuse, particularly incest survivors, may be prone to experience the therapeutic relationship in erotic or sexual terms, regardless of the gender of the therapist. Feeling too ashamed to recognize the actual origins of such reactions, they may be unable to share them until they have achieved a more trusting relationship with the therapist. With some individuals, the clinician may elect to anticipate distortions in the therapeutic relationship without referring explicitly to sexual or erotic reactions that might arise on the part of the client. In a nonspecific way, the therapist may simply ask the client to share any and all reactions to the relationship, however crazy or bizarre they may appear. The therapist should express the hope that the client will share any dreams or fantasies about the relationship, even those which may seem illogical or incoherent.

As treatment progresses, the therapist may suspect that the client is experiencing some reactions to the relationship that for some reason he or she is unable to share. One way for the therapist to stimulate disclosure of the client's reactions is by continually weaving hypotheses about the probable distortions of the therapeutic relationship into discussions of other relationships, particularly those with parents or spouses. *Any time the client can clearly identify cognitive distortions, information-processing errors, or self-defeating coping strategies in other relationships, the therapist should take the opportunity at some point in the discussions to explore, and if necessary, spell out directly, the potential implications for the therapeutic alliance.*

For example, when the client describes the experience of having a parent who could neither nurture her nor protect her, the therapist may comment, "Perhaps when you started seeing me, it was hard for you to see me as someone who had the ability to help. After all, *there was no basis in your experience* to think that someone else would be capable of doing anything for you." Note that the therapist's use of the phrase, "no basis in your experience," is an attempt to remove the stigmatizing elements associated with any distorted perceptions the client may be experiencing by emphasizing that such distortions are the direct outgrowth of powerful learning experiences. Over the course of treatment, the therapist may need to make similar suggestions repeatedly before the client discloses his or her most private reactions to the therapeutic relationship, as the following example illustrates.

Lilly, a rather passive and withdrawn woman in her early 30s, had been raised by a physically and sexually abusive father after her mother abandoned the family. Her childhood experiences had been as bleak and destructive as any the therapist had ever heard. Her husband, although not a violent man, tended to be quite verbally abusive, particularly when he drank. Again and again, the therapist anticipated that Lilly might find herself afraid of being victimized in treatment, just as she had been abused by the other significant men in her life. Such remarks from therapist only seemed to elicit blank looks and bland responses from the client.

After over 18 months of treatment, Lilly impulsively hugged the therapist on her way out of the office after a session. The therapist, who considered anything more than a warm handshake to be inappropriate with his clients, felt quite uncomfortable with the hug and responded rather stiffly to it. While reflecting on the incident later, the therapist had a number of different reactions. At first he wondered if he had done anything to cause the client's behavior, but he realized fairly quickly that he had maintained consistently appropriate boundaries with client. The therapist then remembered that several times in the past, he had felt uncomfortable with Lilly's grip and her gaze when he had shaken hands with her at the end of her sessions. Because these incidents occurred at wide intervals, without any apparent consistency or pre-dictability, the clinician was able to tell himself that his perceptions were simply stray products of his imagination. Although the therapist knew that he had to process the issue with Lilly, he was initially afraid that he would be unable to do so without causing her to feel embar-rassed and rejected. The clinician made a mental note to investigate why he felt so protective of the client, particularly in light of Lilly's generally passive, submissive attitude. Part of him wanted to forget about the whole issue, but he knew he had to address the matter before the end of the next session; otherwise, he would run the risk that Lilly might hug him again. Besides, being able to raise the issue in a forthright manner would give him an opportunity to model effective communicational skills for the client's benefit.

The therapist raised the issue immediately at the next session, centering the discussion on his *own* discomfort and the clinical reasons behind it, rather than on the "badness" of Lilly's actions. Although he suspected that there was an erotic element to her hug, he never directly confronted her with that aspect of the situation but embedded relatively nonthreatening references to it in his discussion. He emphasized that treatment was supposed to focus on the client's needs, not the thera-pist's. He stated that the therapist needed to be content with the fin-ancial rewards and the sense of accomplishment that accompanied working with people. The therapist explained that looking to clients to gratify other wants compromised the therapist's objectivity and under-mined the integrity of the treatment process. Hugging clients raised legitimate questions about who really benefited from such actions and, in his opinion, opened the door to other potentially exploitative phys-ical contact, as well as dangerous misinterpretations all around.

Now the therapist tried to open the door for the client to disclose some of the more threatening or shameful elements of her reactions to him. Even if Lilly had reactions to the therapeutic relationship of a romantic or erotic nature, the therapist said, he knew that her feelings truly were not in response to him *as a real person*. Likewise, he told her that he knew that the "recovering side" of her personality would never want to have any sort of sexual contact with him. The therapist repeated his hope that Lilly would discuss any erotic or romantic thoughts or feelings with him. In his opinion, Lilly had already suffered too much as a result of abusive men and poor boundaries. The therapist told her that he owed it to her, especially given her abusive background, to be clear about the nature of their relationship, so that she could feel safe with him as much as possible. In closing, the therapist acknowledged that since he had found it hard to undertake the discussion with Lilly, he assumed that it had also been quite difficult for her as well. He anticipated that either now or at some point in the future she might perceive his reaction to the hugging episode as a rejection, and he exhorted her to share such reactions with him as they occurred.

Predictably, Lilly's reaction to the therapist's remarks was bland and uninformative. Other than offering a rationale for her behavior ("I guess I just felt real bad and needed a hug"), she failed to respond to most of the points the therapist had raised. The discussion seemed to go nowhere, but the therapist was quite reluctant to move on to some other topic, as Lilly seemed to want. Rather than persist in eliciting reactions from her however, the therapist switched gears and asked her to summarize some of the major points of his discussion, adding that he needed to know that he had communicated effectively with her. Somewhat to the therapist's surprise, Lilly's feedback indicated that she had indeed absorbed the major points.

The therapist reviewed the entire hugging incident with the client during the following session as well. He again solicited Lilly's responses to the episode and the discussion of it that had occurred during the next interview. Lilly finally opened up somewhat regarding her reactions to the therapist. She did acknowledge having felt rejected by the therapist. This admission led to an involved discussion of her relationship with her father, who only expressed affection of any kind when he approached her sexually. She discussed the utter lack of affectionate physical contact in her life, and her ambivalent feelings about seeking out such contact, even in nonsexual spheres. She also described her father badgering her with questions when he had disapproved of her behavior as a child, then beating her when she was too frightened to answer. The therapist asked the client if she ever experienced his questions in a similar manner. She acknowledged that sometimes the therapist's questions frightened her and that once threatened she was likely to freeze up instead of offering a response.

Now the therapist could see clearly why Lilly had always answered so many of his questions with "I don't know" or other equally uninformative replies. In the past, he had not challenged her behavior as strongly as he might have in other cases, since he perceived so many gaps in his knowledge of her. The therapist asked Lilly if he should assume she was "freezing up" whenever she responded with "I don't know" to questions she was fully capable of answering. She replied in the affirmative. Thereafter, whenever the client seemed to be evading his questions, the therapist would ask her to think about what might be making her feel anxious at that instant. As a result of the discussions that would follow, both the therapist and the client were able to achieve a much greater awareness of how her traumatic background influenced her behavior on a moment-to-moment basis.

Lilly also disclosed a dream she had had about the therapist during the first few months of treatment, one she had been afraid to share at the time. She dreamed that she had gone with her 10-year-old daughter to the therapist's office, which now contained a table designed for internal examinations. The therapist, clad in a white lab coat, told her to disrobe and get up on the table, where he intended to examine her. Prior to the examination, he told Lilly to send her daughter out into the waiting room. "She shouldn't see this," he told her. What happened next was no longer clear to Lilly, but she did recall that whatever it was, she had been quite frightened when she awoke.

Lilly was visibly uncomfortable while describing her dream to the therapist. Nonetheless, her disclosure of the dream did facilitate a more frank discussion of her fears of being abused by the therapist. As the discussion progressed, she seemed to overcome much of her embarrassment about the dream and the anxiety it expressed. Thereafter, the therapist found it easier to facilitate discussions of the therapeutic relationship. As the therapist began to understand more about Lilly's relationship with her children, he was also able to identify some of the potential themes associated with the daughter's appearance in the dream. Subsequently, the therapist referred back to Lilly's dream as a means of illustrating various points about the client's sense of worthlessness, her concerns about rejection, and her fears of being victimized again in her relationships.

ANTICIPATING AFFECTIVE/SYMPTOMATIC RESPONSES TO THE TREATMENT PROCESS

Clients often believe that therapy will flow in linear fashion, resulting in a steady and progressive process of symptom reduction. Unfortunately, some of our greatest therapeutic successes involved exacerbations of dysphoric moods and other symptoms, which were directly attributable to the clients' involvement in treatment. In our view, there are various types of individuals who may experience potentially disruptive affective and/or symptomatic reactions to the treatment process:

1. Clients who extensively or exclusively utilize denial processes to cope with relationship problems in their current lives.
2. Clients who undergo a period of trauma revelation.
3. Clients who lack full awareness of their own victimization, either on a contemporary or a historical basis.

4. Clients who are characteristically avoidant in their coping styles, particularly in regard to conflicts with significant others.
5. Clients who have a wide repertoire of fear-based coping strategies, particularly controlling behaviors, which tend to preempt anxious feelings before they can occur.

Clients in the categories listed above may well experience a heightened level of anxiety in the course of treatment with good reason. As we have emphasized repeatedly, emotion is generally a consequence of cognition. When overvigilance decreases, we expect that any associated dysphoric emotions, such as anxiety, will also decrease concomitantly, and the client will experience a sense of relief and increased well-being. On the other hand, a therapeutic assault on the client's denial processes will frequently result in higher levels of dysphoric affect, particularly as the client becomes more aware of previously unacknowledged difficulties in his or her life. Overt panic attacks or phobic reactions may occur, perhaps without immediately apparent connections to ongoing stressors or to the content of treatment. Clients who begin to recognize past or current victimization, and its ramifications, will experience a range of appropriate emotions at different times, including fear, anger, and a powerful sense of loss. Such affective experiences would be profoundly disturbing for anyone, let alone an individual who has learned to be afraid of intense emotions. Clients who have been victims of unacknowledged physical or sexual abuse in childhood may experience intrusive imagery, feelings of panic, and other symptoms suggestive of posttraumatic stress disorder. Such imagery, which can be revolting and/or terrifying, may interrupt sleep, impair concentration on daily activities, or disrupt sexual responsiveness. A client who undergoes a period of trauma revelation during treatment may experience a fear of going to sleep at night, or may find herself unable to participate in sexual relations with her husband.

Therapists have an ethical obligation to forewarn clients regarding potential negative side effects associated with treatment, such as intensification of negative emotions or increased friction with significant others. By educating clients about the vicissitudes of therapy, the therapist normalizes affective and symptom fluctuations, and consequently, enables clients to remain focused on *precipitants* rather than on the actual complaints. Moreover, clients should experience a greater sense of trust and security in the therapeutic relationship if they have been adequately prepared for the more challenging aspects of treatment. Finally, by forewarning clients about symptomatic responses to the treatment process, the therapist sets the stage for reframing periods of turbulence as unique opportunities for learning and growth.

Clients may begin to associate fearful or uncomfortable feelings with the time periods before, during, and after treatment sessions. As a consequence, they may arrive late for their appointments, cancel or miss sessions, or simply avoid mentioning certain threatening topics altogether. Not only may clients dread coming to the office, they may also begin to regard the therapist, either figuratively or literally, as an abusive figure. After all, wasn't it the therapist who opened Pandora's box in the first place? Again, the clinician should inform the client that it would be quite natural to resent the therapist, or want to terminate treatment during a symptomatic period. In the same manner, the therapist should encourage the client to disclose any such reactions should they occur in the future.

The therapist can also insert into ongoing dialogue some direct statements that acknowledge the client's resistance or reservations about treatment, thereby introducing such topics for discussion in a less threatening way. For example, the therapist may say,

"I know that at times, you're pretty sure that you were abused by your grandfather and that some of your relationship problems today seem to relate to that abuse. At other times, though, you start to wonder if maybe I might have brainwashed you to the point where you started believing all these things that are really untrue. Even though part of you wants to go forward and continue working with me, maybe another part wants to get as far away from therapy and your therapist as you can."

Even when the therapist anticipates the likelihood of such affective responses to the treatment process, clients may still be shocked at the intensity of their reactions. As one client put it, "I know you warned me that I might start to feel bad, but I didn't think it would be *this* bad." Reflecting their typical use of denial processes, many clients may have simply dismissed the therapist's warnings at the time. At a later point, they may find themselves sliding downhill for no apparent reason.

When symptomatic reactions to treatment do occur, the therapist should remind the client that such developments are neither unusual nor unexpected. Through an interactive dialogue with the client, the therapist should review carefully the changes in information processing and in belief content that have stimulated the intensification of symptoms and/or dysphoric affect. In this manner, the clinician can begin to relabel an affective or symptomatic reaction as an outgrowth of therapeutic gains *already* achieved by the client.

The therapist should help the client to feel as much control as possible over the discussion of issues that produce high levels of anxiety within the session. Clients need to be told explicitly that they have the right (and the therapist's blessing) to halt any conversation in the session that becomes intolerably uncomfortable for them. Likewise, the therapist should offer frequent reassurances that the client should approach phobic or other anxiety-provoking situations outside of therapy *only* if he or she feels ready to do so, not in response to the perceived expectations of others. It is important to exhort the client to speak up any time he or she experiences pressure from the therapist to say or do anything that arouses excessive anxiety.

The therapist should also insure that other more challenging messages are embedded within the essentially permissive stance taken toward the client's avoidance of anxious feelings and/or anxiety-provoking topics. Although the therapist wants to empathize with and validate the client's discomfort, he or she should scrupulously avoid supporting the client's irrational fears, particularly those that relate to intense affect. Without asking the client to *do* anything differently at that particular time, the therapist needs to find a way to communicate that the experience of anxiety will not lead to insanity, loss of control, or any other anticipated negative consequences. Whereas the therapist may allow the client complete latitude over whether to discuss anxiety-provoking topics, he or she does not need to give any ground on the relevance of the material in question or on the need for its eventual inclusion in treatment. The therapist may say to the client, for example,

"Thanks for letting me know that the discussion was getting to be too much for you. We don't need to talk about this subject any more. I'm sure we'll talk about it more down the road, since you seem to realize that it's very, very important to you. I'm also sure that you'll become more skilled at tolerating anxiety in the future, so that these discussions won't be quite so frightening."

ONGOING AFFIRMATION OF THE CLIENT'S WORTH

As we pointed out in Chapter 3, a belief in one's worthlessness can set up a lifetime of overvigilance for signs of criticism and rejection. Such overvigilance will manifest itself in the therapeutic relationship in a variety of ways. Clients with severe self-esteem difficulties may find it extremely difficult to process new information during treatment sessions because they are continually distracted by questions of blame and feelings of guilt. They may become so overwhelmed by feelings of worthlessness, that they have difficulty sustaining close psychological contact with the therapist, particularly during discussions centering around childhood abuse, sexual experiences, compulsive or acting-out behaviors, and so on. When feeling badly about themselves, these individuals may withdraw, become hostile or defensive, or attempt to provoke rejection by the clinician. Until the therapist restores a sense of collaboration with the client, the issues that had precipitated the sensations of worthlessness cannot be discussed satisfactorily. In such instances, the therapist's best move is to find a way to establish reassuring contact with the client, perhaps by moving away from the topic in question altogether.

It goes without saying that clients who struggle with a sense worthlessness find it extremely hard to tolerate discussions of situations in which their responses may have been questionable in some way. Whether they react defensively or self-punitively, these individuals will often be unable to engage in an open-minded analysis of the situation in question. Consumed by the need to determine whether they have erred or sinned in some way, they may rush to quick, simple judgments about complex situations and interactions. The client who is obsessed with issues of morality or culpability generally has difficulty building skills incrementally by learning from one's experiences. As the client sees it, one either chooses rightly or chooses wrongly. If one chooses wrongly, there is nothing to build upon other than a shaky sense of resolve to act differently in the future. Unfortunately, individuals who become distracted by worthless feelings cannot process detailed information about their responses to difficult situations. As a consequence, they may find it hard to learn much from their past errors. Predictably then, they will keep making the same mistakes over and over again, while remaining stuck in guilt and shame as a consequence.

From the outset of treatment, the clinician should try to determine how each client's difficulties with worthlessness will affect the therapeutic process. As we discussed above, it is useful to forewarn the client regarding potential distortions in the therapeutic relationship. Likewise, right from the beginning of treatment, the therapist should work to affirm the client's worth and to build a foundation for the examination of material that would normally stimulate feelings of worthlessness. We contend that opportunities for the clinician to bolster the client's sense of competence or self-worth occur during each and every session. As the list below and later case examples indicate, the therapist's interventions will involve a mixture of explicit communications and embedded messages. All of the following strategies help to affirm the client's value as a person, while reducing the impact of worthlessness, even during discussions of sensitive material:

> Repeatedly referring to the client's expertise, knowledge, or experience in certain areas while in the process of illustrating an-

other point so that the individual cannot directly disavow the affirming messages.

Allowing the client to teach the therapist something about which he or she may be ignorant.

Asking about an area of the client's competent functioning that sincerely arouses interest or curiosity.

Repeatedly referring to any victories, however small, the client can acknowledge having achieved, at any time in the past, over adversity.

Repeatedly depicting the client's childhood or adolescence as a battle for survival, a struggle against insuperable odds, and so on.

Reviewing current instances of successful coping in a careful, detailed manner with the client and specifically outlining specific cognitive and behavioral changes reflected in the individual's performance.

Repeatedly implying, and demonstrating, that the client is capable of transferring skills from an existing area of competent functioning to master other life difficulties

Highlighting all instances of *incremental skill acquisition* and *gradual change* on the part of the client, in contrast to the individual's all-or-nothing perceptions of self.

When identifying instances of denial or other lapses in judgment, emphasizing contrasts with areas of more effective functioning and asking questions such as "Why would an intelligent (insightful, thoughtful, careful, considerate, etc.) person like you approach a situation like this in such a manner?"

Identifying as a sign of growth or an act of strength the client's willingness to process information that had been denied previously, despite the potential negative repercussions in terms of dysphoric affect and/or increased interpersonal friction.

Whenever appropriate, repeatedly reframing addictive, compulsive, and/or acting out behavior as coping behavior, *usually driven by fear.*

Repeatedly drawing distinctions between *deliberate choices* by the clients and those thoughts and feelings that occur without the individual's conscious control.

Reframing guilty feelings, as opposed to the behaviors that may have stimulated them, as reflective of the individual's *true* motivations or moral values.

Underscoring the client's courage, honesty, commitment to recovery, and so on, particularly when he or she shows a willingness to confront addictions, compulsive behaviors, acting

out, or other potentially shameful areas of functioning in treatment.

Repeatedly highlighting the distinction between productive self-
dissatisfaction, which stimulates attention to new data and acquisition of new skills, and feelings of worthlessness, which only
stimulate repetitive obsessive thinking and dysphoric feelings.

Expressing trust in the client's recovery processes and affirming
confidence in the individual's ability to decide what issues to
confront and when.

Alluding to one's own foibles or irrational experiences but in a way
that does not volunteer overly personal information or otherwise
compromise boundaries with the client.

Confessing ignorance, a lapse in attention or judgment, or an inability to learn new skills readily in a particular area.

After a session or two with a particular client, the therapist should
be able to anticipate with a fair degree of accuracy that topics might be
most threatening to the individual's self-esteem. It may be somewhat
harder to predict how the individual might actually *behave* with the
therapist when he or she is experiencing feelings of worthlessness.
Moreover, it may take even longer for the therapist to learn how to
approach the most sensitive topics with the client without eliciting
defensive reactions. The therapist will often need to formulate *complex*
strategies to facilitate the processing of certain threatening subjects with
particular clients. Such strategies will usually require detailed knowledge of the particular client's typical response tendencies so that the
therapist can attempt to preempt habitual shifts of attention before they
occur. Moreover, such interventions are likely to involve lengthy preliminary groundwork by the clinician, often distributed over a number
of sessions. In Chapters 9 and 11, particularly in the sections on relabeling and confronting acting out, we present some lengthy case examples
that illustrate how the therapist implemented a complex posture that
enabled the client to address extremely threatening material in a productive manner.

STAGES OF CHANGE, CLIENT MOTIVATION, AND THE THERAPIST'S POSTURE

Prochaska and DiClemente (1984) identified four stages in the change
process: precontemplation, contemplation, action, and maintenance.
They discussed at length the problems inherent in working with unmotivated clients, whom they label "precontemplators." These individ-

uals have yet to reach a stage in the change process in which they can focus on their own issues. They typically externalize blame and deny personal problems or any need for change. The active alcoholic is the classic precontemplator. The reader will recall that in Chapter 4, we discussed a number of other diagnostic indicators that we have found to be correlated with poor motivation for treatment, for example, limerance.

When precontemplators present in therapy, they are highly defensive. They typically view themselves as unworthy and incompetent. They often experience family members and friends as critical and controlling. In their interpersonal interactions, they may be fearful that others will attempt to discredit or unmask them. Individuals who have been coerced into therapy by a spouse or by the court will view treatment as a way to pacify others and to take pressure off themselves. In couples or family therapy, the precontemplator may sometimes take the role of a "surrogate therapist," one who is ready and willing to do whatever it takes to help someone else with his or her problems.

To establish a relationship with the precontemplator, the therapist must convey warmth and respect and try not to assume an adversarial posture. The therapist's task is complicated, however, by the precontemplator's heightened state of vigilance for criticism, coercion, and/or scapegoating of any kind. The therapist needs to communicate to the precontemplator that his or her interest lies solely in understanding the presenting problems. By taking a noncontrolling position, the therapist endeavors to lower defensiveness as he or she underscores the message that any personal changes are completely up to the clients themselves. The therapist should also seize opportunities, where appropriate, to reframe the precontemplator's "shameful" behaviors as coping strategies. In couples or family therapy, the precontemplator's spouse will often try to enlist the therapist's support in an effort to change the partner. Should the therapist collude with the spouse, the precontemplator will either retreat further into a defensive posture or simply drop out of treatment. Only when the precontemplator's anxiety has diminished and a measure of safety has been established in the relationship, can the therapist begin orienting the client toward areas of self-dissatisfaction.

The following case illustrates the therapist's approach to working with a couple in which the husband entered treatment fully expecting to be scapegoated as the source of the problem.

Tom and Pat had been married for 16 years when they sought treatment for increasing friction in their relationship. Tom stated that the couple's problems began when his wife refused to support his efforts to confront the defiant behavior of their teenage son. He said he often felt like "the odd man out" in the family, all because he had tried to raise his son, Matthew, in a strict manner. He believed that there was little possibility of change in the family unless his wife stopped being such a "pushover" with Matthew.

According to Pat, Tom was relentlessly critical of Matthew and had never been satisfied with his son's efforts to please him. As a result, she said, there had been no alternative other than to protect her son from her husband's unfair treatment. Prior to their first marital session, the couple had had one consultation with Pat's pastoral counselor, who apparently had confronted Tom and admonished him to "get his act together" or else risk losing his family for good. Not surprisingly, Tom refused to return to his wife's counselor. Tom's defensiveness during the initial interview clearly indicated that he expected the therapist to blame him for the couple's difficulties, just as his wife and her counselor had done previously.

Tom was raised in a poor, immigrant Irish family. Two years older than his sister, Tom had worked from the age of twelve to help support the household. His father was a loner who worked long hours for low wages and drank in solitude at the end of the day. Tom's mother, a housewife, had also worked at a variety of odd jobs for extra money. He described his mother as a critical, rejecting woman who had offered little praise or affection. Tom recalled that his parents always seemed too tired or too busy to spend time with their children. Only a poor grade, a messy room, or an argument between the children seemed to draw their attention. In summing up his childhood, Tom reported with a mixed sense of pride and bitterness that he "always did what was expected" and that he "had worked for everything" he got.

Tom joined the service after high school and pursued a military career. At age 21, he had married Pat, his high school sweetheart. While dating, and prior to the birth of their son, Tom felt cared for and supported by Pat. By his account, she was a solicitous and admiring partner. However, following Matthew's birth, Tom felt as though he had become less of a priority for his wife. Tom's sense of alienation from his wife only intensified after the birth of their daughter. Since Tom found it hard to articulate his painful feelings directly, his growing sense of rejection seemed to have been expressed through the ongoing conflicts over parenting. When Matthew reached his teens, his behavior became more demanding and rebellious. Now the teenager was constantly being triangulated into the marital relationship. He became the focus of many heated arguments, each invariably ending with Pat positioning herself squarely against Tom in support of her son.

As mentioned, Tom clearly expected to be chastised and scapegoated by the therapist. It was apparent that he also felt ashamed about his failing relationships. Moreover, the therapist sensed that despite Tom's rigidity and apparent narcissism, the man had a sincere desire to be a good parent to his children. The client's encounter with his wife's counselor had not only struck a blow to his already fragile self-image, but it had also fueled his perceptions of others as uncaring and untrustworthy. Having received little nurturance and much criticism from his parents, Tom had long ago learned to protect himself from the experience of worthlessness by externalizing blame. From the outset of marital therapy, Tom made it clear he did not intend to be an easy target. His agenda was to insure that treatment would be focused on his son's defiant and provocative behavior and on his wife's unwillingness to confront the problem appropriately, *period.*

To engage Tom, it was first necessary for the therapist to make it clear that he had no interest in assigning blame for problems or in attempting to change anyone. Rather, the therapist stated explicitly to the couple that the aim of treatment was to try to understand the problem from each of their perspectives and to help *them* decide what to do about it. The therapist took pains to validate each spouse's feelings and concerns, all the while assiduously avoiding even the appearance of an alliance with Pat.

The therapist also drew on Tom's family of origin experiences in an effort to forge an alliance. For example, the therapist commented on how difficult it must have been for him to have had to work from an early age, especially since his after-school jobs prevented him from participating in sports and other activities with his peers. The therapist pointed out how, in contrast, Tom had been able to provide *his own son* with many more opportunities "to be a kid" than he ever had. The therapist noted that Tom's childhood experiences had taught him the meaning of responsibility and the value of hard work. The therapist also acknowledged that the client's values had helped him to achieve within the military and to provide well for his family. However, the therapist also suggested that because of Tom's own learning experiences, he might be understandably frustrated, *even resentful,* to see his children having access to privileges when they had not followed through on *their* responsibilities. After all, said the therapist, Tom had worked extremely hard for all he had obtained while growing up.

Tom responded to the therapist's supportive comments with an increased level of openness and self-examination. He acknowledged that perhaps because of his own upbringing he had been too harsh with his son. In response, the therapist wondered aloud whether Tom might well have been afraid that his son might end up paying a price as an adult if he did not learn the value of hard work and responsibility now.

The therapist further speculated that Tom's habitual scrutiny of Matthew's adherence to rules and responsibilities might well have been fear-driven in that this was the client's way of helping his son to *avoid failure.* Tom said that although such an explanation for his behavior had never occurred to him, he thought it might well have merit.

The therapist's reframing of Tom's behavior as fear-driven, coupled with Tom's increased openness to examining his own contribution to the marital problems, enabled Pat to take a far more supportive stance with her husband. The therapist would eventually be able to draw on Pat's family history as a parentified child to explain her own compulsive tendency to protect her son. The reframing of each partner's responses as learned coping behavior allowed Pat and Tom to make far more positive attributions of each other's actions. As a consequence, they eventually were able to work together in a non-blaming fashion to confront their son's difficulties.

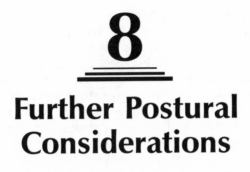

Further Postural Considerations

MAINTAINING APPROPRIATE BOUNDARIES

The therapist is responsible for creating and maintaining clear boundaries in his or her relationship with the client. Certain individuals, particularly those who have been victimized by incest or other forms of sexual abuse, necessitate more careful monitoring of the therapist–client boundary, on an ongoing basis. The therapeutic relationship can provide such clients with a vehicle for learning how to sustain closeness without incurring exploitation, manipulation, loss of selfhood, or other negative consequences in the process. It is vital for the therapist to assume a role that insures that the client will experience a maximal amount of privacy, autonomy, and safety while, at the same time he or she still feels accepted and supported.

The therapist's communications about boundaries should occur on multiple levels, resonating through many types of exchanges with the client. As will be discussed in the following sections, some of the therapist's messages about boundaries will be explicit, whereas others will be embedded in the treatment context.

Nonverbal Communication

Other than offering a supportive handshake to begin or end a session, therapists really have no business initiating physical contact with their clients. We question the motives and/or competence of therapists who insist on using "hands on" techniques of any kind, regardless of the treatment ideologies they might espouse. A moment's reflection should reveal to the reader that there is ultimately nothing that a therapist cannot communicate effectively in a way that avoids touching the client. Why impose such a high-risk therapeutic technique on the client when the possibilities for confusion and misinterpretation are so great?

Indeed, we hope that through the therapeutic process our clients will learn that having feelings and acting them out need not be synonymous. Clinicians too can learn to separate affect and behavior more effectively. The therapist who feels a powerful impulse to nurture the client by initiating physical contact should view such a response not as a call to action, but rather, as a prompt to step back and scan the entire treatment context. The therapist needs to answer the question, "Why am I experiencing these feelings so powerfully *now*, with this particular client?"

At a moment when the therapist might experience a desire to nurture the client in a physical manner, he or she could always choose to make a statement such as the following: "I want you to know how strongly I feel your pain right now. Because of the boundaries of my professional role, it's not appropriate for me to touch my clients. But right now, I am visualizing my hand on your shoulder, supporting you. I hope you can feel that too, and that you can draw some strength from that hand." Here the therapist performs several operations: (1) defining the boundaries of the therapeutic relationship in a supportive context, free of rejecting or punitive undertones; (2) moving powerfully in a caring posture toward the client but in a way that does not contain the intrusive or victimizing elements associated with previous relationships; (3) modeling good communication skills, while underscoring the notion that acknowledging feelings need not involve acting them out; (4) embedding the messages "I care about you," "I'll be there for you," "I believe in you," "I am hopeful about your future," and so on, in a manner that discourages direct refutation by the client.

In addition to avoiding physical contact, therapists frequently need to modulate other nonverbal behaviors, which may be perfectly appropriate under normal circumstances, in order to create safe boundaries for certain clients. For example, therapists who habitually move their chairs forward to express support or to emphasize a point may find that they have inadvertently strayed too far into the "psychological comfort zones" of some clients. Consequently, they may need to use space in the office differently with such individuals. Certain clients may equate increased vocal levels and intensification of affect on the part of the therapist with the anger of an abusive or rejecting parent. Therapists who speak loudly, or use profanity routinely may need to curtail such habits while working with such individuals.

Therapist Self-Disclosure: Some Guidelines

It should be clear to the reader from our case vignettes and our discussion of the therapeutic relationship that we seek to convey a sense of genuineness to our clients. Genuineness does have its limits, however. Therapist self-disclosure with clients who have a documented history of boundary violations should occur only with great deliberation and caution. Such clients may express great curiosity about the therapist's background and current life circumstances, but the interest may stem in part from a history of relationships in which the privacy of the individual was routinely disregarded. Clients who have a tendency to become obsessed with the inner workings of others will be prone to focus on the therapist's material in unproductive ways, often allowing themselves to be diverted from contemplating their own issues. In guarding his or her privacy, the therapist models a vital relationship skill for the client with boundary issues—how to sustain closeness without loss of psychological integrity.

Therapists often disclose personal information to clients in an attempt to normalize various thoughts, feelings, and behaviors. Although there is nothing wrong with showing one's human side to one's clients, we often find that such self-disclosure fails to achieve its intended purpose, that is, helping the client to feel more comfortable about his or her reactions in a particular situation. In our experience, clients often identify with and perceive themselves as similar to the therapist in a variety of significant ways, *but only to a certain degree*. As in their other relationships, clients will perceive many significant differences between themselves and their therapists. For the client, the bottom line may be: "The therapist may think we're alike, but I'm really different from him, and negatively so." Consequently, such perceived differences may ultimately prevent the individual from making beneficial use of the therapist's self-disclosure. In a "worst case scenario," the client may begin to think that the therapist shares some of his or her shameful attributes or difficulties. As a consequence, the client may experience a loss of confidence in the therapist, assuming that if the clinician is also plagued by some of the same problems, treatment will inevitably fail.

There are other ways to utilize the content of the therapist's life experiences in a constructive manner with the client without incurring the potential risks associated with self-disclosure. The therapist may describe his or her own experiences quite accurately—but as if they had happened to someone else. The therapist can also relate anecdotes about others encountered in the course of his or her own lifetime, including friends, family members, and of course, other clients. Although the therapist is speaking from his or her personal direct experience with the individual who is the subject of the anecdote, it is not necessary to disclose threatening personal information in order to share the relevant information with the client. Further, the therapist is free to "customize" the identity of the protagonist, so that it is easier to highlight similarities to the client and to obscure differences that are irrelevant to the discussion.

The following case vignette illustrates how the therapist used self-disclosure in a powerful manner, with a client who had experienced severe boundary violations in childhood. Ironically, however, although it involves a successful intervention, the case also underscores quite forcefully the complex risks associated with self-disclosure by the therapist.

After more than a year of treatment, Buffy told her therapist about an event that had occurred to her when she was 12 or 13 years old. She had been sent by her mother to stay for the summer with an aunt in rural Montana. The youngest of her cousins, a big, powerful young man of 19 or 20, was also living in the aunt's home at the time. Immediately upon Buffy's arrival, he began making sexual advances toward her, in an extremely aggressive, frightening manner, stopping just short of physical coercion. He seemed to follow her everywhere and was particularly fond of cornering her when she walked alone in the woods.

Buffy's parents had minimized or ignored her previous complaints of sexually inappropriate behaviors on the part of various relatives and friends of the family. When the cousin's attacks began, Buffy assumed from her past experiences that neither her aunt nor her parents would take her current complaints seriously. She concluded, and probably rightly so, that no adult was going to protect her. She knew she was stuck at the aunt's house for rest of the summer and that she would have to do something to protect herself from the cousin. Finally, Buffy found an ingenious solution, one which involved prolonged discomfort and considerable physical disfigurement. She found some poison ivy and rubbed her entire body with it, particularly the areas which might most interest the cousin. The consequence, as she put it, was that "I was gross for the rest of the summer." Despite the disfigurement and the physical discomfort Buffy experienced as a result of the poison ivy, she did achieve her objective. The cousin left her alone for the rest of her visit. Moreover, because of the severity of her condition, Buffy was able to return home earlier than had been originally planned.

The therapist was powerfully affected by the image of a vulnerable youngster being driven to take such drastic measures to protect herself from harm. He wanted to share his reactions to the story with the client immediately but stopped short when he saw how uncomfortable she looked after the disclosure. When the therapist asked her what aspect of the story seemed to be upsetting her, Buffy replied that it was the fact that she had deliberately disfigured herself with the poison ivy. Revealing her familiarity with the disparaging terms used in the mental health world, Buffy said, "It was such a borderline thing to do." Not surprisingly, she was concerned that the therapist would view the behavior—and her—in the same light.

The therapist replied that although he had been deeply moved by Buffy's story, he had not been thinking about her actions in the context of personality disorders or any other diagnostic considerations. In fact, he saw her infecting herself with poison ivy as a courageous act in the face of desperate circumstances. He then decided to share his associations to the vignette of the poison ivy. He told the client that her anecdote had reminded him of the story of his grandmother, a survivor of the 1915 Armenian genocide. He explained how his grandmother and her sister were the only ones—among literally scores of family members—to live through the forced deportation marches across the parched deserts of Asia Minor. Since the men had generally been killed first or conscripted into the Turkish army, where they were marked for certain death, the deportees were primarily women, children, and the elderly, all unarmed. Most were sick and starving. At night, the women were considered fair game for the soldiers who guarded the convoys. In order to discourage sexual attacks from the soldiers and the criminal elements who also preyed on the deportees, the therapist's grandmother and her sister would cover themselves each night with ashes, dirt, and even dung. At times they would bury themselves in the dirt from the neck down. The women also cropped their hair to appear less inviting. Another sister, who could not bear to part with her beautiful tresses, had been carried off and was never heard from again. Through these strategies of self-disfigurement, the therapist's grandmother and her sister were able to avoid attack. Somehow they survived the physical and psychological trauma of the massacres and the torturous march across the desert into Syria. The therapist emphasized that he viewed Buffy's actions in the same heroic light as his grandmother's. As he put it, he believed that desperate circumstances often demanded desperate measures. If his grandmother had not used such desperate measures, she might not have survived. Perhaps the same could be said for Buffy as well, he told her.

Buffy thanked the therapist for having shared the story with her. She said, "I guess you're right. It *was* a survival strategy." Although the client seemed to view her own actions in a different light as a result of having heard the therapist's feedback, he was not sure that the intervention had been appropriate. After the session, he had pretty much chalked up the exchange with Buffy as another instance of "self-indulgent therapist self-disclosure." He decided to process the client's reactions to the discussion carefully during their following meetings. Nonetheless, in succeeding sessions, Buffy emphasized that the therapist's story had been vital in changing her perspective on both the poison ivy incident and other instances in which she had used similar means to escape sexual abuse. She now had begun to see herself more clearly as the *victim* in these episodes. Having been trapped in desperate and dangerous situations, without the benefit of adult protection, having to rely only on her wits to defend herself, she, like the therapist's grandmother, had been forced to utilize extreme measures. Buffy now began to see the measures she took as reflecting courage, creativity, determination, and heroism, not psychopathology. Again, she thanked the therapist for having shared such a powerful personal story with her. Even as she was terminating more than a year later, Buffy still referred to the therapist's disclosure as one of the most profound learning experiences she had encountered in the course of treatment.

In retrospect, the therapist's discomfort after the self-disclosure to the client was legitimate and noteworthy on a number of counts. First, although the vignette disclosed was appropriate to the content of treatment at the time, it clearly involved extremely personal material for the therapist, whose family had suffered enormous trauma as a result of the genocide. The therapist believed that the impact of the genocide upon his family of origin played a direct and significant role in many aspects of his own life script, including his choice of vocation. Any discussion of the *personal* ramifications of the grandmother's tale for the therapist was clearly out of bounds with Buffy, who, as a survivor of childhood sexual abuse, needed strong, clear boundaries in treatment. The therapist had consistently and explicitly respected Buffy's privacy, generally allowing her to determine the pace and content of her treatment sessions. He seldom allowed his feedback to the client to stray into areas that were uncomfortable for her, unless he had her explicit permission to do so. Moreover, he had spent considerable time encouraging her to recognize and prevent various boundary violations in her current personal and professional life. Now that she was disclosing such personal information, it was even more important not to blur the boundaries between client and clinician.

Second, the therapist wanted to keep Buffy fully immersed in her own issues, particularly those involving childhood sexual trauma. He did not want to divert her into his material, which was a strong possibility given her tendency to become immersed in things outside herself as a means of dealing with personal discomfort. She was the type of person who might distract herself by reading every book she could find on a subject that involved her personally, rather than spend time pondering her *own* experiences and the consequences thereof. She could easily lose herself in speculating about the therapist and his family dynamics, or in learning more about the tragic history of the Armenians, instead of taking care of her own business.

Third, the therapist knew he was entering an affectively unpredictable area for himself whenever he touched on the events of 1915. His emotional reactions to the subject ranged from sorrow and helplessness, to horror and absolute rage, especially when he was exposed to recurring evidence of historical revisionism by the current Turkish government regarding the genocide. He rarely even raised the topic with anyone other than members of his family and his closest friends, and typically, he felt very vulnerable and uncomfortable when he did. The one time a client had introduced the topic of the genocide, the effect on the therapist had been decidedly negative. A few years previously, a highly educated older male client, with strong business ties to Turkey, had remarked to the therapist, "I don't understand why these Armenians are still so upset. Why can't they forget about all that? It's a different Turkish government now. Besides a lot of Turks died in the war too." At that moment the therapist felt like a pressure cooker about to explode. Later, in a much calmer moment, the therapist was able to realize that rather than being directed against him personally, the client's ignorant remarks only reflected the man's lack of empathy and lifelong inability to sustain constructive relationships. Carefully controlling his anger, the therapist quickly changed subjects with the client and struggled through the remainder of the interview in an unpleasantly altered state of consciousness, looking forward to the moment when he could usher the client out of his office. Although this admittedly represented an extreme scenario, the experience with this particularly insensitive client made the therapist quite reasonably apprehensive about discussing the genocide in a treatment setting.

Fourth, the therapist's desire to share something of such a personal nature reflected the intensity of his response to the anecdote Buffy had shared. Perhaps because he had felt so protective of the little girl in the story, the therapist found it hard to tolerate Buffy's subsequent negative attitude toward herself. Consequently, he may have felt compelled to intervene in a powerful way. We suspect that overprotective urges in therapists often set the stage for impulsive or highly dramatic moves in treatment sessions, many of which turn out to be ineffectual or even destructive. By alluding to his own personal and family material, the therapist may have missed opportunities to address both the content and overpowering emotional impact of his client's tale in other ways.

For example, he could have responded to Buffy's humiliation and self-blame over the poison ivy incident by using Socratic dialogue to help her review the dangerous circumstances that had necessitated her behavior in the first place. Such a patient, disciplined strategy would have been much more consistent with the therapist's approach to Buffy up to that point in treatment.

Fifth, since self-disclosure is a potentially high-risk behavior by the therapist, it should be accompanied by some reasonable soul-searching afterwards. The clinician should attempt to answer the following questions following an episode of self-disclosure:

What were the therapist's cognitions and emotional responses prior to and during the self-disclosure?

Were there signs that the therapist might have acted impulsively, perhaps because of his or her *own* discomfort?

Who was more affectively involved in the exchange, the therapist or the client?

How did the therapist's posture change during and after the self-disclosure? Were such changes consistent with the overall treatment plan?

What is it about the particular individual that stimulates self-disclosure by the clinician, either in terms of the client's issues, the therapist's issues, or, as is most likely, a combination of the two?

Were there reasons, particularly in the therapist's nonprofessional life, why he or she would be thinking of the personal material in question at this particular time? On balance, was the therapist dealing with his or her own material or with the client's?

Did the client truly benefit from the information, or did he or she discount it somehow because it involved the therapist?

Was the level of self-disclosure appropriate with the particular client, particularly in light of any boundary problems he or she might have in relationships?

How will the therapist feel and respond if the client wants to discuss the topic again?

What other interventions might the therapist have attempted instead of the self-disclosure, either directed at the same point or addressing related areas of content?

Could the therapist's material have been used more effectively if it had been reworked into an anecdote about a third party?

In our opinion, therapists who regularly ask themselves such questions after instances of self-disclosure, or address such issues in their consultations with supervisors, will probably remain fairly judicious in the degree of personal material they choose to share with clients. Those clinicians who are not willing to subject themselves to such rigorous questioning, for any reason, will put their clients at risk if they make a habit of regularly using self-disclosure as a treatment strategy.

Fees, Scheduling, and Other Business Arrangements

Fees are part of the organizational structure supporting the professional status of the therapeutic relationship. Business arrangements help the client to differentiate between the unique role of the therapist and those played by friends, lovers, parents, and so on. Unfortunately, many therapists have their own issues about money, particularly when they first enter private practice settings, where clients pay them directly for services. The reader should remember that fee arrangements should not be a vehicle for addressing the therapist's discomfort over the value of the psychotherapeutic services being rendered. If the therapist has re-servations about the quality of the therapy, reducing the cost of treat-ment is not the solution. Poorly focused treatment (or treatment with a poorly motivated client) will not be cost effective at any price. On the other hand, effective psychotherapy produces such wide-ranging im-provements in the quality of life that its actual value will far exceed the monetary cost of the treatment the individual received.

The authors have a strong philosophical commitment to the use of sliding scales and other alternatives to rigid fee structures in psycho-therapy. There is something inherently distasteful about suggesting that a client take out a second mortgage on his or her home in order to pay for treatment, as some therapists have been known to do. However, fee reductions should occur for the right reasons, for example, legitimate need on the part of the individual or family, not because either the client's or the therapist's issues have led the latter to assume an over-protective posture. Moreover, therapists also need to be careful not to victimize themselves or their families by selling their professional ser-vices too cheaply. All too often therapists have offered reduced fees to some clients who, as was later learned, were all too willing to make substantial expenditures for various goods and services of a frivolous nature.

Shoddy business practices and/or poor limit-setting on the part of the therapist can begin to replicate conditions associated with sexual abuse or other forms of victimization. First of all, the therapist's role as a powerful benefactor, even though it occurs within a benign frame-work, defines the client as helpless and inadequate, in short, as a victim. In cases of clear-cut need, the therapist who wishes to lower the fee must find a way to do so that preserves the client's dignity and status as a consumer of services. Totally free services may tend to reduce the client to the status of a supplicant without the ability to question and challenge the therapist in the same way as when money for services had changed hands. Once again because of a shameful circumstance (in this case, lack of money), the client may feel forced to occupy a one-down position in a significant relationship.

Some incest victims receive special privileges or favored treatment in the family as a "reward" for being victimized. The therapist wants to avoid putting the client in a similar position, through neglecting fee arrangements or by failing to confront departures from treatment norms, such as chronic lateness or repeated missed appointments. Likewise, the therapist wishes to avoid colluding with the client to mislead insurance companies in any way, however innocuous. Aside from the obvious legal and ethical reasons for avoiding such actions, the therapist also needs to avoid any billing arrangements that lead to sharing a "guilty secret" with the client. On the other hand, with the ascendance of managed care, all clients, particularly those who have experienced boundary violations in the past, need to be informed about the flow of information between the therapist and the health insurance system and the consequences that might result from such disclosures.

Sensitive Information

The therapist helps to maintain a climate of safety in the treatment hour by encouraging the client to take control over the timing and manner of disclosure of sensitive material. In fact, the therapist at times may even mildly restrain the client from revealing something uncomfortable, saying, "I'm sure you'll find a more comfortable way to talk to me about this," or "You'll tell me about these things when the time is more appropriate for you." Such an intervention does not aim to elicit a so-called "paradoxical" effect. Instead, the therapist wishes to communicate to the client that this is a relationship in which his or her privacy will be respected. Embedded in the therapist's communication is the expectation that currently withheld information will eventually surface in treatment. However, the therapist asks the client to ignore the implicit demands of the treatment situation for now in favor of respecting his or her own legitimate feelings of discomfort. What better way to communicate the necessity of feeling safe and the importance of valuing oneself!

The client needs to know that the therapist's interest in graphic details of childhood sexual abuse or other sexual experiences is clinical, not voyeuristic. At times clients may volunteer information about their sexual encounters a bit too readily, so that the therapist begins to feel discomfort, embarrassment, or the beginnings of "prurient interest." The therapist's discomfort at such moments, which may be quite appropriate, could in fact reflect the client's inability to maintain appropriate boundaries. The client may be enacting issues of worthlessness in the therapeutic relationship by attempting to shock, titillate, and/or court rejection from the clinician.

The therapist should attempt to address sexual abuse or other sensitive topics within the format which the client finds most comfortable. Although a number of clients do experience relief from sharing their painful experiences in considerable detail, the therapist may only need a limited amount of information in order to begin developing hypotheses about the client's issues. Moreover, some clients may be much more comfortable sharing a lengthy narrative with a Twelve-Step sponsor, a member of the clergy, or someone else in a nontherapeutic context. Other clients may also be willing to write about their experiences for the therapist, as long as they do not have to discuss the particulars in great depth.

Katie, a 30-year-old mother of three, had entered treatment during the latter stages of a very bitter and costly divorce. Various elements in her history had suggested to the therapist that she may have been a victim of childhood sexual abuse, for example, sexual assaults in her marriage, chronic self-mutilative wishes, and a family of origin environment marked by physical abuse and neglect. Also consistent with the presence of traumatic material, was the way in which Katie needed to control the content and direction of her treatment sessions. She always came to therapy with an agenda, which in most instances would be a positive prognostic sign. However, Katie seldom allowed the therapist to discuss a potentially uncomfortable topic for two sessions in a row. She invariably seemed to find a more pressing matter that simply had to be discussed. The therapist was not entirely satisfied with the lack of continuity in treatment but found it difficult to enable Katie to address the anxiety that triggered much of her controlling behavior. In the meantime, the material she offered did continue to be clinically relevant.

Although she had spent nearly 2 years in treatment, Katie maintained considerable distance from the therapist, as evidenced by her attempts to control their discussions and by her habit of maintaining long intervals between appointments. Katie's level of distress had dropped considerably in the course of treatment, and she seemed to have difficulty coming up with meaningful agenda items for her sessions. When the therapist shared his observations with her, Katie acknowledged that she had been considering ending treatment soon. She and the therapist decided on a termination process that involved four final appointments, scheduled at 3-month intervals.

To the therapist's surprise, midway through the termination process, Katie started to open up in a much more powerful way. She now described her avoidance of men, which she had previously depicted as a simple matter of personal preference, as a phobic response, based on feelings of sheer terror. Sensing the change in her self-presentation, the therapist enthusiastically agreed with Katie's request to postpone termination in order to work on her fear of intimacy. Unlike her earlier approach to treatment, the client now wanted to schedule frequent, regular appointments.

Like some other clients who find it difficult to acknowledge childhood sexual abuse, Katie began to introduce the topic by spontaneously sharing dream material with the therapist. During several sessions, she referred to one particularly upsetting dream but clearly indicated that she was too uncomfortable to discuss it. She also alluded to an entry in her journal that had been stimulated by the dream, but did not bring it with her to the session. Katie began as well to recall and disclose new details of her childhood history, which led the therapist to conclude that there were several potential perpetrators of sexual abuse in the client's extended family.

Katie was also now able to acknowledge and discuss her need to control the content of her sessions. Although she recognized that she was afraid to let the therapist take command of the treatment process, she was not able to identify the reasons for her style of interaction. The therapist was concerned that, acting out of a sense of embarrassment, Katie might invest more energy in suppressing her controlling behavior than in investigating the sources of it. Consequently, the therapist urged her not to try to "control her control" but, rather, to watch it happen and learn from it. Her response to this suggestion by the therapist could only be described as a laugh of recognition.

The therapist was in no hurry to hear about the trauma-related dream and/or related content. Instead, he wanted to facilitate a new style of processing material in the session, one which enabled Katie to relax her need to control the interaction in a rigid manner. The therapist now assumed that Katie's need to orchestrate the sessions, and the underlying anxiety which had stimulated such efforts on her part, were directly connected to traumatic incidents in childhood. Consequently, it seemed desirable to deepen the treatment relationship before any extensive disclosures took place. Until this change was accomplished, the therapist suspected that the client would thwart his efforts to explore any trauma-related material in greater detail beyond what she offered herself. Moreover, Katie seemed like the type of individual who might proclaim that a serious issue was resolved after only a cursory examination. The therapist wanted to have the opportunity to offer extensive feedback on any traumatic material, ideally over a period of many sessions. Unless the client was comfortable, she would want to move him off the subject quickly, just as she had done with other topics in the past. Further, in view of the boundary violations involved in sexual abuse, it made sense to allow Katie to explore the traumatic material on her own schedule. The therapist did not wish to replicate any features of the original trauma by violating Katie's carefully guarded privacy. It was important that she not feel pressured, manipulated, or cajoled into disclosing secrets.

The therapist acknowledged Katie's reluctance to share the dream and the journal entry on several occasions over the two sessions following her mention of the material. During each brief comment, the therapist emphasized his wish that the client only discuss the traumatic issues with him when she felt absolutely safe to do so. Reaffirming his desire to avoid even the *appearance* of hurrying her along, the clinician asked Katie to tell him if it ever seemed as if he were pressuring her. He also expressed the opinion that she was obviously involved in a period of psychological growth and offered several pieces of data to support his point of view. The therapist told Katie that, in his experience, clients caught up in such a growth cycle tend to continue inexorable forward movement, even if they experience setbacks, fearfulness, and resistance in the process. He reiterated his confidence in the client's recovery process and his belief that she would do things *in the right sequence for herself*.

After the second time the therapist ran through the points detailed above, Katie said in a firm tone of voice, "I don't know if I like that." When asked to explain, she stated that maybe on some level, she *did* want to be pushed. The therapist remembered that, earlier in the interview, the client had described having been frustrated with her difficulties in recalling and disclosing information. She told him that she had thought before the session, "How can he be so nice to me? Why can't he just slap me across the face and tell me to shape up?" From his notes, the therapist read Katie the direct quotes of her earlier statements, wondering aloud whether there was a parallel between being treated in such an abusive manner and being pressured to disclose material prematurely. The therapist asked Katie if she was really saying that she believed that she deserved to be punished. The therapist's remarks struck a responsive chord with Katie, as evidenced by another laugh of recognition, this time accompanied by the exclamation, "That feels right!" The therapist's last comment on the matter was that he did not want to become yet another man who abused her and violated her boundaries. "You've had too much of that. You don't need any more disrespect," he said, as he held eye contact with her. There was no laugh this time from Katie, only a sigh, and the comment, "I never looked at it that way."

THERAPIST FLEXIBILITY

Since many of our clients think in black or white, all-or-nothing terms about a wide range of significant issues, it is not surprising that they come across as rigid at times. Often the therapist's goal with such clients is to stimulate more flexible patterns of thinking and behavior. It is important for the therapist also to avoid becoming locked into rigid modes of thinking and behaving. Through his or her approach to treatment, the therapist should seek to *model* flexibility in addition to attempt to stimulate it within the client.

Often therapists worry needlessly about having made errors with clients, believing somehow that their mistakes have irrevocably altered the future course of treatment. We therapists do not need to remain locked into prior mistakes in judgment forever after. As long as the client continues on in treatment, the therapist always has the opportunity to reverse a prior position or interpretation, change direction or emphasis, confront an attempt to deceive or manipulate, renegotiate the therapeutic contract, or simply apologize for past errors. Such moves demonstrate forcefully to the client that the therapist is willing to look carefully at new data about the individual and the treatment process and, where appropriate, to revise his or her perspective accordingly.

The client will not necessarily lose faith in the therapist who acknowledges an error or changes direction in treatment. Clients want competent, honest therapists, not omniscient ones. How threatening it must be to have to interact with someone with no discernible faults or foibles, someone who always turns in a peak performance, someone who never loses focus or objectivity, someone who remains unswervingly rational and efficient! The therapist's job is to mirror reality, not to create the illusion of perfection. Moreover, a therapist who embodies perfection might make the client can feel even more worthless and inadequate by comparison. We believe that, in the long run, the therapist who is secure enough to acknowledge mistakes or misperceptions will earn *greater* levels of trust and respect from his or her clients. In our view, such acknowledgments only serve to build the therapist's credibility with the client because they reflect humility, candor, and self-awareness on the part of the clinician.

The therapist may introduce a change in therapeutic direction with a statement such as "I was reviewing our last session," "I've been thinking about some of the things we've been working on," "I kept hearing your words from last time," "I found myself feeling uneasy about something I said during our last meeting," and so on. Although some clients might begin to brace themselves to receive bad news on hearing the therapist make such statements, many will feel curious and perhaps somewhat flattered as well. Wouldn't most of us want to see a therapist who does homework between sessions? The client will experience less anxiety about changing some aspect of treatment if he or she truly understands the therapist's rationale. The therapist should walk the client through the pertinent data and the inferences drawn from them, making sure that the client follows the chain of reasoning every step of the way. If the clinician is apologizing or acknowledging errors, then it is important to block the client from using denial strategies to exonerate the therapist or otherwise minimize the importance of the topic under discussion.

The following case illustrates typical circumstances under which the therapist had to reverse or "undo" previous treatment efforts. During a previous session, the therapist behaved in a way that was unnecessarily upsetting to his client. By processing the incident extensively with the client during succeeding sessions, the therapist was able to repair the breach in the therapeutic relationship and to address in an immediate, powerful manner, a number of issues that were central to the individual's distress. The client's reaction to the therapist's apology, which mirrored her responses in other relationships, was to serve in turn as a powerful learning vehicle during subsequent sessions.

After 2½ years in treatment, Lena had made exciting progress on a number of fronts. In addition to her individual sessions, which she attended twice monthly, she had participated in two time-limited groups, one for Adult Children of Alcoholics, the other for battered women. She had a good grasp on the ways in which her childhood in a physically and sexually abusive family had set her up to remain a victim in her adult life. Lena had overcome powerful feelings of worthlessness, particularly in connection with her functioning as a spouse and as a parent. She had begun to repair estranged relationships with two of her children. She successfully resisted exploitative treatment at work, which she had previously tolerated because of a sense of fearfulness and unworthiness. Most importantly, Lena had reached the point where she could now confront her husband, Mario, regarding the episodes of physical abuse and intimidation that had taken place in the marriage over the years.

Originally, Lena had been highly resistant to participating in couples treatment with Mario, out of a fear that the marital therapist would blame all the relationship problems on her. Through her work in individual treatment, she eventually overcame her irrational fear of being blamed and, as a result, demanded that Mario accompany her to couples sessions with another therapist. She more than held her own in the marital treatment, to the point where Mario actually began to acknowledge some of his own personal issues. She reported that for the first time in years, she no longer felt unsafe with her husband, even when he seemed angry or irritated. Lena's impressive self-transformation did not happen by magic—it was the result of hard work on a number of fronts. The therapist had generally taken a very supportive role with Lena, remaining low-key and nonconfrontational, while avoiding behavioral prescriptions of any kind, particularly when discussing the husband. All the significant changes Lena made had been entirely of her own invention.

Sometimes therapists refuse to be satisfied with success. One day, the therapist kept Lena waiting for an appointment while he was handling a crisis call from the father of an alcoholic adolescent. Quite appropriately, the therapist exhorted the father in loud, forceful tones to take command of the son's situation. The father subsequently behaved as the therapist had requested, thereby facilitating the son's recovery. Unfortunately, the therapist carried the same attitude and the same tone into the session with Lena. Such an approach had never been necessary or appropriate with her in the past. The therapist began in a rushed manner, neglecting to review notes of previous sessions or otherwise take his bearings with the client.

Early in the session, Lena described friction with her husband that had taken place over some duties she had performed in his business. The therapist persisted in questioning why Lena continued to serve as her husband's part-time employee, despite a history of conflicts over the job, implying that he thought she was setting herself up for mistreatment. Rejecting her assertion that she continued in the job because the money was good, the therapist continued to challenge the client to identify the motives behind her behavior. As the therapist persisted in his mode of questioning, Lena looked more and more distressed, although she continued to respond to his questions and comments. Finally, the therapist realized his error when the client said, "I feel backed into a corner." The therapist immediately apologized for perseverating on the topic and thanked her for giving him such clear feedback. Lena and the therapist switched to other subjects for the remainder of the session. She gave no outward indication that the earlier discussion had produced any enduring negative effects.

After the session, the therapist felt a sense of sadness over the interaction with Lena that persisted somewhat into the following day. The therapist realized that he had pushed his client much too hard and had hurt her feelings without a valid clinical justification. The therapist had been "on a roll" from his previous phone call when the session started and was too grandiose and full of himself to listen to the client effectively. In retrospect, the whole interaction appeared to the therapist to be a replication of other abusive experiences Lena had endured.

The therapist discussed the entire episode with Lena during the next session and the one that followed as well. He reiterated his regrets over the incident and encouraged the client to describe her reactions to it. Lena acknowledged that she had felt attacked and cornered by the therapist. She readily agreed when the therapist drew parallels between the incident and other instances in which she had been bullied by others, particularly her husband. However, Lena was quick to offer up explanations for the therapist's actions. "I know you were on the phone dealing with another case before my session. *That* must have affected you," she said. Without addressing the accuracy of her perceptions, the therapist pointed out that Lena was *excusing* his actions, much as she once had excused her husband's abusive behaviors in the past. "I don't want you to take me off the hook or take care of me," he told her. "Regardless of *why* I behaved that way, I still hurt you unnecessarily," he reminded her. With the therapist's prompting, Lena was able to recognize a very familiar pattern. Once she excused the behavior of the other person, then she would soon begin to tell herself that she had no right to be upset. Then if she continued to have negative reactions to the incident or the individual, Lena would typically accuse herself of being self-pitying or mean-spirited, thereby triggering off strong feelings of worthlessness.

The therapist told Lena that the incident might produce a breach in the relationship that would not heal immediately. He reminded her of how Mario's abusive behavior had frequently stimulated lingering feelings of mistrust on her part in the past. The therapist urged the client to monitor her reactions and share them with him. Indeed, Lena reported that she did not want to come for the next session. She acknowledged that at times she had still experienced angry thoughts about the incident, even to the point of contemplating termination because of it. The therapist consistently labeled these reactions as appropriate given the kind of intense pressure she had experienced during the episode in question. These discussions gave the therapist a direct opportunity to work with Lena's responses to victimization while he restrained her from drifting into an enabling posture toward him. By freely acknowledging his wrongdoing and resisting her efforts to assuage his guilty feelings, the therapist helped to keep the client focused on her own reactions of hurt and mistrust. Moreover, he provided Lena with further exposure to the kind of relationship in which *both* parties assumed full responsibility for their errors in judgment, their distorted perceptions, and their hurtful behaviors.

THE THERAPIST'S ISSUES

The therapist was raised within a small Greek-American community. Like other such communities, it was founded in the early 1900s by immigrant men, who worked long hours at low-paying factory jobs until they could save enough money to arrange for family members and relatives to join them. These first-generation arrivals imbued their off-spring with an intense work ethic and a passion for success, born out of earlier experiences of struggle, pain, and prejudice. Many of this second generation indeed made their parents proud, achieving in a variety of business settings, as well as in the fields of education, law, and politics. In contrast to many of their contemporaries, the therapist's own parents did not attain such occupational heights. They did not acquire the trappings of success which seemed, to a child at the time, to be so common among the other families. The therapist sensed as a child that he and his family were alienated from the community mainstream. He felt as though his family were outsiders looking in, publicly accepted, but privately derided for their failure to climb the socioeconomic ladder.

The therapist experienced particularly acute feelings of shame on Sunday mornings when he could almost always be found playing basketball on the playground neighboring the Greek church. Few other families would allow their children to miss church services, especially not for the purpose of practicing their jump shots in full view of the entire congregation. The therapist was clearly in violation of accepted community practices. Moreover, he imagined that each of the dutiful parishioners filing past him into the church was shaking his or her head in contempt, not only for him, but for his family as well.

The therapist recalled these boyhood experiences as he pondered his intense reaction to the parents of a 14-year-old boy he had been seeing for several weeks. The boy was on the verge of flunking out of a prestigious private high school. He had been abusing alcohol and marijuana, ignoring curfews, neglecting household chores, and refusing to do homework. The boy's parents were attractive, well-dressed, and articulate. They came from upper-class families, possessed degrees from elite universities, and had become accomplished professionals. They seemed fairly reasonable and responsible—at least on superficial inspection. The conflicts between the boy and his parents were severe, however, with each incident usually culminating in an episode of acting out on the son's part. Perhaps wisely, the son completely refused to meet jointly with his parents in the therapist's office.

Although the parents acknowledged some of the son's problems, they showed clear signs of denial with respect to the boy's most significant difficulties. Their descriptions of their son seemed to focus exclusively on his *badness* rather than on issues such as self-esteem. Moreover, they habitually attempted to delegate their parental responsibilities to mental health professionals and other adults who came into contact with the young man. As evidenced by their descriptions of several previous treatment experiences, the parents had no qualms about scapegoating other clinicians when things went wrong with their son. From the outset, they demanded answers from the therapist in an aggressive manner, yet consistently took exception to the ideas he offered to them. Although they rejected sensible input, the parents managed to convey the consistent threat that they might blame the therapist if the son's difficulties persisted. They also never stopped questioning the therapist's competence, both implicitly and explicitly. In the meantime, the son's symptoms, and the severe family conflicts, continued on unabated.

Prior to and during each meeting with the parents, the therapist found himself unusually anxious and uncomfortable. After the sessions, the therapist invariably obsessed about his performance. It was not until the therapist discussed the case with his colleague that he became aware that the boy's parents were eliciting the same feelings and self-deprecating thoughts that had been stimulated on those Sunday mornings in his childhood. Feeling threatened and inadequate, the therapist had become unduly concerned about being criticized and/or "fired" by the parents. Consequently, he had been unable to exert consistent pressure for changes in the family structure. Instead of challenging or confronting the family system, the therapist had become inducted into it, so that now *he* felt a sense of direct responsibility for the son's behaviors.

With this awareness in hand, the therapist could now concentrate more fully on the task of transferring the anxiety *he* had been carrying back to its rightful owners. After all, it was not the *therapist's* child who, while ostensibly under his parents' supervision, had become so seriously out of control. The therapist was now better able to carry out *his* treatment plan without being unduly distracted by the threat of being scapegoated by the parents. Since he felt less threatened by the parents, the therapist was also able to develop a more realistic picture of their individual strengths and limitations. A greater understanding of the parents' issues enabled the therapist to join more effectively with them and to anticipate when they might react in a demanding or otherwise defensive manner to him. He found it easier both to deflect their demands for behavioral prescriptions, and to redirect their attention to data about their son who demanded greater involvement and leadership from *them* as parents.

The therapist's experience with this case enabled him to reexamine some long-standing assumptions of his own. Did any of those parishioners *really care* that he was playing basketball on Sunday mornings? Were they really drawing such awful conclusions about him and about his family? Since the therapist had later come to know many of these individuals as well-meaning and family-oriented, he suspected that he had been understandably but seriously mistaken in his earlier perceptions. What was probable, however, was that most of the therapist's *own* peers, suffocatingly stuffed into suits and dresses, *were* eyeing him on those Sunday mornings, but most likely with envy and *not* with contempt.

How can an individual practice psychotherapy for a living without encountering one's own issues again and again in the process? Is it possible to find a mental health professional whose own family of origin issues did *not* play a role in his or her vocational choice? According to Fussell and Bonney (1990), there have been few methodologically sound investigations of the childhood experiences of psychotherapists. Their own study, a carefully designed comparative analysis of the family of origin experiences of male psychologists (all practicing therapists) and male physicists, lends support to the contention that therapists become oriented toward their chosen profession as a function of predisposing family circumstances. Specifically, Fussell and Bonney found that therapists (1) viewed their families of origin as generally less happy and less healthy, (2) were more likely to describe themselves as having assumed caretaking roles as children, and (3) perceived a greater degree of ambiguous communication in the home during their formative years. Finally, when compared to physicists, therapists were found to have experienced a higher incidence of childhood trauma and emotional deprivation.

If the findings we summarized above are valid even to a modest degree, then it would appear that a substantial number of therapists might stand to benefit from treatment themselves. Indeed, we find it astonishing that some mental health professionals treat clients year after year without ever having experienced the therapeutic process themselves. A therapist who has never been in treatment may shortchange, or even jeopardize, the client from sheer ignorance of the way in which his or her issues play themselves out in the consulting room.

The responsible therapist, in our opinion, should assume that both current concerns and historical issues will *always* influence his or her clinical responses to some degree. Ongoing self-examination, consultations with supervisors or colleagues, and personal therapy experiences all help to minimize the impact of the therapist's issues on the quality of the treatment process. A reasonably aware, well-functioning therapist should be able to identify several vulnerable personal areas that have the potential to create problems clinically. The therapist's therapist should be the resource for examining the larger implications of such vulnerable areas, whereas the supervisor or consultant should address the clinical manifestations.

It makes the authors nervous when they hear clinicians say they don't always know the difference between supervision and therapy. We believe that mental health professionals ought to be very clear on the distinctions. Supervisors must respect the boundaries of supervisees, just as therapists need to respect the boundaries of their clients. The supervisor has far too much power and too many conflicting interests and loyalties (such as to the clients whom the therapist treats), to be entrusted with the kind of intimate material that is associated with formal treatment. No supervisee should have to make him- or herself so vulnerable with a supervisor. The authors find it hard to believe that it is not *always* a boundary violation for a supervisor to put any pressure, however subtle, on the supervisee to disclose highly personal material as part of a case consultation.

Naturally, the supervisor has a responsibility to recommend treatment to the supervisee when it seems to be indicated. Such a recommendation might be appropriate, for example, when the therapist seems to be falling into the same self-defeating pattern again and again with certain clients. However, the supervisor should not, and does not really have the capacity to, help the supervisee achieve an integrated understanding of why such a pattern might occur. The supervisor *can*, however, help the therapist to find some new ways to think about and interact with the clients in question. If truly necessary, the supervisor may ask the therapist to consider relinquishing responsibility for the case so that someone better positioned to offer a beneficial therapeutic experience can see the client(s).

On the other hand, when mental health professionals are in therapy, they should not have to worry about whether their professional skills are being evaluated. Most mental health professionals whom we have seen in treatment were afraid at some point that we would begin to question their clinical abilities. Unless the therapist hears clear evidence that the mental health practitioner has specific performance problems on the job, or cannot work because of a more global psychiatric impairment, the professional who is in treatment deserves the same presumption of competence we extend to clients who are "civilians." In instances of actual work disability, the therapist should indicate to the client that it still remains the supervisor's job to evaluate the individual's professional competence. The therapist's job is to facilitate recovery—not to supervise the client's treatment cases. Aside from the occasional situation when the mental health professional merely wants some support and perhaps an opportunity to ventilate, discussions of the practitioner's cases during the treatment hour should probably only occur if they bear directly on recurring personal issues. If it appears that there is not adequate ongoing supervision of the mental health professional, the therapist does have a responsibility to encourage the clinician to secure it at once, so that no harm will be done to his or her clients.

Therapy can produce reactive effects for the mental health professional who is in treatment just as it might for any other client. Some of the reactive effects may show up directly in the therapist's work with clients or interactions with colleagues. Therapists may find themselves unable or unwilling to work with certain kinds of cases, which may evoke much more powerful negative reactions than ever before. In some instances, mental health professionals who begin to lift the veils of their own denial may decide that they no longer wish to work in certain settings, or with certain populations, whereas in the past they might have tolerated stressful conditions on the job without experiencing substantial distress. Indeed, some of our therapist–clients have realized in the course of treatment that they no longer wished to work in human services at all. Unless we saw evidence that such decisions were made impulsively, or were based on a fear of failure, we usually found it easy to support our clients from the helping professions who chose to change their careers.

THE OVERLY RESPONSIBLE THERAPIST

The majority of the therapists we know seem to have been parentified children. The structure of the family of origin required the young therapist-to-be to play an overly responsible, nurturant role, perhaps with strong enabling components, toward parents and/or siblings. Consequently, each therapist has the capacity to replicate an enabling or overprotective parental role with certain types of clients, thereby choking off the capacity for growth in those individuals. Often the therapist's struggle with a particular client will mirror that client's struggle with his or her significant others, in that both must learn how to nurture and help without becoming controlling or otherwise hindering progress.

Below are a number of typical signs that may suggest that a therapist has assumed an overly responsible posture with a particular client:

1. *The therapist tolerates a high rate of dependent behaviors on the part of the client that do not appear tied to discrete environmental stressors.* Indices of excessive dependency include repeated phone calls between appointments, prolonged sessions, frequent need for additional visits, requests for the therapist's advice on inappropriate matters, statements that idealize the therapist ("You're the only one who understands") and so on.

2. *The therapist tolerates persistent noncompliance with treatment norms, such as missed appointments, chronic lateness, failures to complete homework assignments, unpaid bills, and so on.* The therapist may tolerate such behaviors inappropriately with certain clients, while finding it uncharacteristically difficult to confront the noncompliance effectively.

3. *The therapist tolerates regressed or childish behaviors, particularly in the treatment session itself* (e.g., answering fairly neutral questions repeatedly with, "I don't know").

4. *The therapist makes unusually liberal fee arrangements or engages in lax fee collection.* Therapists whose concern for their fellow humans prevents them from being rigid about fees must carefully scrutinize the special arrangements they make with certain individuals to insure that they are being fair to themselves and expecting enough from their clients. Setting extremely low fees, or waiving them entirely, may devalue treatment and, perhaps even worse, may discourage the client from assuming a more responsible position.

5. *The therapist works too hard to "sell" treatment to a clearly symptomatic client or becomes too invested in preventing a premature termination.* Aside from life-threatening situations, we assume that the best time for the client to be in treatment is when he or she is truly motivated. The therapist who tries too hard to hold on to a poorly motivated client will insure a poor treatment outcome.

6. *The therapist works too hard in the treatment sessions.* The therapist should provide structure, direction, and plenty of feedback, but the client who is chronically passive and inactive during the therapy hour may be abdicating his or her responsibilities while placing an unreasonable burden on the clinician.

7. *The therapist becomes unduly anxious or depressed about the client's situation, overly invested in the solution of specific problems, or too narrowly focused on changing certain client behaviors.* Therapists cannot control how clients think, feel, or behave either during sessions or between appointments. Clinicians who spend a great deal of time giving advice to clients are attempting to *control*, not to facilitate, change. In the process, they

can violate boundaries and give unintended negative messages regarding the client's competence. They also may ignore the level of the *client's* own motivation, which might not be strong enough to support substantial changes in lifestyle or behavior. On the other hand, we consistently find that individuals who have removed the appropriate psychological roadblocks will find all sorts of creative solutions to their problems, solutions which turn out to be far more effective than any we might have proposed.

The following case included many of the classic indicators of an overly responsible posture on the part of the therapist. The therapist's excessively responsible stance was a joint product of his own family of origin issues and the intense difficulties experienced by the client. The personal growth that the clinician achieved as a result his own treatment clearly helped him to understand and control his reactions to the client, and to assume a far more effective therapeutic posture with the case.

Donna, a 50-year-old homemaker, presented a complex array of symptoms. In addition to a history of depressive episodes, she experienced a wide range of medical problems, several of which had potential psychological effects. At one time, Donna had had a large network of friends and an active social life. As her various symptoms worsened, Donna's life had became more and more circumscribed, to the point where she rarely ventured out of her home except to attend her many medical appointments. A few of her remaining friends had questioned the validity of her physical complaints, prompting Donna to spend even less time with them. Moreover, her chronic sleep problems kept her locked into a nocturnal schedule, which only increased her sense of alienation from the rest of the world.

Donna's husband, Jeff, was as cold and detached as she was warm and personable. Several years before, he had abruptly terminated marital therapy after four or five sessions. From that point on, his interest in the marriage seemed to have stopped. Although there was an absence of overt conflict, most forms of intimate contact between the couple, including sex, had disappeared. Occasionally Donna told the therapist that she thought Jeff was having an affair, but she resisted any of the clinician's attempts to explore the matter further.

Donna acknowledged that her father and many other males in her family had drunk to excess during her formative years. She recalled having been beaten on numerous occasions by both parents, usually for minor infractions. She described physical assaults from an older brother, occurring as late as her senior year of high school. Donna's mother scapegoated her, while she infantilized the younger sister and enabled the older brother. The mother had harbored a deep mistrust of anyone outside the immediate family to the point of outright paranoia on some occasions. She enforced her rules, especially those involving family secrecy, not only with physical abuse but also by terrifying her children with dark, superstitious religious imagery. Naturally gregarious as a youngster and a teenager, Donna particularly angered her mother by maintaining a variety of relationships outside the family.

Donna found it difficult to discuss her family of origin in treatment. She experienced her recollections as if through a haze, often saying to the therapist "I may be making this up." She had trouble recalling discussions from previous sessions, particularly those which involved her childhood and adolescence. When she spoke about her parents during the therapy hour, she often experienced both fear of their potential retaliation and guilt over having betrayed them to the therapist. In a variety of situations, she frequently found herself thinking "If I get better, I'm going to die." The therapist's attempts to label her childhood as traumatic seemed plausible to Donna only for fleeting moments. Once she left the session, she would begin to think of counterarguments to the therapist's observations. She would wonder if she had made up stories about her family for the therapist's benefit. Eventually she would say to herself "He's wrong. I'm the one to blame, not my parents."

Donna did appear to derive a variety of secondary gains from her symptoms. She routinely avoided social events and other activities that might make her uncomfortable. She repeatedly told the therapist that she could not even begin to think about the sorry state of her marriage, or her husband's possible infidelity, "until I'm feeling better." Donna missed many meetings with the therapist allegedly because of illness. Many times it seemed to the therapist that she was most likely to cancel out following a session in which she had discussed a topic she preferred to avoid, such as her marriage. Donna formed highly dependent attachments to a number of doctors, particularly her primary care physician. It was not uncommon for her to see him several times a week. In addition to the office visits, there were also frequent phone conversations between Donna and her physician, often on a daily basis during difficult periods. That she idealized the man was obvious. At times, Donna was taking as many as nine medications concurrently, including an addictive minor tranquilizer, an antidepressant, a synthetic estrogen replacement, a synthetic thyroid replacement, a narcotic painkiller, and an antiinflammatory drug. A brief inspection of the *Physician's Desk Reference* was sufficient to convince the therapist that with respect to side effects alone, the medication situation was out of the physician's control. Unfortunately, Donna demonstrated the same kind of anxious loyalty to her physician that she showed toward her parents. She frequently expressed fears about being dropped as a patient by him, and never failed to remind the therapist how much the physician had done for her.

Although Donna was always quite courteous and respectful, the therapist often found himself uncomfortable with her. The client never completed a homework assignment and resisted recommendations aimed at increasing her level of activity or social contact. Donna seemed content to use her treatment sessions to dwell at length on her numerous physical symptoms. Even if all of her medical complaints were legitimate, the therapist was convinced that there were still many significant attitudes and behaviors Donna *could* change. Long discussions of Donna's health problems always seemed to make the therapist feel helpless and somewhat angry at the client. He found it hard to address her passivity and her avoidant lifestyle in a supportive manner without conveying the irritation he felt toward her. The therapist also had difficulty addressing the secondary gains associated with her medical problems without eliciting defensive reactions from Donna. He was convinced that she was being overmedicated by her primary care physician but had to be careful not to threaten the client by attacking the relationship or to commit an ethical violation by expressing a medical opinion. Overall, the therapist felt responsible for Donna's lack of progress and guilty for the negative feelings he experienced toward her.

As the therapist reflected on this client, he recognized that treating older women who experienced significant health complaints had always made him somewhat uneasy. In fact, he had to admit to himself that being around physically ill adults had made him anxious, to an unreasonable degree, for as long as he could remember. In analyzing his reactions further, the therapist realized that he would typically experience feelings of helplessness and agitation in such situations, coupled with a strong sense of responsibility for the other person. The therapist's reactions to Donna were rooted in his own family of origin experiences.

For several years during the therapist's adolescence, his mother's physical health had been quite poor. In fact, her very survival had been at stake. When the therapist was 12 years old, his mother had undergone the first of two operations for malignant tumors. The initial surgery had required a long hospital stay and a lengthy convalescence at home. The second operation, which had occurred nearly 2 years later, involved a much larger tumor, more serious and intrusive surgical procedures, and a more complicated recovery. Although his mother responded positively to the radiation treatments she had received, she was prone to develop worrisome growths in the same region of her body for many years thereafter.

Quite serendipitously, the therapist had himself entered treatment about the same time he began seeing Donna. He discussed his reactions to her with his own therapist, and with a valued senior colleague. Until he began to examine his reactions to working with Donna, the therapist would never have described his mother's illness as a seminal event in his life. If pressed, he even might have maintained that he had been too preoccupied at the time with the emerging issues of adolescence to have been affected significantly by his mother's bouts with cancer. Such a contention would of course have been ludicrous. In retrospect, there were many indications that his mother's illness had been a powerful stressor during the therapist's early adolescence. The therapist recalled having seen his mother in the hospital shortly after one of her operations. Her ghostly appearance then had been terrifying to him. Although she had been a healthy and vigorous woman before the operation, not yet 40 years old, the therapist remembered thinking that his mother looked old and frail in her hospital bed, almost as if she had been damaged beyond repair.

Like Donna, his mother's life had been filled for many years with doctors and medical treatments. Like Donna, his mother had idealized her physician. Like Donna, his mother had been a heavy smoker and coffee drinker, despite repeated warnings that these habits might exacerbate her ill health. The therapist recalled feeling angry at his mother during his adolescence, when he thought that she was smoking too much or letting herself become overly fatigued. Expressing these concerns had always elicited angry, defensive reactions from his mother. He remembered thinking on several occasions that she surely would not live very long at the rate she was going. Paradoxically, during his adolescence, the therapist had also viewed his mother as a hypochondriac, telling himself that she complained of physical problems in order to obtain sympathy and other secondary gains. These thoughts, which he had never shared with anyone at the time, had not only made him feel angry as a teenager, but they also led him to view himself as selfish, mean-spirited, and disloyal. Now the therapist realized that his anger at his mother stemmed from his *anxiety* about her health. Moreover, as a young adolescent, it was probably less stressful for him to believe that his mother could control her health by eliminating her bad habits, or indeed that she really wasn't so sick in the first place, than to live with the intense fear he had experienced that day in her hospital room. Only from his experiences in adulthood as a psychologist had the therapist realized that his reactions to his mother's illness, including his anger, had been entirely appropriate.

The therapist had assumed a parentified role long before his mother's illness, as it turned out. In fact, his parentification was the product of multiple factors. As the oldest child, he was always strongly encouraged, particularly by his mother, to assume a protective role toward his younger siblings. Like many of his clients, the therapist discovered one of the most powerful sources of his parentification quite serendipitously while he was in the process of coping with a seemingly unrelated issue. The therapist's 10-year-old son had recently been diagnosed with a neurological disorder. During a discussion about the potential genetic background for the disorder, the therapist's mother recalled some problems of unknown origin experienced by the therapist's younger sister many years before. She reminded the therapist of how, while only a toddler, his sister had undergone episodic loss of motor control, so that she was rendered unable to raise her head or support her neck. The malady continued from the time the sister was a year old until she was nearly 3 years, departing as mysteriously as it had arrived. The therapist spontaneously remembered his response to his younger sister's unexplained illness, which had taken place when he was between 3 and 5 years. As he recalled, he had been fond of playing "buttercup" or tickling his sister under the chin. Sometimes he became a little forceful in the process, or persisted in the behavior when she wanted him to stop. When the sister's symptoms had started, the therapist clearly remembered thinking that he must have done something to "break" her neck. The sense of shame and responsibility that accompanied the therapist's reaction to his sister's difficulties persisted for decades, influencing many aspects of his life, including his vocational choice.

Having been cognizant for some time of the material that involved his sister, the therapist was better able to understand his reactions to his mother's illness when was an adolescent. Moreover, having worked extensively on the parentification issues related to his sister, it was relatively easy for him to shed himself of feelings of responsibility for his mother's situation and, in turn, for the plight of his client Donna. *In looking back at his responses as an adolescent, he saw himself not as a miniature adult, but as he really had been, young, scared, vulnerable, and basically good.* The therapist came to realize that his mother's illness *had* affected him as a teenager in a powerful manner that had been essentially beyond his control. He had not *chosen* to be angry at his mother or to distance himself from her when she was ill any more than he had chosen to minimize the severity of her illness. As he thought about his experiences more and more, therapist felt a chronic burden of guilt begin to lift. He realized that he had felt neutralized by Donna because he had been assuming a position of blameworthiness with her, just as he had done for many years with his mother. He began to feel much more relaxed with his mother, and much more competent with Donna.

It was vital for the therapist to find a way to sustain empathy with Donna's health problems and her sense of helplessness without experiencing either anxiety or anger. On the other hand, there was a need for the therapist to confront Donna's passivity, her dependency, the secondary gains associated with her physical complaints, and the behaviors she engaged in, such as smoking, which actively sabotaged her health. Donna's previous therapists had failed to address these issues adequately, whereas her medical doctors merely became angry and scapegoated her for calling too often or not taking proper care of herself. The therapist had to overcome the sense of pessimism about Donna that seemed to be rooted in those failed confrontations that had occurred with his own mother so many years before. He reminded himself repeatedly, that *he* was the legitimate authority figure in the exchange now and that Donna was paying him for his feedback. The therapist tried to keep in mind that he had never seen any evidence of the kind of defensiveness on Donna's part which he had experienced previously with his mother. Moreover, even if the client became hostile, it was unlikely that her anger could hurt him the way a parent's anger had.

The therapist began to make significant adjustments in his posture with Donna, taking care to do so in a gradual manner, so as to avoid threatening the client. Slowly, he demanded that Donna assume a more competent role with him in a number of ways. He asked her to bring a notebook with her to each session so that she could take notes on what they discussed. He told the client that since he needed to keep her focused on the issues he could help her with, he was going to limit the discussions of her physical symptoms. On the other hand, when she did mention her physical complaints, the therapist now began a long and careful campaign aimed at prying her loose from her symbiotic relationship with the primary-care physician. Whenever Donna complained that various medications or treatment strategies were ineffective, the therapist gently but persistently encouraged the client to consult specialists for additional opinions. The therapist vowed to himself that he would end his sessions with Donna on time and stuck to his promise. Although he did not question her practice of canceling appointments when she felt ill, he restricted his phone conversations with her to perfunctory matters, so that their significant discussions only took place in his office. Rather than allow an unpaid balance to build up indefinitely, the therapist negotiated a reduced fee with Donna that she was expected to pay him every week. He began to insert phrases into their conversations such as, "After all, even people who are terminally ill have a right to use their time productively," and so on.

Ironically enough, the therapist's mother, now in her late 60s, underwent another health crisis during his work with Donna, again with a positive outcome. This time the therapist was able to articulate his reactions to his mother's illness and share them with those closest to him. Although he struggled with justifiable worries regarding his mother's health, since he felt no need to distance himself from her this time, the therapist found it easy to behave in a supportive manner. In the meantime, his mother's resiliency, her optimistic attitude, her sense of humor, and her unwillingness to relinquish any ground to her illness, all stood out in dramatic counterpoint to the way in which Donna was responding to her own far less serious health problems. At this point the enormous differences between the two women could not have been more obvious. Now more than ever, the therapist knew that he could continue to confront Donna in a supportive context without allowing his own issues to interfere with the process.

Later, the therapist supervised a case in which an adolescent girl seemed to show no reaction at all to her father's terminal illness. The treating clinician, already dismayed by the teenager's oppositional behavior in the family, wondered if the girl's lack of discomfort reflected narcissistic, or worse, antisocial tendencies on her part. It was clear that the clinician's empathic connection with the adolescent had been damaged, despite the fact that the teenager had behaved in a fairly normal and cooperative manner previously. After describing the reactions he had as a teenager to own his mother's illness, the therapist encouraged the clinician to view the girl's nonresponsive condition as a reflection of denial mechanisms at work, not as a reflection of more serious personality problems. This denial-oriented formulation provided the clinician with a fresh and workable perspective on the case. No longer irritated or dismayed with the girl's lack of response to her father's illness, the clinician was now able to play a supportive role in the adolescent's life.

9

Promoting Awareness of Family of Origin Issues

The aim of this chapter is to describe how the therapist can promote the client's awareness of basic schemas and information-processing styles without damaging the therapeutic relationship and impeding progress. We emphasize that many individuals enter treatment with little if any awareness of their core beliefs. As awareness grows, clients still tend to regard their beliefs not as tentative hypotheses but, rather, as facts. The therapist and client together must build a data base that can be referred to *repeatedly* over time in order to demonstrate the day-to-day operation of family of origin issues and to challenge faulty beliefs and information processing errors. The therapist helps the client build the data base gradually, by orchestrating learning experiences that expose distortions in thinking. Each successful learning experience can provide the foundation for future interventions with the client.

AN OVERVIEW OF STRATEGIES FOR PROMOTING AWARENESS

We believe that, above all, enhanced awareness is the foundation of meaningful long-term change in the client's life. To characterize our treatment model as "insight-oriented," however, invites comparisons to therapeutic approaches that do not share our explicit educative focus. When we speak of "promoting awareness," "raising consciousness," or "building insight," our goals are probably more ambitious and complex than those of our colleagues who come from other treatment orientations. In essence, we would like our clients to *internalize the model* we outlined in Chapters 1, 2, 3, and 5 as it applies to their own particular life experiences. An "internalized model" implies a kinetic, expanding base of knowledge, one that enhances the client's self-awareness on a moment-to-moment basis. Clients who are able to internalize a model of their difficulties will, in the long run, find themselves able to interrupt and correct long-standing patterns of thinking and behavior *as they occur in process*, without necessarily enlisting the aid of a therapist or anyone else. In the same manner, armed with a road map of their own vulnerabilities, they will be better able to anticipate and avoid potential difficulties in the future.

Below are a number of specific items that we would like to bring to the client's awareness:

Details of dysfunctional characteristics of family of origin, including impaired parenting, parentification of children, boundary violations, traumatic experiences, chronic rejection, cognitive distortions, and distorted communications.

Details of traumatic and/or victimizing experiences in childhood and adolescence.

An understanding of the impact of dysfunctional family circumstances, and other victimization experiences, upon oneself as a developing child.

An understanding of one's basic beliefs about the self, about others and the world, and about relationships, and the manner in which such schemas developed in the family of origin.

An understanding of how past and current cognitive distortions relate to basic schemas.

An understanding of how basic coping strategies, including information-processing styles, evolved in direct response to stressors in childhood and adolescence

An understanding of the model of coping represented by "Solomon's dogs," and how it applies to one's own past and current coping strategies.

An awareness of the operation of denial strategies in one's past and current experiences.

An awareness of manifestations of overvigilance and how such mechanisms relate to basic beliefs, and experiences in childhood and adolescence.

An awareness of how habits of denial and overvigilance are stimulated by stressors in one's life.

An awareness of the cognitive underpinning of addictive, compulsive, or other self-defeating behaviors and how such beliefs and actions connect to experiences in one's family of origin.

An awareness of the cognitive and behavioral components associated with recurring relationship patterns and the connections between those components and circumstances in the family of origin.

An awareness of how personal issues resonate with those of significant others, particularly one's partners.

An understanding of how, through cognitive distortions and information-processing errors, one has allowed or perpetuated victimization in past or current relationships.

An inventory of the kinds of thinking patterns, information-processing mechanisms, and behavioral tendencies that will demand one's attention in the future, perhaps throughout one's life span.

No doubt most therapists find it easier to work with clients who are highly intelligent, well-educated, and psychologically minded. Nonetheless, we do not find that the client's intellectual and/or educational level has to be a barrier to developing greater awareness of the mechanisms listed. Many of our clients with limited educational backgrounds and modest intellectual abilities have become "star pupils" in treatment. Such individuals succeeded in internalizing much of what they learned in their sessions, probably because they were strongly motivated, and because their therapists were able to conduct treatment in terms that were meaningful and comprehensible to the client. We consistently find that variables such as externalization of blame are far more likely to limit the success of treatment outcome than a comparative lack of intelligence or education.

We utilize all of the following strategies to build awareness of family of origin issues:

1. *Orienting.* This term refers to basic therapeutic operations that aim to focus the client's attention on pertinent data. We discuss orienting strategies in detail in the next section.

2. *Socratic Dialogue.* As many of our readers know, Socratic dialogue is the foundation of the cognitive therapy approach developed by Beck and his colleagues. Later in this chapter, we illustrate how we use Socratic techniques specifically to build awareness of family of origin issues.

3. *Analyses of "Found Distortions."* The therapist has a golden opportunity to create a powerful learning experience for the client any time the individual *spontaneously* recognizes and/or corrects previous cognitive distortions or simply expresses beliefs that contradict ideas expressed at another time. The alert clinician should not let such changes in the client's thinking go by without elucidating and underscoring the mechanisms involved. The therapist needs to highlight the

contrasting ideas of the client so that he or she can fully appreciate both the presence and the power of cognitive distortions. In similar fashion, the therapist needs to walk the client through the reasoning process that led to the cognitive changes and to assist the individual to spell out concretely how the new ideation can be used to counter similar cognitive distortions in the future.

We want our clients to be amazed by (but not ashamed of) the disruptions in reality testing that they experience in certain situations. The longer they remain amazed or distressed by such disturbances the better, since they will experience a greater level of motivation and a clearer sense of focus in treatment as a result. "Found Distortions" provide the therapist with an ideal opportunity to stimulate and encourage the client's curiosity regarding the possible origins of such disturbances in thinking. The therapist can begin to offer hypotheses about why the distortions occur based on what is currently known about the client's family of origin and developmental history.

4. *Analyses of Critical Incidents, Both Historical and Contemporary.* Throughout this volume, our case examples illustrate in various ways how the therapist's analysis of clients' early memories helps to establish the links between family history and current distress. The client's recollections from childhood or adolescence provide the therapist with an opportunity to underscore how such experiences may have led to the development of particular core beliefs and coping strategies. As we discuss in Chapter 11 (p. 290) in a section on "Accessing the Inner Child," such recollections also enable the therapist to educate the client about the reactions of a typical youngster to specific stressful situations.

Understandably, clients typically want to use treatment sessions to discuss stressful situations in their current lives. The therapist attempts to stimulate and maintain forward momentum in two directions simultaneously during such discussions. The first dimension involves always moving the client from dealing with specific current concerns toward confronting more pervasive and significant personal issues. The therapist must become adept at extracting from critical incidents those elements that connect back to the client's basic beliefs and coping strategies and to the family of origin. The second dimension involves shifting from content involving lower levels of degree of belief to those that involve higher degrees of belief, greater cognitive constriction, and increased emotional arousal. As treatment progresses, more and more of the analysis of any given incident will also be devoted to building conceptual bridges to other treatment discussions, as well as other experiences in the client's history.

5. *Analyses of Events Within the Therapeutic Relationship.* It should be clear by now to the reader that like other cognitive therapists (e.g.,

Safran & Segal, 1990), we view the therapeutic relationship as a primary source of data regarding the client's interpersonal style and the belief systems that support it. Case examples throughout the remainder of the volume also illustrate various ways in which we have utilized events within the therapeutic relationship to strengthen the client's awareness of the impact of family of origin material on current functioning.

6. *Analyses of Instances of Successful Coping.* The therapist has another unique opportunity to orchestrate a rich learning experience whenever the client spontaneously acknowledges an instance of successful coping. Through Socratic dialogue, the client may also come to identify a particular experience as a successful one essentially as a result of the therapist's prompting. In Chapter 12, we discuss in detail how the therapist can approach an instance of successful coping on the part of the client.

7. *Analyses of Imagery and Dreams.* The client's spontaneous imagery not only reveals much about the underlying cognitive structure, but it also discloses a great deal about the family of origin experiences that gave rise to basic beliefs and coping strategies. One of the authors (R.B.), stubbornly (and rather ignorantly, given the embryonic stage of his career at the time) refused any professional offerings from a psychoanalytic perspective. Consequently, for a number of years, he never used dream material for any purpose in treatment. At one time he would jokingly tell clients "Sorry, I don't do dreams." However, over the years, it became apparent to him, albeit somewhat belatedly, that certain clients seemed to want to communicate in treatment through sharing dream material. As we discuss in Chapter 11 in a section on "Trauma Revelation Processes," we often find it essential to work extensively with dream material, particularly when we treat individuals who experienced severe physical and/or sexual abuse in childhood.

8. *Repetitive Presentation of Formulations and Summaries.* As much as possible, clients need to be able to grasp some sort of "big picture" of themselves, their difficulties in life, and the effects of their formative experiences. Without explicit assistance from the therapist, many clients find it hard to keep such an overview in mind. The therapist must remain alert for opportunities to point out multiple manifestations of the mechanisms under consideration at any given time. Awareness of multiple iterations of a particular theme or response pattern can provide clients with a sense of intellectual integration and an appreciation of the power and pervasiveness of particular issues. *A client who begins to recognize how frequently and reflexively certain reactions occur will also begin to grasp why change takes time and practice.* Moreover, clients who appreciate the intensity and complexity of their reactions will find it easier to remain committed to treatment and recovery.

The therapist's ability to integrate information from diverse parts of the client's life, past and present, helps to provide both continuity and a powerful sense of immediacy in therapy, even during discussions which center on events in childhood or adolescence. The therapist who can keep *both* the past and the present alive during the session will prevent therapy from becoming either a dry rehash of history or a frantic review of current symptoms. It is necessary to remind the client constantly of the connections between family of origin experiences and the presenting complaints. The therapist will also look for specific opportunities to link events within the therapeutic relationship with any significant topics under discussion.

The therapist also needs to provide the client with a framework for understanding where they are in the recovery process. Frequent, updated reviews of treatment by the therapist provide the client with a sense of continuity and accomplishment while they strengthen the conceptual foundation on which long-term recovery will rest. Moreover, such reviews provide an opportunity for the therapist to gauge the current fit between his or her perceptions of what has occurred in treatment with those of the client.

No doubt nearly all of our readers have heard the song, "The Twelve Days of Christmas," in which the gifts given by the singer's true love for each previous day are enumerated once again in every verse. Although it may become tiresome hearing "a partridge in a pear tree" so many times over the course of the song, most listeners would agree nonetheless that it's very hard to forget that particular gift, given the twelve repetitions it receives. We often find ourselves enumerating pieces of data in such a fashion with our clients, as we accumulate multiple instances of cognitive distortions, dysfunctional basic beliefs, information-processing phenomena, or other coping strategies. Each time the therapist walks the client through the formulations and the relevant data that support them, there is an opportunity to strengthen new beliefs through the integration of new information, as well as through sheer repetition. The therapist can also use the presentation of the formulations as a means of drawing attention to important questions about the client that perhaps have not yet been answered, for example, "We still don't really understand what has made it so hard for you to end a relationship that you say has nothing to offer you."

When reviewing treatment or alluding to insights achieved in previous sessions, it is vital for the clinician to incorporate the client's unique imagery, symbolism, and vocabulary. Any descriptive phrases or terminology that the client picks up from the therapist and begins to use spontaneously also merit continued, frequent repetition in subsequent discussions. The therapist and client who work together on a long-term basis may develop a shared shorthand that they both utilize for a variety of purposes, for example, to create a sense of continuity in treatment. The therapist may reach the point where he or she can say, "This story reminds me of the 'Pie Episode' and the 'Motel Incident' " and be reasonably sure that the client will know that the underlying issue is an irrational fear of being rejected by her parents.

It is generally desirable for the therapist to begin each session with a capsule review of the mechanisms that were discussed during the previous interview, with a particular emphasis on establishing connections to the ongoing themes of treatment, and to the presenting complaints. This practice is particularly important for clients with pervasive denial mechanisms, clients who tend to "shut down" between sessions. It is also important for the therapist to establish a strong sense of continuity in treatment with clients who live in a state of constant uproar drifting from one problem or symptom to another. We recommend that the therapist often read verbatim quotations from the client as part of such a review, particularly if the verbalizations in question reflect new insights or more functional attitudes.

9. *Listening to Audiotapes of Treatment Sessions.* In our model of treatment, a lot goes on during each session. The therapist is likely to offer the client detailed feedback at critical junctures several times during a typical interview. Many of our clients will report that they have difficulty recalling the content of their treatment sessions, let alone retaining new perspectives that might emerge during interviews. The taping of sessions allows the client to go over pertinent material several times. The therapist may direct the client to review specific parts of a particular session, typically with the goal of increasing the individual's awareness of key mechanisms. In fact, the therapist may include some remarks in a session that can only be absorbed by the client through repeated listenings. Since most cars are equipped with cassette decks, clients generally have opportunities to listen to their session tapes in private. Needless to say, some clients find it too threatening to have to listen to themselves speaking for extended periods of time. Although the therapist should attempt to reassure the client that the sense of discomfort over one's voice and diction may fade over time as he or she gets in the habit of listening to session tapes, the clinician should be respectful of the individual's right to say no. As an alternative, clients may be willing to take notes during their sessions. One of our clients, no doubt foreshadowing a future trend, brings a laptop computer with him to record pertinent thoughts during his sessions!

10. *Journal Writing, Thought Recording, and Other Self-Monitoring Assignments.* Our clients often need to develop a keen appreciation for the way in which family of origin issues manifest themselves on a

day-to-day, moment-to-moment basis. As we discuss in a subsequent chapter, homework assignments help clients to sustain awareness of key mechanisms between sessions and thereby facilitate transfer of learning. Almost *any* time the client identifies a significant cognitive distortion, dysfunctional belief, information-processing error, or self-defeating coping strategy in a session, he or she should be instructed to watch for additional manifestations of the mechanism in question over the weeks that follow.

11. *Bibliotherapy, Group Experiences, and Other Educational Resources.* Educational resources keep the client immersed in material relevant to current symptoms and/or family of origin dynamics. Except where particular clinical considerations lead the therapist to seek a greater degree of control over the flow of information in treatment, it is desirable to encourage the client to seek exposure to a broad range of materials. The therapist needs to elicit the client's specific reactions to any educational materials or experiences encountered in the course of treatment. Global reviews by the client are not sufficient, since the therapist will want to identify as precisely as possible those elements of the materials in question that seemed most relevant or helpful to the individual. We were able to learn a great deal about certain clients, who were unable to tell us much about themselves directly, by asking them to highlight the passages in self-help books that they had found to be most meaningful. The therapist should then try to build directly on the ideas that have *already* captured the client's attention.

ORIENTING

Without some outside intervention, long-established habits of over-vigilance lead the client back toward the same old inferences and ruminations. Similarly, denial strategies habitually direct the client away from important data of all sorts. Successful treatment often requires the therapist to refocus the client's attention away from habitual and/or obsessive patterns of thinking, toward new data. As revealed by transcripts and recordings of sessions, even a "nondirective" therapist such as Carl Rogers seems to be constantly orienting clients, in an unobtrusive manner, toward "deeper" thoughts and feelings simply through the use of highly attuned reflections and paraphrasings. In an active, strongly educative style of treatment such as ours, the therapist constantly seeks to capture and direct the client's attention.

Orienting strategies all aim at keeping the client focused on a particular area of information that the therapist views as relevant to the individual's difficulties. When the therapist is performing an orienting function, he or she will avoid "telegraphing" his or her viewpoint on the material at hand to the client. In fact at times, the therapist who is performing the orienting function may not have a particular viewpoint at all but instead simply recognizes a need to keep the client focused on a certain body of data. Although the therapist may behave in a curious or amazed manner, the goal at all times is to move the client away from the clinician's reactions, back toward the data at hand.

The therapist needs to monitor carefully all failures to capture and hold the client's attention. Why was the client unable to sustain concentration on a particular topic? Where did the client's attention go? Was there evidence of dissociative processes at work? Did issues such as family loyalty or intense feelings of worthlessness prevent the client from continuing to consider the matter at hand? To what extent did the dynamics of the therapeutic relationship interfere with the client's ability to attend to the relevant material?

A great of deal of orienting work in treatment requires the therapist to keep the client's attention focused on a rather narrow, highly selective *bandwidth* of information. For example, suppose a client has described a series of dreams and recollections that suggest that she may have been sexually abused by her father. She feels understandably revolted by the imagery she has experienced and frightened by the potential implications. She tells herself and the therapist that although her father had his problems, among them chronic alcoholism, he could not possibly have molested his daughters. Despite her fears however, the client continues to experience and disclose the imagery in question. She wants to understand what, if anything, happened to her, and with whom it occurred.

Among other goals (see Chapter 11 on "Trauma Revelation Processes"), the therapist at this point will want to investigate several key areas in much greater detail than he or she might have previously. The therapist will want to learn more about the household routine when the client was growing up. Who performed caretaking functions, when, and under what circumstances? Where was the father when he was drinking? The therapist will also question the client more intensively regarding family norms in areas such as bathing and nudity and other topics relating to sexuality. Additionally, the therapist will want to take a detailed sexual history from the client herself, including her experiences and behavior in adulthood. Such questions will generate usable data only if the therapist can keep the client very narrowly focused. If the client continues to experience intense feelings of disloyalty toward her father, she may respond in a noninformative way to therapeutic inquiries, out of a need to protect him. If the client is frightened off by the imagery and the affect associated with it, she may become panicked, perhaps to the point of developing an anxiety reaction, or she may simply close down processing of the information at hand. If she feels terribly ashamed of something that happened in childhood or adult life, she may be too overcome by feelings of worthlessness to address other aspects of her own victimization. Each of these issues is compeling, and eminently worthy of lengthy exploration, probably at some other time. Because highly charged topics such as loyalty and worthlessness so readily usurp the client's attention, they can easily interfere with the therapist's ability even to obtain information, let alone change long-standing beliefs. Consequently the therapist will need to devise strategies for preempting attentional shifts in response to these issues or in handling such shifts when they occur. In Chapter 7, we discussed various ways in which the therapist might engage in such "preemptive maneuvers," primarily through the use of embedded messages.

The therapist must help to anchor the client's attention through the use of compelling language, intonation, and nonverbal gestures. For some clients it may be desirable to raise the volume almost to a shout, whereas for other clients, the therapist will be far more captivating if he or she speaks in only a whisper. It may be helpful for the therapist to use space and stage gestures much like an actor, so that a trip to the tissue box while speaking might be used as an opportunity to recapture the client's attention, by stimulating visual tracking of the clinician. We refer the reader to the trance induction work of Milton Erickson (Haley, 1967, 1971) for an inspirational collection of techniques for capturing and narrowing the client's attention.

The case of Craig presented below exemplifies the use of reflections and paraphrasings, the employment of questions in the context of history taking, and the expression of curiosity as orienting strategies. As illustrated, orienting strategies are not only tools for promoting awareness but serve as *probes* for testing clients' receptiveness to exploring potentially threatening content or themes. The subsequent dialogue with Craig demonstrates that one of the key orienting strategies, particularly with clients who might resist more direct approaches, involves amplifying incongruities in the client's ideas and feeding them back to the individual. Although the therapist may appear pensive, curious, or confused, his or her demeanor should not become so striking that it becomes the focal point of the session, since it is used to draw the client's attention back to the material in question.

Craig was a 20-year-old student at a local college who lived with his parents. On the verge of flunking out of school for the second time, Craig entered treatment for help with depression. He reported a history of poor school performance despite a documented high IQ and no apparent learning problems. Craig told the therapist his history of underachievement stemmed from a long-standing pattern of low motivation, irresponsibility, and outright laziness on his part. He stated explicitly that not only did his parents concur with his explanation for the school failures but that *they had been telling him the same thing* since he was a young child. In response to the client's statement, the therapist wondered to himself why this particular explanation for Craig's difficulties had been so repeatedly offered by his parents. Since Craig had not previously received help for his "motivation" problems, the therapist suspected that perhaps this particular labeling of Craig's problems reflected other problems in the family system. Perhaps his "incompetence" and "irresponsibility" rendered him unable to leave home, thereby providing his parents with a distraction away from more threatening issues.

Inquiring more closely about symptoms, the therapist learned that Craig was not clinically depressed. Moreover, it appeared that he had not suffered extensive symptoms of depression in the past either. Interestingly, Craig had been diagnosed as depressed by the psychiatrist who was also treating the client's father for an affective disorder. Craig had begun seeing the psychiatrist at his parents' behest. The fact that Craig had been treated by his father's therapist supported the therapist's suspicions about diffuse boundaries in the family. In a seemingly bold move, however, Craig had told his parents he wanted to have his own therapist, someone who wasn't already involved with the family. The therapist asked Craig what it was like telling his parents that he wanted to seek out his own therapist.

Craig: I usually just go along to get along, but this time I thought it was important enough to speak up. I really didn't get the feeling that Dr. Oliver was going to help me. I felt like he already had his mind made up about me.

Th: So normally you go along to get along. A bit later, I'd like to learn more about how that has worked out for you over the years. In this situation, however, you chose to speak up to your parents because you really didn't think you were going to be helped by Dr. Oliver. What went through your mind when you first considered telling your parents that you wanted a different therapist?

Craig: I honestly didn't know what to expect. I was a little nervous, I guess.

Th: What you were afraid might happen by speaking up?

Craig: I though it might turn into a hassle, you know, and get my mother and father started with each other. Then they'd be upset with me and on and on and on. It usually just isn't worth it.

Th: So if I understand correctly, the usual reaction to challenging your parents is a big fuss. They get upset with each other and then *you get dragged in* as well.

Craig: You've got it.

Th: *Pulled right into the middle* of a conflict between them.

Craig: Yeah, and I hate it, so I've learned to stay out of it.

The therapist discovers in this interchange that Craig appears open to the idea that he has a role in detouring conflict away from his parents. The therapist used simple reflective statements to orient Craig to this theme. The therapist also embedded phrases (in italics above) that highlighted the theme in more powerful terms. Since Craig did not seem to object to such comments, the therapist would now continue to use them repeatedly.

Apart from the use of reflections and paraphrasings, the most innocuous orienting strategy is the simple question. Done in the context of history taking, the therapist is in an uniquely opportune position to ask probing questions under the guise of "standard operating procedure." At a later point in treatment, such questions might well arouse suspicion and defensiveness, particularly if the therapist has failed to establish a rationale for the particular line of inquiry.

Craig dated the onset of his depression to the time he had gone away to college two years earlier. The therapist, who was curious about how issues of separation and individuation played out in Craig's family, decided to explore in greater detail the client's experiences living away from home at that time.

Th: You said that you first felt depressed during orientation. Can you describe what happened in more detail?

Craig: I guess I just felt really homesick.

Th: Do you remember anything about the kinds of thoughts you were having when you were feeling homesick?

Craig: Yeah, I remember thinking "I'm not strong enough to handle this."

The therapist focuses here on Craig's specific report of *homesickness* as a means for highlighting separation difficulties and for exploring the cognitive underpinnings of his reaction. The therapist discovers that Craig's explanation for his homesickness ("I'm not strong enough") was generally consistent with his explanation for his academic problems

("I'm lazy and irresponsible"). In both cases, Craig's attributions reflect themes of personal inadequacy and self-blame.

The therapist followed up on the above exchange with an inquiry about whether there were other examples of situations in which Craig had become homesick or otherwise had difficulty being away from home. Craig related several important experiences. First, Craig's mother had been hospitalized for a "nervous breakdown" when he was in kindergarten. Craig recalled experiencing tremendous anxiety during this time, since he was not able to visit his mother and received almost no information about her condition. He did not express his fears, however, because he sensed that he was not supposed to talk about his mother's absence. Craig's mother would have two more hospitalizations over the next 10 years, ostensibly for recurrent depressions, for which she remained medicated. Still, she managed a full-time job and the household responsibilities during the bulk of Craig's childhood and adolescence. Craig did not view his mother as seriously impaired, although he recalled worrying a great deal that she might become too stressed and again require hospitalization. As a consequence, he remembered "trying to help out as much as possible."

Craig also reported a history of school phobia. He recalled that he had never felt relaxed in school and was intimidated by many teachers. He remembered having been "humiliated" on several occasions when he found himself unable to answer a question in class. As a result, he often feigned illness to avoid going to school. Craig rarely involved himself in team sports or other outside activities during his school years. Apart from taking piano lessons and participating in recitals, Craig tried only one group activity, the Boy Scouts, with disastrous consequences. Shortly after joining the scouts, Craig went on an overnight camping trip with his troop. He became so anxious, however, that special arrangements had to be made to return him home the next morning. This event also caused him considerable humiliation and embarrassment. When the therapist asked about his thought process prior to and during the camping trip, Craig remembered thinking, "I'm not like these other kids. I don't have what it takes."

The therapist asked Craig about his parents' reactions to his history of physical complaints and to his academic and social failures. On the one hand, his parents habitually minimized the significance of such events and suggested that they were not worth getting too upset about. On the other hand, both parents also reminded Craig again and again that his susceptibility to illness and lack of "toughness" reflected some constitutional or characterological weakness.

The therapist was uncomfortable with the ease with which Craig accepted his parents' communications. More to the point, he was growing angry with Craig's parents for the history of debilitating messages they had delivered to their son. The therapist reminded himself, however, that both parents experienced significant psychiatric problems of their own. They were unlikely to have had much insight into the effects of their parenting. Moreover, since they probably saw themselves as incompetent, it was predictable that they also would have viewed their son as weak or defective in some way. The therapist also assumed that Craig's parents were unable to address issues directly with one another. The parents might have denied their own relationship problems and, instead, focused obsessively on their troubled son. Given a stronger alliance with the client, the therapist might have attempted to focus Craig's attention on his reaction (or lack thereof) to his parents' communications. With only the seeds of a therapeutic alliance in hand, however, the therapist did not want to risk inducing a loyalty conflict for Craig by asking him to "question" or to "criticize" his parents. Consequently, the therapist thus chose simply to express *curiosity* about what Craig had just described. The expression of curiosity allowed the therapist to demonstrate a benign or naive interest in the subject at hand, while it conveyed in a nonthreatening manner the message, "There *is* something worth paying attention to here."

Th: So your parents gave you two different messages about these situations. One was, "Don't worry about it. No big deal." The other was, "We pretty much expect you to have these kinds of problems since, by nature, you're not someone who is likely to handle challenging situations very well." Is that right?

Craig: Yeah, that's about right.

Th: And when your parents would react this way, let's say for example, to the camping trip, what did you think about their reaction?

Craig: I don't think I ever thought too much about it. I guess it didn't surprise me. That was kind of just their way.

Th: I'm curious [Pauses and looks away momentarily to ensure that he will capture Craig's attention]. Did you ever wish that they might have reacted differently at times—when it was hard for you to handle the anxiety of being away from home?

Craig: *I never really thought about it.*

Th: I wonder if you might have wished they'd have pushed you a bit, you know, to hang in there, to encourage you to try to stick it out?

Here the therapist spoke to two issues. First, the therapist implied that he would expect that *any* parents would encourage their child to persevere when confronted with a challenging situation. Second, the therapist suggested that Craig would need to understand the ramifications of his parents *not* having encouraged more assertive responses.

Craig: That *definitely* was not their way. They weren't very aggressive themselves, and I suppose they didn't instill much aggressiveness in me. I think they just didn't want me to get hurt or upset.

Th: I'm sure that was the case. It sounds like they've been very concerned about you and have tried to figure out how best to help you.

The therapist wanted to avoid any appearance of blaming Craig's parents. He offered a conciliatory statement about them as Craig began to defend them. The therapist did decide subsequently to try one more probe.

Th: Let's say for a moment that they *had* pushed more at those times when you wanted to avoid a scary situation. What do you think that would have been like for you?

Craig: Well, on the one hand, I probably would have gotten more upset because I can remember on the camping trip, for example, just wanting to go home as soon as possible. On the other hand, who knows? Maybe it would have done me some good. I guess they made it pretty easy for me get out of things I didn't like.

The therapist noted that although Craig continued to respond to the line of questioning, the client's tone and manner suggested he was beginning to feel disloyal to his parents. Although the therapist would address Craig's discomfort at a later point in treatment, he decided to "play it safe" for the time being, by moving on to other historical topics.

The therapist began the second session in standard fashion by asking whether Craig had had any reactions to the initial meeting that he wished to share. The client's responses to such an inquiry provide the therapist with various types of information. For example, the therapist can assume that denial mechanisms are operative when clients report either that they remembered little of the previous session or that they had reflected upon it only briefly. Should the client return increasingly symptomatic and/or more intensely focused on perseverative themes, the therapist may suspect that the prior discussion(s) had been at least moderately threatening and will need to develop a posture to respond to the client's discomfort. On the other hand, the therapist receives an "open invitation" to revisit or explore anew core themes when the client reports having spent time reflecting upon them.

Craig reported no particular negative reaction to his first session. He said that he was comfortable with the therapist's style and that he had some increased optimism about the prospects for change. The therapist heard the client's response as permission to expand upon a variety of themes that had surfaced in the initial meeting. These themes included separation difficulties, triangulation and parentification, the effects of parental messages on self-image, the effects of parental impairment on their ability to nurture and protect, denial on Craig's part and in the family system, and so on.

The therapist asked the client to describe his parents' relationship. The client's nonverbal response to the question suggested that he rarely thought about his parents in *relationship to one another*. Craig described a state of constant conflict and alienation in his parent's marriage. The client revealed that he frequently functioned as companion and confidante for his mother, whom he considered his best friend. Unfortunately, Craig did not find it unusual that he spent all his leisure time with his mother instead of with young people his own age, nor was he apparently uncomfortable being privy to so much information about his parents' personal lives. Consequently, the therapist had to be careful to limit his activities during this discussion to information gathering. Only later in treatment was Craig open to examining the negative effects of his parentified role in the family, the enmeshed relationship with his mother, and his chronic involvement in the parental conflicts.

SOCRATIC DIALOGUE

As illustrated in a number of classic texts on cognitive therapy (Beck et al., 1979; Beck & Emery, 1985) and rational emotive therapy (Walen, DiGiuseppe, & Wessler, 1971), Socratic dialogue aims to lead the client through a body of data that underscore cognitive distortions. In Socratic dialogue, the therapist leads the client with a series of probing questions but assumes a fairly neutral, investigatory stance, so that the individual can more easily remain focused on the information at hand. The therapist underscores anomalies or inherent contradictions in the client's responses as he or she gently encourages the individual to reconsider interpretations in light of such data.

The effectiveness of Socratic dialogue often depends on the therapist's ability to elicit the *specific* data that form the basis of the client's conclusions and interpretations. Inevitably the therapist will attempt to zero in on inconsistencies or other "soft spots" in the client's thinking about a particular subject or incident. The clinician must learn how to pursue a line of questioning in a fairly persistent manner without making the client feel as if he or she is being grilled. The therapist also needs to become skilled at asking for more detail about the client's reasoning processes without sending blaming or invalidating messages. In our experience, fairly subtle differences in wording and intonation can turn a seemingly neutral question into a more threatening one, particularly with clients who are inordinately sensitive to blame or criticism of any kind. Moreover, a line of questioning will probably be less threatening if the therapist has taken the time to make empathic reflective statements to the client *first* (e.g., "It sounds like it was a very lonely and painful evening for you") before attempting to dissect the individual's reactions.

Successful implementation of Socratic dialogue enables the client to recognize that the cognitions in question are irrational or erroneous in some manner. Recognition of the irrational nature of particular cognitions is only part of the therapeutic battle, however, particularly when long-term recovery is the goal of treatment. Once the client can recognize the irrational cognitions, he or she then needs to understand how the ideation in question relates to basic schema and information-processing strategies. In family of origin work, the therapist will seek whenever possible to forge a strong link between the current distortions and the client's developmental history.

In our treatment approach, we utilize Socratic dialogue to achieve multiple additional goals with clients over and above the recognition of current cognitive distortions. The therapist may want to employ a Socratic approach to heighten the client's awareness of any or all of the mechanisms we listed at the beginning of this chapter. In some cases, particularly with clients who lack psychological mindedness, or who suffer from pervasive use of denial mechanisms, the therapist may use Socratic dialogue to establish and reinforce the most basic assumption underlying treatment, that family of origin conditions have the power to influence the individual's past and current functioning.

For example, Gary entered treatment shortly after his wife asked him to leave the home. His wife complained of his rigid, perfectionistic attitudes about order and cleanliness, his tendency to abuse her verbally when he was frustrated, and his recurring bouts of irrational jealousy. During his initial interview, Gary described having grown up with two physically abusive parents, who themselves were quite obsessed with order and cleanliness. Although he tolerated the therapist's attempts to obtain a history, it was clear that the client viewed the family of origin material as irrelevant with respect to his current pressing difficulties. Gary certainly remembered having been unhappy growing up in an abusive family; however, he seemed to view himself as not having been affected by his early experiences in any significant or enduring manner. Not surprisingly, he drew a complete blank during the initial interview when the therapist asked him questions such as, "How did the treatment you received from your parents affect your self-image when you were growing up?" In a subsequent session, the therapist returned to the subject of Gary's early family history by initiating the dialogue which follows:

Th: If you don't mind, I want to go back over some of the things you told me about your family history, in order to understand better some of the experiences you described, and to see whether there are any connections between your background and the problems in your marriage. Will you begin by describing to me some of the typical ways in which your parents responded when you or your siblings acted up?

Gary: My father worked long hours, so he usually wasn't around when things actually happened. When he got home though, he would spank us on the butt with a belt if my mother told him we needed it.

Th: Did he ever hit you on other places besides your bottom?

Gary: Not too often. Once in a while he might backhand somebody in the mouth if they started getting fresh.

Th: Did he ever hit you with any objects other than a belt, or with his fists instead of the back of his hand?

Gary: Not that I can remember. My mother, though, when she got pissed off, she'd grab anything that was handy. She might hit you with some kind of stick or throw a pan at you. One time, she threw a plate at me so hard that it shattered and opened up a big gash on my face. I actually had to go to the hospital and have stitches that time. The doctors thought I had some kind of concussion, so they made me stay overnight there.

Th: Were your mother's violent outbursts predictable at all?

Gary: Sure, if one of us screwed up in a big way, we knew we'd be getting a beating, from her, and probably from him too, when he got home. Sometimes though, she would flip out over something really small, sometimes for no reason at all. You never knew what she was going to do.

Th: I'm wondering if there was also a lot of verbal abuse in your house when you were growing up. How did your parents talk to you when they were irritated or angry?

Gary: The yelling and the name-calling were constant. It seemed like they called us "asshole" or "shithead" all the time.

Th: So your parents, especially your mother, could be extremely violent, at times in an unpredictable way. In addition to beatings, there was constant verbal abuse in your house when you were growing up. How did you learn to protect yourself?

Gary: (Laughs derisively.) I learned to stay away from my mother, especially if she had anything sharp or heavy in her hand. I also tried to keep a low profile when I was around the house.

Th: Did those strategies help you to avoid beatings?

Gary: Not really. Since I was the oldest, I always got blamed for everything that happened anyway. As soon as I was old enough, I got a job so I didn't have to go right home after school. By the time I was 16, I had saved enough money to buy a car. Then I spent even less time at home.

Th: Do you recall feeling afraid of your mother?

Gary: Not really. I just stayed away from her as much as I could.

Th: I realize you don't remember actually *feeling* afraid of your mother, but I think you'd agree that your efforts to distance yourself from her certainly sound like they were motivated by a desire for self-preservation, which is really another way of saying they were motivated by fear. I'd like you to think about something. How would you predict *another* kid would begin to feel toward a parent who subjected him to violent beatings on an unpredictable basis?

Gary: I think he'd be scared—and maybe pretty angry too.

Th: I agree. Do you think those unpredictable beatings might make him distrustful as well, maybe even toward people other than his parents?

Gary: Sure. He might start to have a chip on his shoulder or something.

Th: Can you think of a reason why you would react differently from any other kid under similar circumstances?

Gary: It seems like I might have been different, but I really can't think of any reasons why that might have been true.

Th: I'm also having trouble thinking of any reason why you wouldn't have been scared by the violence in the household, much like any other little boy. I think we should assume for now that you were. It's interesting to me that you also mentioned the idea of becoming angry in response to physical abuse. You may not realize it, but anger and fear are very closely related in that they are both reactions to threat. I'm reminded that Val has complained that you are tense and angry all the time with her. I can't help but think that the similarity between your behavior in the marriage and the behavior of your parents toward you isn't a coincidence. After all, the family is where kids learn the basics about relationships. This may seem like an unrelated question, but, do you hit your kids?

Gary: No way!

Th: Why not?

Gary: I don't want to screw them up, or hurt them the way I was hurt.

Th: Listen for a minute to what you just said. "I don't want to screw them up or hurt them the way I was hurt." Your philosophy of raising children is another acknowledgment of how strongly your parents' behaviors affected you when you were growing up. You had trouble answering me before when I asked you how the physical and verbal abuse you experienced affected your self-image. Let's think about that question again, this time from the standpoint of Gary Junior. Suppose that in addition to hitting him regularly, you also kept calling him "asshole" and "shithead" all the time. Suppose you never ever apologized for what you said or did to him. Remember that your son loves you and respects you. Right now he thinks you know all there is to know. Would he think *you* had a problem, or would he begin to think that maybe he *deserved* to be abused?

Gary: He wouldn't know enough to realize that I had a problem. He can't even understand why Val and I are separated.

Th: How do you think your son would begin to feel about himself after years of abusive treatment from you?

Gary: When you put it like that, I guess he would begin to feel pretty lousy about himself. It makes me feel glad I don't hit my kids.

Th: Let me summarize our discussion so far. By your description, the conditions in your family during your childhood were very stressful, perhaps more stressful than you realized. You were a victim of constant verbal abuse and frequent, unpredictable physical abuse. You tried to learn strategies to avoid being beaten, but were only partially successful, at least until you were old enough to spend much of your time out of the house. Your actions as a child suggest that you were afraid much of the time and probably angry as well. You acknowledge that any other child would have reacted in a similar manner. As you think about your own children, you can see the possibility that the abuse you received also had a profound effect on your self-esteem. I have pointed out that there seem to be some similar themes playing out in your behavior with Val, although at this time I am not sure exactly how your family of origin experiences and your marital experiences are connected.

The reader should note that in the above example, the therapist stuck very closely to the raw data that the client provided as he patiently built a case for the notion that Gary's abusive childhood may have had a lasting impact on him. As we discuss in greater detail below, the therapist attempted to shift the perspective at several points in the dialogue by asking Gary to imagine the likely effects on other children exposed to similar circumstances. Because Gary showed so little insight into the effects of his family of origin on his functioning as a child and an adolescent, the therapist was careful not to speculate extensively on the possible connections between the client's early experiences and his current marital difficulties. The therapist offered frequent capsule summaries during the dialogue using direct quotations from the client whenever possible. As the therapist delivered the summary statements, he maintained continuous eye contact with Gary. If he had seen signs of confusion on Gary's part, he would have solicited feedback from him immediately, perhaps by asking the client to summarize what he had heard up to that point.

Many of our clients are adept at anticipating, and delivering, what others appear to expect from them. They are prone to sense the "demand characteristics" of an interpersonal situation, and they play along accordingly, without verbalizing or otherwise revealing their inner reactions to the interaction. Clients with extensive trauma in their histories may simply "space out" and go through the motions. Similarly, some clients may try to get the therapist off a threatening topic by behaving as cooperatively as possible in the hopes of thereby bringing the discussion to a more speedy conclusion. An overly aggressive attempt at Socratic dialogue with such individuals may appear on the surface to result in attitude change or increased insight on the part of the client, when in fact it only produces acquiescence or capitulation to the perceived expectations of the therapist. If a Socratic dialogue is going "too well," then the therapist needs to back off and attempt to assess the nature of the client's involvement in the process, probably by inquiring specifically about some of the mechanisms described above. The therapist may open the discussion with comments such as:

- Are you thinking about what I expect from you right now?
- I'm concerned that you might disagree with me on some level but don't want to show it, maybe for fear of letting me down or making me angry? Have you had any thoughts along those lines?
- I'm wondering if maybe you really would like this part of the conversation to end as soon as possible but can't tell me

you feel that way. Am I totally off the mark, or am I in the ballpark?

- I'm worried that you might let me tell you how you think and feel just the way some of the other people in your life do. I think I might be doing that inadvertently right now, and it's not how I want to act in here with you. Were you starting to feel as though you were talking to your mother (father, husband, wife, etc.) ?
- You've told me that sometimes you space out when people are pressuring you or giving you a hard time in some way. I wonder if maybe you were doing that just now. How would I know if you started spacing out during one of our discussions?

The therapist may need to preempt or address the shame or embarrassment on the client's part that may well accompany recognition of cognitive distortions. Otherwise, instead of utilizing the therapeutic exchange as a learning experience, the client may simply feel stupid or defective. The client may feel particularly uncomfortable as a result of identifying a recurring cognitive distortion, especially one which has occupied center stage in treatment previously. The client may express the attitude "See! There I go again!" The therapist needs to remind the client continually that he or she *expects* to encounter the same kind of distortions again and again and, indeed, *welcomes* the opportunity to address the same underlying issues repeatedly. The therapist should emphasize that the recurrent nature of distortions is a reflection of the strength of the underlying mechanisms not of the client's incompetence or stupidity.

At times the therapist may utilize Socratic dialogue more effectively with a particular client if he or she changes the content or the perspective of the discussion somewhat. For example, suppose a woman reports having been repeatedly sexually abused by a man in her neighborhood when she was between the ages of eleven and thirteen. She sees the sexual relationship as having been consensual, as opposed to abusive or exploitative. She maintains that she knew the relationship was wrong, but came back for more again and again, because she wanted the attention. The client states these ideas with an air of absolute conviction, making it clear through her demeanor that she is not likely to consider alternative viewpoints. Despite the client's high degree of belief in the ideas she has expressed about herself, the therapist suspects that she will at least tolerate further discussion on the topics in question without becoming defensive or otherwise uncooperative. Consequently, the therapist decides to back up and approach the issue of child sexual abuse from another pathway, one which might involve ideas associated with a more moderate degree of belief on the part of the client. The therapist has a number of potential options available at this point:

1. Address the sexual abuse of *another* child, not the client. The therapist may center the discussion on a hypothetical child, another client, the client's child, or even his or her own child. To make the discussion more powerful, the therapist may hold up a picture of the client's child, or even his or her own child, pointing to it frequently, while repeatedly asking the client to respond to the hypothetical sexual abuse of this particular youngster.

2. Move the discussion to another type of abuse or victimization of a child, involving either the client or someone else. What happens when an adult involves a child in prostitution, burglary, or other criminal activities? Who assumes culpability or criminal responsibility? In this manner, the therapist may set up a straw man, particularly if he or she knows in advance that the client will not blame the victim.

3. Address more general aspects of sexual abuse and sexuality in childhood. When is it a crime for an adult to have sexual contact with a minor? Can it be a crime even if no force is involved, or if the child initiates the contact? At what age can a child give his or her consent to sexual relationships with adults? At what age does a child truly understand all the ramifications associated with engaging in sexual relations? What if the adult uses his or her superior power or cunning to manipulate the child? The therapist may also ask the client if he or she is aware that the legal system would consider sexual contact between an adult and a child to be *rape*. The therapist may continue to use the designation of rape as he or she probes for the client's reactions to this new, more powerful label. In the meantime, the therapist's use of such a forceful term sends a strong metacommunicative message to the client about the degree of his or her victimization.

Even when the therapist addresses the issue at hand through an alternative pathway, the client may still arrive at the same self-defeating conclusions. Likewise, the client may address the matter of abuse quite differently in a less personally relevant context, only to cap the discussion by stating "That may be true for someone else, but it's still a different story when it involves me." The therapist should not become overly discouraged by such developments. First of all, as we preach repeatedly to our clients, the changing of long-standing beliefs takes time, practice, and repetition. *Remember that our treatment goal is to build and strengthen new beliefs that will eventually compete successfully with more strongly held, well-established ideas on the client's part.* Gradually, the alternative viewpoints the therapist helps to develop through Socratic

dialogue and other means may begin to insinuate themselves permanently into the client's frame of reference. It will be necessary to go over
the same ground many times with the client before the therapist can
legitimately conclude that efforts to change certain ideas will be futile.
*As long as the client tolerates the discussion without becoming defensive or
otherwise resistant, then the therapist has accomplished an important goal,
namely providing the client with an opportunity to process alternative data.* As
long as the client does not feel pressured by the therapist in the process,
each segment of Socratic dialogue can help to provide a foundation for
long-term change, even if the immediate results are not dramatic.

Like our hypothetical client described above, Betsy had been repeatedly
sexually abused by several older men when she was between the ages
of 10 and 13. However, she did not view herself as having been victimized. Instead, she emphasized the fact that she had consistently
initiated contact with the individuals involved, knowing that sexual
activities would occur, and fully realizing that such activities were
wrong. In some instances, she saw herself, not the man, as having been
the one who performed the seduction. As she put it, "I wanted the
attention, and I was willing to do whatever I had to do to get it." Betsy's
convictions about her childhood sexual victimization seemed to be
utterly unshakable. She experienced such overpowering feelings of
worthlessness associated with these cognitions that she could only tolerate very limited discussions of the subject during her treatment sessions. If she became too uncomfortable, Betsy would be unable to maintain eye contact with the therapist for the remainder of the interview.
    The therapist continued to address the subject of childhood sexual
abuse with Betsy, but he did so for shorter periods of time, all the while
monitoring the client's reactions very closely. He quickly changed topics if Betsy appeared to grow increasingly uncomfortable and encouraged her to ask him to terminate a particular line of conversation any
time he failed to notice her discomfort in time. He frequently adjusted
the content and perspective of their discussions, as described earlier in
this section, often centering the dialogue on other children and other
types of childhood victimization. The therapist also spoke a great deal
to Betsy about the experiences and reactions of other clients who had
been sexually abused in childhood. He encouraged her to think about
the actions and motives of perpetrators who had abused other children.
Through the use of Socratic dialogue, he also directed her to think in a
more general, abstract way about the sequelae of childhood sexual
abuse, again as manifested in the lives of other individuals. All the
while the therapist tended to refer very lightly, if at all, to the actual
details of Betsy's experiences.

Although Betsy's core beliefs about her own experiences appeared to be as immutable as they ever had been, after many months of treatment, there were other, more subtle indications that the therapist's efforts with her were yielding some results. She began to tolerate their discussions of sexual abuse for far longer periods and with less overt anxiety. She sustained eye contact with the therapist much more consistently during their sessions. Instead of simply becoming silent and withdrawn, Betsy was more often able to articulate her reactions when she did begin to feel overwhelmed by feelings of worthlessness. In her day-to-day life, she also seemed less withdrawn with people. Despite her chronic feelings of alienation, she continued to increase her degree of social involvement with peers. Betsy also began dating for the first time in years, although, predictably, she found the sexual aspect of her relationships with men to be extremely uncomfortable. Instead of describing amorphous feelings of terror or depression that threatened to overpower her, she now referred to "that core feeling of being no good." Although she still was unable to view herself as having been victimized, Betsy no longer objected to the therapist's contention that she had been adversely affected by her childhood sexual experiences. Instead of objecting to the idea that she needed to work on the issue of childhood sexual abuse, the client now expressed a desire to get it over with as soon as possible. Perhaps the most significant indication of the impact of treatment involved Betsy's responses to a close friend who was struggling with new recollections of having been abused by her stepfather. In an effort to help her friend, Betsy had repeated many of the therapist's remarks from previous sessions, practically verbatim. She had not simply parroted the therapist's statements however. It was clear that she not only had internalized the therapist's words about sexual abuse but had also absorbed and understood the underlying *concepts* with a high degree of sophistication. As Betsy described the interaction with her friend, the therapist felt a buoyant sense of optimism about the client's prospects for recovery.

RELABELING OR REFRAMING MANEUVERS

The client who has grown up in a chaotic, rejecting, abusive, or otherwise dysfunctional environment will show distorted attributional processes in many ways. Clients frequently frame personal problems in ways that permit no workable solutions yet lead to recurring feelings of helplessness and worthlessness. A man who has experienced chronic school and work underachievement, for example, will say "I've failed because I am lazy." All he can do with such a label is resolve to work harder, and of course, beat himself up even more when he fails to work hard enough. To the extent that the client views "laziness" as an immutable personal trait, he will experience a sense of futility and hopelessness as he contemplates the future. If the man seeks treatment for the chronic underachievement, the therapist will probably need to help the client reframe the problem in some manner. Otherwise, the client is likely to continue the same cycle of avoidance behaviors and self-recrimination, only now feeling that he has also failed the therapist (or vice versa). In our experience, an incremental behavioral approach, although eminently sensible, will not prove to be effective in a case of chronic avoidance, at least not until the therapist helps the client to identify the cognitive underpinnings of the problem.

With the therapist's assistance, the client may come to recognize that a fear of failure (and a fear of the feelings of worthlessness which will result from failure), not inherent laziness, is the true source of his problem. Moreover, the client may also eventually understand how chronic abuse and rejection in his family of origin discouraged initiative and robbed him of the self-confidence that enables an individual to risk failure. This new framework begins to open up new pathways for the solution of the client's problem. Most of us probably feel much less stigmatized or shameful viewing ourselves as "fearful" as opposed to "lazy," particularly if we can trace the origin of such feelings back to events in childhood over which we truly had no control. Laziness is an all-or-nothing problem, in that either one manifests it or one doesn't. On the other hand, an individual *can* begin to overcome fear *gradually*, particularly if he or she develops a trusting relationship with a knowledgeable therapist.

Over the course of treatment, the cognitive therapist will help the client to affix new labels to a wide range of thoughts, feelings, behaviors, and interpersonal experiences. Relabeling or reframing maneuvers are of course essential to many other approaches to individual, marital, and family treatment (e.g., Watzlawick, Weakland, & Fisch, 1974). However, in cognitively oriented treatment, the therapist's goal is not only to provide a temporary frame for facilitating behavior change or restructuring the family system, but also to change a client's attributions in an *enduring* way, thereby providing a more lasting foundation for the relief of symptoms. Enduring changes in beliefs require repeated interventions by the therapist and most likely practice and homework on the part of the client. Moreover, in our treatment model, our attempts to reframe or relabel client experiences will typically include explicit references to the individual's family of origin.

For example, Ann accumulated thousands of dollars in credit card expenses feeding her insatiable desire for stylish clothing. She described herself to the therapist as "vain, selfish, and materialistic." Ann reported with some embarrassment that she had enough clothing in her closet to wear a different outfit to work each day for 8 or 9 weeks before having to repeat herself! She experienced a flood of guilty feelings as she described how she had often lied to her husband to conceal her expenditures. "Now the whole family has to suffer financially for the rest of the year to pay for my expensive, disgusting habits," she told the therapist. The solution as she saw it, was simple: Stop the compulsive behavior. Unable to stop the shopping and spending for more than a few weeks at a time, however, Ann had no "fall back position" and remained stuck in a repetitive cycle of compulsive behaviors and self-denigration. Ann wondered aloud how motivated she *really* was to stop the problem, accusing herself of not wanting to change.

Ann's parents were Holocaust survivors from Eastern Europe. Immigrating to the United States in the late 1940s, they had worked hard at factory jobs for several years in order to save sufficient funds to purchase a modest house. When Ann was 5, her mother contracted polio and remained severely disabled until her death 12 years later. From a young age, Ann had been entrusted with many of the household responsibilities, including much of the care of her mother. In the meantime, the father, who probably suffered from posttraumatic stress disorder himself, began to decompensate following the onset of his wife's illness. He drank heavily and became increasingly secretive and paranoid, hoarding most of what little money he managed to earn. Ann recalled how her father's miserliness reduced the family to a threadbare, poverty-stricken existence. Moreover, the father was frequently and unpredictably abusive toward her, both verbally and physically.

Being poor, Jewish, and the child of foreign-born parents conferred no social advantages in the affluent suburb where Ann grew up. In grade school, she was clearly more shabbily dressed than the other children. Because of her father's increasingly bizarre behavior, she stopped inviting classmates to her house. Paradoxically, Ann found her greatest satisfactions outside the home, where her diligence and seriousness seemed to produce positive results. From an early age, she worked at a variety of jobs. Somehow she always managed to squirrel away enough money to buy "presentable" clothes for herself, so that she could at least feel that she no longer stood out as different from her peers. Ann's excellent academic performance earned her a full scholarship to college. Shortly after her mother's death, Ann left home and never looked back.

During the first few treatment sessions, Ann found it very painful to reveal her family history. She also seemed extremely embarrassed about having cried in front of the therapist as she discussed her parents. At one point, she began to question the relevance of such historical data with respect to her presenting problems, although at another juncture in the conversation she also said, "I guess there are some things I have to face, but I don't know if I can do that right now." Thinking that he had sufficient background information on the client at this point, the therapist vowed to himself to keep historical discussions well contained for the time being, particularly until Ann could see more clearly the potential benefits associated with such conversations.

The therapist performed a number of relabeling maneuvers with the client's compulsive shopping and her obsession with clothing. Over a number of sessions, the therapist engaged in a series of Socratic dialogues with Ann, directed toward several goals. First, he tried to underscore the *driven* nature of the problem. The therapist asked Ann about her previous attempts to stop the behavior, attempts in which good intentions repeatedly ran aground. Ann readily acknowledged that the thoughts, feelings, and behaviors associated with this problem were in their own way out of control in that they occurred despite her resolutions to the contrary. The therapist told the client that he wanted to explore her discomfort over the compulsive shopping in greater detail.

Th: You said a while ago that maybe you really don't want to stop the compulsive shopping. If that's so, why aren't you simply able to enjoy your new clothes without feeling so guilty?

Ann: Because my obsession has hurt myself and other people.

Th: Is that contrary to your values?

Ann: Yes it is, even though maybe I don't always show it.

Th: From everything you've said about yourself, and the way you've acted in here, I *can* believe that hurting others is very much against your moral code. I would suspect that deception of any kind is unacceptable to you as well. Am I right?

Ann: Sure. I *hate* having to lie about the money I spend.

Th: I believe you do. That's an important point to consider when you think about the relationship between the compulsive shopping and who you really are as a person. It's clear that deceiving and hurting other people makes you feel *awful* about yourself. I think that says something about where your real values are. Otherwise, why would your conscience bother you? You would only be distressed if you happened to get caught.

Notice that in a fairly unobtrusive way, the therapist began to restore some of the client's self-respect, by relabeling her guilt in more positive terms, as a reflection of her well-developed sense of morality. The therapist would make similar interventions many times during subsequent sessions with Ann. Now the therapist sought to explore the client's own attributions for her compulsive behaviors and to lay the foundation for alternate explanations.

Ann: If what you say is true, why can't I stop doing it?

Th: I think that's an excellent question, one that I think we're going to be able to answer together. First of all, I assume that there must be an *extremely powerful force* motivating you to do things that so clearly violate your own ethical principles. Why do you think you buy clothes so compulsively?

Ann: I think it's because I want to look better than everyone else in the office. I guess I just need a lot of approval from other people.

Th: Do you buy a lot of really expensive clothing, clothing that looks like "money" to the other women at the office?

Ann: Not necessarily. I do a lot of shopping at outlets. I look for things on sale too, believe it or not. I'm not obsessed with designer stuff, either. I just buy a *lot* of merchandise, a lot of the time.

Th: I guess if the motivation was to look better than others, I'd have expected you to be a lot more status conscious in what you picked out. What about jewelry? Isn't wearing a lot of expensive jewelry a typical way that women attempt to outclass one another? I notice you're only wearing a bracelet and a wedding ring.

Ann: (Glances at her wrist and chuckles) Well, I guess jewelry never really turned me on.

Th: But if your goal was to make a big splash, to feel superior, why would you pass up the chance to wear a lot of gold or a big diamond?

Ann: I don't know. I guess it doesn't make sense.

Th: Maybe that's because some other issues are motivating your behavior.

The therapist wanted to have the client picture a vulnerable, insecure, frightened woman buying all those clothes, rather than a vain, spoiled, twisted one. To facilitate such a transformation, the therapist needed to introduce the idea that Ann was driven not by the need to look good to everyone *but by the fear of looking badly*. With some trepidation, he referred back to the client's history.

Th: I'm remembering what you told me about your high school years.

How important it was for you look "presentable." Were you trying to look better than everyone else or were you just trying to fit in?

Ann: I was just trying to fit in.

Th: And why was that important to you?

Ann: I was tired of looking shabby, like a refugee. I used to throw away my school pictures as soon as I got them. I didn't even bring them home. My teachers and my friends' parents all looked at me like they felt sorry for me. I could feel it. I hated that.

Th: Can you recall how all that made you feel about yourself?

Ann: Awful, just awful. When I walked into the bathroom or the locker room with other girls, I hated seeing my reflection in the mirror next to theirs.

Th: Think about what you just told me. Not having proper clothes to wear made you feel awful about yourself, worthless. *That's* the problem that I think the compulsive shopping attempts to solve. It's a way to prevent you from experiencing feelings of worthlessness. I know I don't have to explain to you how painful those feelings can be. Ironically enough, the shopping ends up creating the problem it attempts to solve, because it ultimately makes you feel lousy about yourself.

The therapist told Ann that in his experience, people fought almost as hard to avoid a sense of worthlessness as they did to sustain the basics of life itself. He reminded her that many glamorous and famous individuals, such as Marilyn Monroe, sought fame and public adulation, not to feel superior to others, but to achieve a basic sense of self-worth. For the time being at least, Ann seemed to concur with the therapist's analysis. Moreover, she was able to acknowledge that she experienced recurring intense fears about her own competence and attractiveness, fears she could temporarily quell at times by buying new clothes.

Using the same model of compulsive shopping as a coping strategy, the therapist walked the client through an explanation of why her frequent attempts to stop the behaviors were accompanied by equally frequent relapses. At some point, her guilty feelings, which had led to resolutions to stop the compulsive behaviors, would begin to subside only to be overtaken by the client's fears about her own worth, particularly in the eyes of others. Beginning in adolescence, Ann had been able to achieve relief, albeit temporary, from feelings of intimidation and inferiority by buying a new outfit. No wonder the frequent resolutions to stop the problem behaviors never achieved any results! Without her preferred coping strategy, the client was left defenseless against mounting anxiety about her own worth. The therapist again reminded Ann of a bitter irony: One of the few things that made her feel good enough about herself to be able to interact constructively with other people ended up having a huge price tag of guilt and, ultimately, worthlessness, associated with it. The therapist used the example of Solomon's dogs to demonstrate to Ann how a coping strategy can persist in the face of self-defeating consequences.

Over several months, the therapist looked for repeated opportunities to review his model of the compulsive shopping with the client. Instead of seeing herself driven by vanity, or by some narcissistic desire to be the center of attention, Ann slowly began to adopt an alternative conceptualization, one that pictured her as pursuing a desperate solution to the desolate feelings of worthlessness, a solution which was ultimately self-defeating. By no means was she fully convinced of this alternative conceptualization, however. Consequently, the therapist walked her through the pertinent data again and again, until her degree of belief in the new viewpoint seemed to remain consistently high.

In the meantime, the therapist tried to redirect the client's attention continually away from the compulsive behaviors, and the efforts to control them, back toward the precipitating factors. Since Ann was now more willing to tolerate a detailed examination of her family history, the therapist was able to focus on how her father's abusive behavior had affected her self-image. With the therapist's assistance, Ann was able to recognize the historical origins of her perfectionistic, self-critical attitudes.

The therapist explicitly disavowed any interest for the time being in helping Ann find a way to control the shopping and spending. The therapist told her, "In order to help you do a better job of controling these behaviors, we need to learn much more about what triggers them off. I suspect that even you are not fully aware of the extent to which the fear of being seen as worthless affects your behavior. I think you're going to find that it's much more of an issue than you realized, on a day by day, moment-to-moment basis." The therapist asked Ann to monitor thoughts about her appearance and her body and encouraged her to pay close attention to the cognitions, emotions, and behaviors that occurred immediately after such thoughts. During another period, the therapist also asked the client to keep a log of social situations in which she felt at all uncomfortable about herself. Through self-monitoring, Ann herself was able to trace the connections between her insecure thoughts and the impulse to buy new clothes. As she became aware of these connections, she achieved a high level of control over her compulsive shopping. She stabilized her behavior without explicit involvement or intervention on the part of the therapist. Ann also learned over time to "talk back" to many of the negative cognitions about herself, thereby improving her overall morale and sense of competence.

WAYS OF STIMULATING RECOLLECTIONS

The client's recollections of childhood constitute the raw material that the therapist uses to build awareness of family of origin issues. It is frequently necessary for the therapist to go beyond the type of initial history taking we described in Chapter 6, particularly when working with clients whose early memories are sparse or with individuals who are trauma survivors. In fact, there may be a need at *several* points in the therapeutic process for the clinician to invest considerable time stimulating and discussing client recollections. Needless to say, individuals who experience a process of trauma revelation may completely rewrite their personal histories before they are finished with treatment.

The more detailed the client's memories, the more accurate the therapist's hypotheses regarding the effects of early experiences on current functioning. Well-articulated recollections enable the therapist to create and present more *credible* formulations, which are firmly rooted in the client's experience. Moreover, detailed memories give the therapist much greater access to the client's unique imagery and phraseology, so that the clinician can incorporate more of these highly personal words and symbols into his or her treatment interventions. Most experienced therapists have developed their own unique methods for eliciting memories from clients. Below are a number of methods of stimulating recollections we have found to be useful:

1. Encouraging the client to visualize: the floor plan of the family home; the interiors of specific rooms; sleeping quarters; being in bed; the yard, the garage and other outbuildings; comparable details of the houses of extended family, particularly if the client stayed there overnight; the neighborhood, woods, or other areas where unsupervised play occurred; the daily journey to and from school; church and other significant structures in the community.

2. Encouraging the client to think about specific events: birthdays, holidays, graduations, sports, or other childhood activities where adults might be present, religious observances, parents' parties in the home, being caught for a particular infraction, bringing home report cards.

3. Surveying with the client the adults and older children with whom he or she interacted during childhood and adolescence, including extended family members, partners of parents or other family members, neighbors, teachers, clergy, babysitters, and so on.

4. Asking the client to review, alone and/or with the therapist, old photos, diaries, letters, yearbooks, and other mementos.

5. Requesting that the client revisit places associated with childhood, and where appropriate and *safe*, seek pertinent information from old friends, family members, and/or other adult authority figures (e.g., priest, teacher, and so on).

6. Utilizing the experiences of another child as a means of anchoring their recollections or perceptions of childhood.

7. Facilitating the client's exposure to high quality "projective materials," including self-help texts, novels, plays, films, poetry, music, and visual arts, and building upon the individual's responses to such stimuli.

8. Encouraging the client to attend group treatment, Twelve-Step or other self-help groups, lectures, or workshops on relevant family of origin topics, and so on.

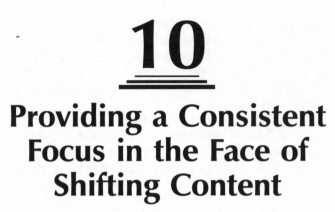

10

Providing a Consistent Focus in the Face of Shifting Content

THE IMPORTANCE OF CONTINUITY IN TREATMENT

Many of our clients live turbulent and disjointed lives in which the turmoil of the current moment always seems to occupy the foreground. They may find themselves encountering an endless series of threatening events, which prevent them from sustaining attention to ongoing personal issues, practicing new responses, or planning in a positive way for the future. Marked shifts in content from one session to another, which reflect the difficulties clients have in establishing and maintaining priorities, are to be expected. Without the therapist's guidance, these clients may allow the treatment itself to become as fragmented and chaotic as their day-to-day lives. The therapist must establish a consistent focus and a sense of continuity in treatment despite changes in the material presented by the client. Again and again, the therapist must identify the core beliefs and coping strategies revealed in the current distress and return the client's attention away from the "uproar," back toward recurring themes and enduring personal issues.

ANALYZING CRITICAL INCIDENTS IN THE CLIENT'S CURRENT LIFE

Since most of our clients are more concerned about today's distress than they are about yesterday's hardships, they generally want to use their sessions to discuss critical incidents from their current lives. By responding to the individual's current concerns in an empathic manner, the therapist helps to sustain a spirit of collaboration in treatment. The treatment plan should define the overall direction of therapy and provide a "menu" that enables the therapist to extract and expand upon key elements of the material the client presents at any given time. The therapist will consistently try to move the client from focusing on relatively narrow and/or specific current concerns toward considering and confronting the larger personal issues that may be involved. Moreover, the therapist always needs to determine if and how the current material is connected with the client's family of origin experiences.

Some clients consistently present material that makes it relatively easy for the therapist to identify cognitive distortions, information-processing errors, and self-defeating coping strategies and to highlight the links between such mechanisms and family of origin experiences. Other individuals, particularly those who lack insight or habitually externalize blame, make it more difficult for the therapist to perform such tasks. These clients may present fairly consistent themes in treatment, but they do so in a manner that prevents the therapist from isolating and/or confronting workable issues. They may resist the therapist's attempts to reframe difficulties in terms of inner mechanisms as opposed to external stressors. In such instances, the therapist might have to be content to wait patiently but alertly for the individual to provide a suitable opening. In the meantime, the clinician can continue to build the kind of therapeutic relationship that will support more intensive examination of the client's most significant issues.

Other than when the client experiences random traumatic or victimizing events, the therapist should start with the assumption that *any* content the individual volunteers has relevance for the treatment, either because of a connection with family of origin issues or as a statement on the therapeutic process itself. If the therapist cannot find the links between current content and broader issues in the client's life, he or she should then investigate the potential implications. The clinician may still not understand the client's basic patterns of thinking and behavior or the related family of origin circumstances that spawned them. Until the therapist gets to know the client better, he or she will not be able make constructive use of the material the individual presents. Another possibility is that the client has become anxious about the direction therapy has taken and is circling back to some better known territory in order to feel a greater sense of control over the proceedings. It will be necessary for the therapist to identify the source of the client's resistance to treatment *first*, before attempting to change the focus of the sessions. Content that involves obsessive thinking also may be peripheral to the client's real issues, but the exacerbation of such ruminations may signal the presence of another source of discomfort in the individual's life. In such instances the therapist will have to take careful steps to deemphasize the material the client has offered.

The following case involves a client who had stymied her therapist for a long time, because of a number of factors. The client finally recounted a critical incident that enabled the therapist to address new themes involving mechanisms central to the individual's distress. Exploiting the opportunity, the clinician lingered on the incident for several sessions. The therapist based several homework assignments for the client on the themes that emerged from the incident. He also continued to use various aspects of the critical incident in sessions with the client for many months thereafter. As a result, the therapist was able to change the entire focus of treatment with the client and to provide a workable vehicle for her recovery.

Isabelle sought treatment for a chronic low-grade depression. Although the client reported lifelong difficulties with self-esteem, her symptoms seemed to have intensified after her children entered school. The client had grown up with a paranoid, physically abusive mother, who overprotected and idealized her sons while scapegoating her daughters. As the eldest child, Isabelle was a particular target for her mother's rage. She also was expected to take care of the house and her younger siblings. The parents, trapped in a chronically unhappy marriage, consistently attempted to recruit the children into their conflicts. Keeping secrets was a way of life for everyone in the household. Although the father's managerial job accorded the family a solid middle-class status, both parents utilized money as a means of control, depriving the children of all but the bare necessities in the process. Despite the fact that Isabelle excelled academically, she received neither praise nor encouragement for her achievements. In fact, she recalled that her parents had actively discouraged her from attending college.

From all outward appearances, Isabelle and her husband, a highly placed executive in a large insurance company, had ventured far from the shabby West Virginia hill town where she had grown up. Although Isabelle had a wide range of artistic and intellectual interests, she struggled with interpersonal isolation and a lack of meaning in her day-to-day life. She complained of chronic loneliness, but she maintained that the women who lived in her small suburban town only wanted to talk about their children, instead of discussing more appealing topics such as art and literature. She aspired to develop a new career but was completely unable to take the first steps. A very limited number of jobs seemed to appeal to her. She was becoming increasingly compulsive about housekeeping, so that, like her mother, she found herself creating a tense and angry atmosphere in the household. It was the escalating conflicts with her husband and sons that seemed to have pushed Isabelle to seek treatment.

The therapist found it difficult to keep his discussions with Isabelle focused on her own issues. Unlike most of the depressed clients the therapist had seen, Isabelle typically externalized the blame for her negative feelings, onto places, situations, and other persons. Her complaints about her marriage typically centered on her husband's passivity about organizing leisure time activities for the couple and his failures to commemorate special events such as her birthday with the proper flourish. Isabelle usually managed to sound demanding and entitled whenever she discussed her marriage. At times, the client appeared as if she wanted to be pampered by her husband , much as a spoiled child might be treated by a parent. In other instances, the therapist observed that the client and her husband seemed to argue with one another as if they were siblings, vying over the use of a favorite toy or the right to sit in the front seat of the car. Despite the fact that the husband seemed generally supportive of Isabelle, the therapist did suspect that there might be some significant problems in the marriage. However, he had difficulty extracting meaningful content from the client's accounts of various interactions with her husband. Isabelle reacted defensively to any suggestions that she might need to examine her expectations of her husband or that it might be necessary for her to assume a greater degree of responsibility for her own happiness. She was also minimally responsive to the therapist's efforts to highlight connections between her reactions to married life and her deprived, abusive childhood.

Although she was prone to agonize over her every flaw and failure, Isabelle also seemed to consider herself more intellectual and sophisticated than most of the other women she met. The clinician suspected that the chic protective coloration Isabelle had assumed probably turned other people off at times. He could easily picture her appearing snobbish and condescending, particularly with some of her less cosmopolitan peers. It was also clear to the therapist that the client failed to appreciate the positive qualities of many of the people she encountered in her everyday life. Although on one level she appeared to be open to new ideas and new experiences, in her own way Isabelle was quite repressed and inhibited, enslaved by trends and fashions. The therapist believed that Isabelle *felt compelled* to read the latest trendy books, go to the critics' favorite foreign films, and dress like a wealthy Parisian not to feel superior to others *but to experience a basic sense of self-worth*. Unfortunately, the clinician could not find a suitable vehicle for raising these issues with the client without making her feel as if he were criticizing her.

Although she had remained in the home since the birth of her first child, Isabelle had extremely ambivalent feelings about motherhood. She told the therapist she was relieved that she had borne only sons, since she was convinced that she would have been too critical and punitive with daughters, much as her mother had been with her. Isabelle often complained of being neglected and unappreciated by her sons, much as she voiced similar concerns about her husband. She frequently expressed her resentment over the fact that her husband and her sons seemed to share so many interests and activities in common. Isabelle viewed her older son as unemotional, distant, and self-sufficient, a carbon copy of her husband. On the other hand, she described her younger boy as sentimental and insecure, a smaller version of herself. Various efforts on the therapist's part to challenge the client's perceptions of her children had met with little success.

In sum, the therapist found it difficult to translate the material Isabelle presented into workable therapeutic issues. The client's cognitive distortions, although fairly obvious at times, were difficult for the therapist to confront without eliciting defensive reactions. Similarly, the clinician also found it hard to focus on Isabelle's relationship problems without coming across as blaming or critical. Finally, although the therapist was fairly certain that the client's family of origin experiences played an influential role in her presenting complaints, he was generally unable to bring the connections alive for her between historical material and current distress. Nonetheless, the client consistently perceived the clinician as caring and supportive, and continued to come to treatment, week after week.

2/26/92

After many months of treatment, Isabelle arrived for a session in a visibly agitated state. "I've had a miserable 2 weeks," she told the therapist as she sat down. Her distressed facial expression contrasted with her typically well-controlled demeanor. She usually came to her appointments looking stylish and "put together." Today it was clear that she had taken less interest in her appearance. Although the therapist was concerned to see the client in pain, he sensed that he might have an opportunity to strengthen his understanding of her and thereby promote greater self-awareness as a result. Consequently, he settled back and allowed Isabelle to recount the events of the past 2 weeks.

First of all, Isabelle noted that her mother had phoned her from West Virginia just after the last session. At one point in the conversation, the mother had blurted out, "If I say anything that's wrong, I'm sorry." For many years, Isabelle had carefully limited her interactions with both parents so as to avoid being hurt. Isabelle had never known her mother to acknowledge *any* wrongdoing in the past. "I don't like that," she told the therapist, "She doesn't know me and I don't want her to know me. I'm more comfortable being bitter." The therapist was sorely tempted to jump into the subject of the mother's call with both feet but restrained himself because it was obvious that the client had a *series* of events she wanted to share with him.

Isabelle then reminded the therapist that she had predicted her husband would fail to commemorate Valentine's Day properly. As it turned out, his sole acknowledgment of the occasion had been to present her with a humorous get well card, which made no reference at all to their relationship. Isabelle responded angrily, announcing that she would not be giving *him* the gifts she had purchased.

Following the Valentine's Day fiasco, Isabelle had driven off with her husband and two sons to spend what she would later describe as the worst vacation of her life. At the husband's urging, the family had booked a week at a ski area in rural Maine. Since she was not a skier, Isabelle had absolutely nothing to do there all day long while the rest of the family was on the slopes. Predictably—at least from the therapist's point of view—by the end of the first day she had become bored, restless, and angry. Having envisioned dinner at an upscale gourmet restaurant and perhaps some companionship with her husband later, Isabelle was disappointed when the three skiers returned at the end of the day in an exhausted state. Although Isabelle was ready for an evening's entertainment, the others all seemed content to stay in the room, eat take-out food, watch sporting events on television, and retire early. As Isabelle put it, "Here I was with these people who didn't want to do anything for me. I was there because they wanted me to be there. They had nothing planned for me." She added in an indignant tone that she had been "good" on the drive up to the ski area, meaning that she had not complained about anything.

Before the first evening at the ski resort was over, Isabelle had initiated two angry confrontations with her family. By her own account, her behavior that night had been childish and demanding. Moreover, she had addressed her husband and her middle-school aged sons together as a unit, implying that both her spouse *and* her children had a responsibility to make her happy. She evidently had singled out her older son in particular, who, like his father, had failed to show her enough affection. From Isabelle's description, it was clear to the therapist that the boys had experienced considerable guilt and a sense of responsibility in response to their mother's outbursts. It sounded as if both the sons and the husband, upset by the client's behavior, had quickly rushed in to placate her.

Realizing that she would continue to be miserable if she stayed another 6 days at the ski resort, Isabelle came up with what sounded to the therapist like a fairly sensible plan. She wanted to drive home and come back to pick the rest of the family up at the end of their vacation. She had no qualms about making the 4 hour trip by herself, nor was she reluctant to spend the rest of the week alone. Unfortunately, her husband was uncomfortable with her plan. He told her that he would "worry too much" about her if she were to drive all the way home by herself. Instead, he suggested that she travel to the nearest city, Portland, Maine, which was about 75 miles away. The client's husband essentially planned the entire excursion for her by selecting a hotel, recommending restaurants, suggesting places to shop, and so on. Isabelle dutifully followed her husband's itinerary. She spent several days in Portland and returned to the ski area to drive home with the family.

The client next described an incident that occurred the night the family returned from the ill-fated skiing trip. As was their habit, both she and her husband ended the day by reading in bed. At some point, the husband announced that he was ready to go to sleep and asked Isabelle to turn off the light. When she refused, he made an angry comment and stormed off to sleep in the guest room. Such displays on the husband's part had almost never occurred in the history of the relationship. Likewise, the husband had never engaged in any sort of violent or threatening behavior toward his wife. Nonetheless, Isabelle reported that when her husband had jumped out of bed and stalked off, she had been seized by a powerful fear that he was going to hit her. Although she was able to recognize that her fear had been irrational, Isabelle still felt the aftereffects of her feelings of terror for several days. She added, "I never know if someone's going to get mad at me. I'm a nervous wreck. Am I doing this wrong? Am I doing that wrong? *I feel like I never left home.*"

It had taken Isabelle nearly the entire session to recount her experiences. The therapist had taken copious notes, interrupting the client only when he wanted her to clarify or expand on certain points in her narrative. He was immensely pleased with the material she had shared, since he had identified a number of potentially fruitful areas of exploration. Moreover, he felt certain that he could use the content Isabelle had presented in a manner that would keep her attention productively focused on her own issues. Unfortunately, the therapist only had time left in the session to tell the client that he firmly believed that they would be able to make constructive use of the experiences she had shared. In support of his contention, he held up a list of topics he had just written down, which he planned to cover during the next session. Isabelle was seated too far away to read the list, which the therapist chose not to enumerate. The clinician had merely wanted to stimulate the client's optimism and her curiosity without opening up more content with her. The therapist ended the session on an upbeat note by saying to Isabelle as she left, "I realize you feel overwhelmed right now, but I want you to know that I'm confident we're going to learn a great deal from the experiences you've just shared with me."

The therapist had compiled the following list of items he wanted to revisit during the next session:

1. Setting self up for victimization—agreeing to go on the ski trip. Role of denial.
2. Fear of husband when he became angry—"I never know if someone's going to get mad at me."
3. Putting self in childlike, dependent role—shopping trip to Portland.
4. Lumping the kids together with her husband—parentification.
5. Boundary issues—closeness and intrusiveness. How her husband uses planning/other controlling behavior.

3/4/92

The therapist planned to start the session by encouraging the client to examine her motives for going along on the vacation in the first place. He knew about the history of the family's previous skiing trips. Since she had no interest in the sport, Isabelle had been understandably unenthusiastic when her husband had proposed similar vacations in the past. Feeling pressured and/or manipulated, she had accompanied him on ski excursions two or three times with consistently negative results for all concerned. Consequently, the therapist had been surprised when the client had told him earlier in the winter that she had consented to go along on another skiing vacation. When he had questioned Isabelle prior to the trip, she had dismissed his concerns, emphasizing some superficial differences between their upcoming vacation and previous ones. Although the therapist was not convinced by her reasoning, he did not think it would be productive to explore the subject further. Since he expected that the trip would be an unpleasant one for Isabelle, the therapist had assumed he would have an opportunity to process the entire matter on her return.

The therapist reminded the client of how surprised he had been to hear that she had agreed to go on the vacation in the first place. He reviewed the difficulties she had experienced on skiing trips in the past. He asked Isabelle to explain why she had thought that this excursion would turn out any better than the previous ones. "I thought it would be like Europe, that there would be plenty to do around there," she replied. The therapist stated in response "As I'm listening to you, I'm reminding myself that you're a seasoned world traveler, with a much better sense of geography than most people. What made you think that *rural Maine* would be like Europe?" The therapist's question produced at first a blank expression on the client's face, followed by a look of recognition. Isabelle acknowledged that she had not really thought much about where she was going or what she would do with her time there. The therapist summarized the discussion as follows:

"So despite being well aware of the problems on previous trips, you really didn't think through the details of this vacation the way you normally would. A few sessions ago, when I reminded you of the problems that had occurred when you went skiing before, you were very quick to downplay the concerns I raised. Both of these points indicate the use of denial mechanisms, in that you steered yourself away from certain information. Now I'm wondering whether denial processes might not create problems for you in other situations as well. We'll come back to the topic of denial later. We need to understand why it was necessary for you to use denial in this instance. Let's see if we can establish what you were trying to accomplish by going on the trip in the first place."

At a later point in treatment, the therapist asked the client to keep a journal of positive distortions and other manifestations of denial in her everyday life.

The therapist said he did not understand why it had been necessary for the client to go along on the vacation at all, since her husband could have easily taken the boys skiing on his own. The trip would have been ideal as a father–son outing, he told the client, particularly since she didn't ski in the first place. The therapist asked Isabelle to think back to the time when she had agreed initially to participate in the skiing trip. What made her agree in the first place? The client replied, "They *wanted* me there. When I don't go, they call me at home twice a day. I went because they wanted me to go. I *had* to go. If I didn't go they would have made me feel guilty." Isabelle's response not only alerted the therapist to her vulnerability to guilt induction, but it also made him think that a fear of her husband's anger, which she had described in the previous session, might have played a role in her decision to go along with the vacation plans.

Isabelle had already described to the therapist how her mother used to make her feel guilty and ashamed as a child, often by blaming her for other problems in the family. Reminding the client of her childhood recollections, the therapist said, "I don't have to tell you what a devastating experience it can be to feel guilty or ashamed. Even now, your mother still has the potential to trigger similar reactions in you. I think that's one of the reasons why you didn't want to hear her apologize a few weeks ago." Isabelle agreed with the therapist's remarks. The therapist also told the Isabelle that given her childhood history and the intensity of her self-reproach, he could readily understand how vulnerable she would be to guilt induction on the part of her husband or her sons. Parenthetically, he added that he still didn't understand why the rest of the family found it so necessary to have her along, but stated that he wanted to postpone consideration of that topic for another time.

The therapist told Isabelle that he wondered if guilt were not the only factor in her willingness to participate in the ski trip. He asked the client to recall the feelings of terror she had experienced when her husband stormed out of the bedroom.

Th: You recognized shortly after that incident that you had no reason to be so terrified of your husband. I do think there was a reason for the way you responded to his anger however. Who else in your life caused you to feel so afraid?

Isabelle: My mother. She was completely unpredictable, especially when my father was at work.

Th: What did she do to frighten you?

Isabelle: I've told you most of it. Slapping us, throwing things around, screaming at the top of her lungs. One time she got so mad that she took off into the woods at the end of the street. She was gone for hours. We thought that she was never coming back. Can you blame me for not wanting to hear her apologize for anything now?

Th: No, I can't blame you. Those kinds of experiences have to be terrifying for a child. I can easily understand why you would be afraid now to let down your guard with her, and *maybe with other people as well*. But that's a topic we'll save for another time. Can you see the connection now between your fear of your mother and the way you responded to your husband a few weeks ago?

Isabelle: Yes.

Th: Good. I think we're going to learn more about that connection as time goes on. Let's think about how you learned to cope with your mother's anger. What did you do in an effort to avoid being abused?

Isabelle: I guess I kept my mouth shut and did what she wanted. I tried not to give her any reason to get mad at me. I was like her little slave around the house. I was always a good student. I kept out of trouble. For all the good it did me!

Th: Kids do their best to prevent frightening things from happening to them. So you worked very hard to avoid doing things that might make your mother angry. It became a way of life for you, probably something you did more or less automatically. Can you see how all this might figure into why you went along on the ski trip?

Isabelle: I can't stand to have any of them angry at me. Doing what they want is the safest way. No one's mad at me then.

Th: That sounds right on target to me. You were *afraid* not to go, not only because they might have made you feel guilty, but also because they might have become angry. I think that's why you didn't really want to hear any of my concerns. Maybe now you can see how fear sets up the denial strategies. You went on the trip in an attempt to protect yourself. You had no desire to risk upsetting your husband and your children. I believe that once you decided to go, you no longer wanted to think about the problems that had occurred during similar vacations in the past. Naturally, you didn't want to hear any of my reservations about the trip either. I think you can also appreciate now just how powerful denial can be, how it sets people up to make the same mistakes again and again.

The therapist asked the client to think about how she typically behaved when she allowed herself to be pressured into certain activities by other family members. Just the fact that Isabelle described herself as having been "good" on the drive up to the ski resort indicated that she was already struggling with feelings of resentment at the start of the trip, the therapist said. The client acknowledged that she *had* expected some sort of payback, from her husband and her sons, for her willingness to accompany them on the vacation. The therapist added that ironically enough, it was *Isabelle* who had become enraged over the trip. Likewise, she ended up feeling guilty, just as she had dreaded, not in response to comments from the rest of the family but as a reaction to her *own* angry outbursts. The therapist asked the client to observe her thoughts, feelings, and behaviors carefully in the future whenever she felt pressured or manipulated into doing things for others. He predicted that many of the same features that characterized the ski trip (e.g., feelings of resentment, a sense of entitlement, angry interactions with others) would recur in similar situations in the future.

Since the hour was nearly over, the therapist summarized what they had covered in the session thus far, while Isabelle took notes on the major themes. He asked the client to write down any questions or associations she might have in response to the material they had discussed. The therapist also suggested that she keep a running log for several weeks of any instances where she experienced a fear of her husband's anger or disapproval. He told the client that he would cover the rest of his agenda items from the previous interview during the next session.

3/11/92

The therapist began by reviewing the last session, item by item. During his review, the therapist read a number of direct quotations from the client back to her from his case notes. Isabelle stated that on reflection over the past few days she found that the conclusions of the previous week continued to make sense to her. She offered little in the way of elaboration on the points of the previous week and reported that she had no questions to ask of the therapist. Moreover, she claimed that she had not been able to log any instances in which she had experienced fear of her husband's anger or disapproval. The client's rather passive response indicated to the therapist that she had not yet absorbed enough of the material to make good use of the concepts involved. He concluded that it would be necessary to cover the same ground many times before Isabelle would be able to put what she learned in treatment to any significant use between sessions.

Now the therapist returned to his unfinished agenda items from the previous sessions. He began by discussing the client's failed efforts to return home from the ski area and the trip to Portland her husband had proposed to her as an alternative. Isabelle indicated that a now-familiar combination of guilt and fear had kept her from going home as she had originally wanted to do. The therapist expressed his astonishment that already having felt pressured into the ski trip, the client allowed her husband to plan yet another excursion for her, *this time down to the smallest details*. As in an earlier discussion, Isabelle's first response to the therapist's probe reflected denial mechanisms at work. She began by telling the therapist how skillful her husband was at planning excursions for them.

Th: I'm still amazed at how you ended up going to Portland. Someone might have predicted that, after all the fuss over the skiing trip, the last thing you would have done would be to follow your husband's instructions the way you did. How did that come about?

Isabelle: He's great at planning trips. Whenever we go somewhere in Europe he figures out our itinerary each day.

Th: Yes, but this trip was only to Portland, Maine. How complex could it be? You've described many trips that you've taken by yourself. Besides, I thought the point of this excursion was supposed to be shopping. Aren't *you* the expert on that subject?

Isabelle: I didn't have really a preference either way.

Th: I think we discovered last session that those kind of statements may not always be accurate. Think about it for a minute. You certainly had a preference to return home, since that's what you had originally proposed. Are you saying you didn't care how you spent your time in Portland.

Isabelle: It was just easier to let him decide for me. That way he wouldn't be upset. I felt bad for him. I didn't want to spoil his vacation. I wouldn't have gone to Portland on my own. I didn't see anything there I wanted to buy.

Th: How did you feel about yourself while he was planning the trip for you and while you were in Portland?

Isabelle: It's funny. I thought of you while Joe was planning my trip for me. I had a feeling you might think it was a bad idea. Then I thought of you again when I was driving to Portland.

Th: Why did you think I might disapprove of the idea?

Isabelle: I thought you'd say that I let him treat me like a baby instead of standing up for myself. To tell you the truth, I did feel a little bit silly in that hotel room, although I managed to have a decent time there.

Th: I believe that you thought of me, not because of how I might react, but because *you* were beginning to feel uncomfortable about the way things were going. I think we're finding out that whenever you sacrifice your autonomy, your right to determine your own choices, it bothers you much more than you may acknowledge at the time. I believe that you instinctively dislike it when anyone, including your mother, your husband, or your therapist, tries to make decisions for you.

The therapist then spent time reviewing the concept of boundaries with Isabelle. He explained to her that many of his clients who had been abused as children found it hard to sustain intimacy without losing a sense of autonomy or selfhood in the process. Isabelle was able to recognize how the act of one adult making decisions for another could be considered a boundary violation. She also acknowledged that at times she was the one who actually abdicated responsibility for herself. The therapist emphasized throughout the discussion that, in his view, her husband was merely misguided, not ill-intentioned. Nonetheless, the therapist also stressed that since it was so easy for Isabelle to sacrifice her self-determination in an intimate relationship, it was inevitable that she would then experience her husband as intrusive, coercive, and perhaps ultimately abusive.

For many years, Isabelle had approached sexual intimacy with her husband as a duty, sometimes engaging in physical relations with him when she felt uncomfortable, out of a sense of obligation. Earlier in treatment, the therapist had encouraged her to share her true feelings about sex with her husband. Somewhat uncharacteristically, Isabelle had been candid with her husband on the subject. The husband had proven to be quite understanding and supportive of her. Once she had initiated dialogue with her spouse, Isabelle quickly learned that she could decline her husband's advances or terminate any sexual activity whenever she felt uncomfortable. As a result, Isabelle became more sexually responsive, and the couple's sexual relationship had improved accordingly. Now the therapist briefly reviewed with the client all the remarkable changes she had made in the sexual relationship with her husband. He told Isabelle that, given her past performance, he fully expected her to make progress on other boundary issues in the marriage as well. The therapist planned to review the whole subject of boundaries repeatedly during subsequent sessions.

Having noted Isabelle's comment on how she thought he would respond to her Portland excursion, the therapist stressed that he did not want to become yet another authority figure in her life. He then asked her a series of questions aimed at eliciting potential distortions in the therapeutic relationship. Despite the thoughts she had experienced about him in Maine, the client denied worrying that the therapist would behave in a critical or rejecting manner toward her. She also emphasized that she had not felt afraid that the therapist would become angry with her at some point. Given the client's history and the cognitions about him she had already reported, the therapist was not entirely comfortable with the responses she gave to his questions. Nonetheless, the therapist simply asked Isabelle to keep him informed of any reactions she might have to him and moved off the topic for the time being.

The therapist now wanted to help Isabelle achieve a better understanding of her husband's behavior during the ill-fated vacation. The client had described her husband's family as emotionally distant and noncommunicative, particularly when it came to matters which involved conflict. Not surprisingly, Isabelle described several episodes that illustrated her husband's difficulties communicating in a direct manner, particularly during periods of conflict. "It's second nature for him to cover up," she said. The therapist suspected that the husband, whom he had met on two occasions, was very uncomfortable with powerful affect of any kind, particularly the intense anger directed at him by his wife from time to time. The therapist told the client "I think that your husband behaves as if he's nearly as afraid of your anger as you are of his." In support of the therapist's contention, Isabelle then described how her husband would typically respond to conflict by attempting to minimize her concerns or placate her with unrealistic promises. The husband would also try to invalidate her perceptions of their interactions, sometimes by simply refusing to admit that he had made certain statements. Such denial strategies only succeeding in making Isabelle even more angry. The therapist pointed out that it would be very difficult for someone like Isabelle, who already found conflict quite threatening, to sustain a belief in her own perceptions in the face of such invalidating messages. At a later point in treatment, the client found it helpful to keep a log of situations in which her husband's remarks led her to doubt the validity of her position. This self-monitoring task helped her to become more confident in the accuracy of her perceptions.

A frank, objective appraisal of her husband's limitations was a new experience for Isabelle, who tended to idealize her spouse. Despite periods of anger and disappointment with her husband, she generally felt inferior to him. She usually viewed her husband as the calm, reasonable member of the couple, whereas she was the crazy, destructive one. Recognizing that her husband had some legitimate communicational difficulties of his own enabled the client to see herself in somewhat more favorable terms. Understandably, Isabelle found it hard to pin her husband down when he failed to communicate in a clear or direct manner. It was much easier for her to rail at him for skimping on a birthday gift than to call him on his evasiveness. As treatment progressed, the therapist found it easier to keep Isabelle focused on the effects of her husband's ambiguous and sometimes misleading communications. He encouraged the client to develop gentle but persistent methods of confronting the issues in her marriage. As she became more skillful at confronting her husband, he seemed to become more considerate and collaborative in his approach to her.

The therapist's last agenda item for the session involved the client's relationship with her children. The therapist did not think Isabelle was ready to use treatment to examine either the attitudes or the behaviors associated with parenting. In fact he seemed to be much more concerned than the client was about the impact of the vacation events on the children. Rather than explore the underlying issues, the therapist decided to help the client behave as any concerned parent would under similar circumstances. He commented that in her account of the vacation, Isabelle had a tendency to lump her sons and her husband together, *as if they functioned as a unit*. The therapist asked the client's permission to alert her if she referred to the children in a similar manner in the future. He told her that he assumed that she did *not* hold her sons responsible for the unsatisfying vacation plans or for the communication problems within the marriage. Moreover, he said he knew that she felt badly for having involved them in the conflicts with her husband during the trip. The therapist stated that he believed Isabelle could take steps to reduce the negative effects of her behavior on the children. Consequently, he recommended that the client speak directly to each one of the boys, apologizing for her actions and specifically absolving them from blame for any of the difficulties that had occurred during the vacation. The therapist assumed that parenting issues would demand close attention at some point in the client's treatment. The therapist could only hope that the client would take his expectations seriously and attempt to implement his recommendations in some manner. For the time being, however, he doubted that he could go further on the subject without eliciting a defensive response from her.

The therapist ended the session by asking Isabelle to work on what would become standing homework assignments for some time. First, he asked her to keep looking for situations in which she was motivated by a fear of her husband's anger. Her work on this assignment did yield more useful results. Second, the therapist also requested that the client keep a log of positive distortions and other manifestations of denial.

3/18/92

The therapist began the next session by asking the client's permission to go back over all the material associated with the skiing trip. Isabelle seemed to tolerate his rather lengthy review of the entire vacation episode in good humor. After what may have seemed to the client like an interminable length of time, the therapist did move on to other topics.

The therapist referred to various aspects of the ski trip many times during subsequent sessions with this client. In fact, the therapist also privately reviewed the notes from the sessions of 3/4 and 3/11 at several different points when he felt unsure about the direction the treatment seemed to be taking. He found that, by reviewing the data discussed above, he was able to keep the treatment focused more effectively on the client's most central issues.

THE USE OF SESSION NOTES

Consistency in treatment depends directly on the therapist's ability to recall and utilize an array of pertinent data regarding the client, the treatment plan, and the content of previous interviews. In order to be most effective on a moment-to-moment basis in each session, the therapist needs to have as much of the pertinent data as possible "on screen" and available during every interaction with the individual. Consequently, the therapist must develop successful strategies for encoding, rehearsing, and recalling large amounts of information on each client. We find that detailed session notes are essential in our efforts to organize and retain data over the course of treatment.

Except for some very rare and thankfully unusual circumstances, there is no reason not to take extensive notes during sessions. The vast majority of our clients have never objected in any significant way to our taking notes during the treatment hour. In fact, most clients come to value the alert, businesslike approach taking notes represents. The notion that note-taking will inhibit the client is, in our view, essentially an anachronism from a time when therapists were concerned about blocking the flow of the client's free associations. All of the case material presented in this volume was obtained from clients whose therapists took copious notes right from the outset of treatment. It would appear that even the most doctrinaire psychodynamic reader will grant that our case studies show no lack of "preconscious," "unconscious," and/or "primary process material," material that clearly flowed directly from our work with clients.

We assume that notes taken during the session do a better job of capturing the client's flow of ideas than do process notations done some time afterward. Unless the therapist spends incredible amounts of time on record keeping, notes taken during the session will always be much more detailed than those written later. Moreover, we often want to be able to confront the client in subsequent sessions, not with general impressions of previous cognitive distortions, but with direct quotations. Direct quotations, as read from the session notes, are evocative and powerful, in part because they keep clients focused on *themselves*, not on the therapist or anyone else. When an individual tends to present scattered or very sparse content, it is often useful for the therapist to perform an orienting function at the beginning of each session by reading notes of the previous interview aloud to the client before settling on an agenda.

We would impart this advice to beginning therapists: Learn to write unobtrusively during the session, possibly with your head up if you find it comfortable. The client's eyes generally remain focused on your face anyway. However, it is always wise to pause temporarily from your note-taking when it appears that the client is disclosing some sensitive information or traumatic content until you know more about the data in question. Don't get caught relying on your memory when it comes to your clients. Review your notes religiously. Read over your intake notes and notes from any other session in which you obtained significant historical data until you have all the pertinent data encoded and accessible in memory. Keep rehearsing these data as long as you know the client. As treatment progresses, make sure that before each treatment hour you read over the notes of at least the past two or three sessions. Go even further back in time if you don't have a clear picture of where you are headed with a particular client. Your clients will be pleased, flattered, and impressed by the amount of personal information you have retained about them. They will also perceive you as smarter and more well-organized. They want to know that you have some kind of game plan in mind for them. When you appear both knowledgeable about them and consistent in your focus, it communicates caring, safety, and best of all, hope to your clients.

Below are a number of pertinent classes of information that the therapist should include in the notes taken during treatment sessions: (1) historical and genealogical details about the client and the client's family; (2) verbatim quotations that reflect cognitive distortions operating in the present moment that the client might be better able to process and acknowledge at a later date; (3) predictions made by the client for the future, which the therapist would like to review later in the light of subsequent objective data; (4) statements made by the client reflecting spontaneous recognition of cognitive distortions, information-processing deficits, compulsive behaviors, and/or relationship difficulties; (5) hostile or defensive reactions to the therapist that will be more profitable to discuss in a later session; (6) major themes developed by the therapist; (7) interventions attempted by the therapist and the client's responses to them; (8) quotations or other evidence of changes in the client's perspective that occur as a direct result of the therapist's interventions; (9) any other evidence of positive changes that have taken place in the client's affect, thinking, or behavior; (10) specific homework assignments; (11) specific themes to revisit explicitly with the client during subsequent sessions; (12) Client issues or behaviors the therapist needs to monitor, perhaps silently; (13) "CYA" variables, for example, items such as the assessment of suicide potential.

THE DOUBLE-EDGED SWORD OF SYMPTOM FOCUS

Therapists with cognitive-behavioral training inevitably become known to referral sources and to the general public for their active, comparatively straightforward approach to problems such as anxiety and depression. People in distress, their significant others, and their professional caregivers may become overly encouraged by reports of direct, quick treatment methods for various psychological problems. Consequently, both referral sources and potential clients may expect treatment to produce relief quickly, generally through symptom-oriented interventions.

Clinicians from all orientations can become victims of their successes. Former clients who have had positive treatment experiences often become enthusiastic referral sources. Unfortunately, they may also encourage unrealistic expectations on the part of the individuals whom they send to their former therapists. To be sure, the clinician who comes so highly recommended has an enormous advantage in terms of respect and credibility during the early phases of treatment. However, the therapist's initial "halo" will tarnish quickly unless he or she insures that the client's expectations about the speed and efficacy of treatment are realistic.

In the authors' experience, it is not uncommon for therapists from other orientations to refer clients for cognitive treatment when they are threatened by the intensity or complexity of the symptom picture or when they encounter a frustrating lack of insight. We suspect that some of these therapists consider cognitive therapy to be superficial and excessively symptom-oriented, in essence, a stopgap solution for clients who are too stupid, rigid, naive, ignorant, or problem-ridden to benefit from the real thing. Unless out-and-out dumping of disruptive clients is involved, we cheerfully accept such referrals and try to tolerate the unfair characterization of our therapeutic work as best we can. It is necessary, however, to provide clients with realistic expectations, particularly if they have been led to believe that cognitive therapy will *not* involve examination of family of origin experiences or other personal material.

Some individuals *do* respond positively and quickly to symptom-oriented interventions, at times quite dramatically so. With certain clients, particularly those whose difficulties have a strong situational component, a brief, symptom-oriented or supportive approach may be appropriate and entirely sufficient for immediate relief of the presenting problems. Likewise, we assume that acute onset, nonrecurrent conditions will be more amenable to symptom-oriented treatment. The traditional cognitive and behavioral literature contains many useful techniques for helping clients manage symptoms associated with a wide range of psychiatric disorders (e.g., Barlow, 1985; Beck & Emery, 1985; Beck et al., 1979). In our view, despite the potential limitations of such techniques, they *do* belong in the armamentarium of every clinician.

Symptom reduction can add immeasurably to the larger process of recovery. Many of our clients need to feel back in control of themselves before they can focus productively on larger issues. Loss of control, or the fear of losing control, over one's thoughts, feelings, and behaviors is a frightening experience for anyone. Once clients can feel as if their symptoms will get no worse, they will be less obsessed with losing control of themselves. Consequently, we are usually open to exploring *any* techniques to facilitate symptom reduction, such as medication, although we do have a preference for methods that allow clients to credit themselves for improvements. Improvements in symptoms never hurt the therapist's potential credibility on other issues. Moreover, certain clients will respond to the immense relief associated with symptom reduction by taking positive steps in areas of life never even explicitly discussed with the therapist. Finally, since symptom reduction improves morale, energy, self-confidence, and the ability to concentrate, it also puts the client in a vastly more favorable position to benefit from other aspects of treatment, provided the individual remains strongly motivated to examine broader issues.

However, some clients do not respond favorably to symptom-oriented interventions. Others may exhibit transient symptom relief, only to experience relapses on a recurring basis. Some clients, who seem to recover from their presenting complaints during one series of treatment sessions, may return to the therapist at a later date with what may appear at first glance to be a new set of problems. Finally, certain individuals, particularly those with an extensive history of childhood trauma, present such a bewildering array of difficulties that it would take most of the therapist's lifetime to address all the symptoms involved. On the other hand, the therapist may find that the same cognitive mechanisms are responsible for the entire package of symptoms the client experiences. As we discuss in greater detail in our discussion of trauma revelation, serious distortions in the therapeutic relationship may also occur when symptoms emerge in response to recollections of abuse. It can be a difficult task to keep the client's sense of optimism and motivation for treatment alive when things seem to be getting worse. Understandably, just as the therapist's credibility can soar when symptoms improve, so can it also crash and burn when the client's symptoms continue, intensify, or proliferate.

As we discussed in Chapter 3, many of our clients present mixed patterns of maladaptive overvigilance and denial in that they characteristically obsess over peripheral or unproductive topics while they ignore or minimize other serious problems. In similar fashion, certain clients may present dramatic symptoms for treatment, such as anxiety attacks, while they fail to acknowledge even more dramatic difficulties in other areas of their lives—perhaps involving relationships with significant others. Without the therapist's assistance, the client may remain stuck in a very narrow definition of "the problem." Certain individuals may become so distracted by a *series* of symptoms that unless the therapist intervenes forcefully, the underlying psychological mechanisms will never even be discussed in the treatment sessions. Clients with chronic or recurring symptoms need to learn how such difficulties are connected with larger *issues* in their lives. In fact, they often have to use the occurrence or exacerbation of their characteristic symptoms as a *cue*, signalling the need to confront other problems or stressors. Through self-monitoring, many of our clients encounter first-hand evidence that symptoms such as panic attacks, obsessive thoughts, and various compulsive behaviors are closely related to other issues, for example, worthlessness, interpersonal conflicts, boundary problems, and so on. As a consequence, clients may develop a new set of "attentional priorities," in which symptoms might begin to assume a less significant position. These clients learn how to maintain an issue focus, not only during their treatment sessions, but in their daily lives as well.

The majority of clients from dysfunctional family backgrounds seem to need more from treatment than symptom-control strategies. Unless they change basic beliefs and coping strategies, they will remain vulnerable to the development of symptoms, particularly when they encounter certain life stresses. The therapist should present the client who needs symptom-reduction strategies with a *decision-tree*, in which several treatment options could be investigated either simultaneously or in sequence. In most instances, we prefer to work on symptoms, basic beliefs and coping strategies, and historical material *simultaneously* from the outset of treatment. However, if the client appears to be resistant to such a multilayered approach, the therapist may decide to place more threatening procedures (e.g., work on traumatic childhood experiences) out of reach temporarily by stressing the need to explore less intrusive treatment options first. The clinician may inform the client that if symptoms persist or recur, there will be a need to confront broader issues. The therapist also may need to warn the client who wants to terminate as soon as he or she experiences symptom relief that the presenting difficulties are likely to return unless more fundamental changes in thinking and behavior occur.

GETTING STUCK IN TRYING TO CHANGE THE CLIENT'S BEHAVIORS

Although the long-term goal of treatment unquestionably involves the modification of self-defeating behavioral patterns, the therapist needs to resist feeling responsible for choices the client makes along the way. We therapists must accept that, in the final analysis, we are helpless to change our clients' behaviors. Unfortunately, many of our clients will continue to make self-defeating decisions, some with ramifications that will persist over many years, *until changes occur in the cognitive processes which produce such choices.* In the meantime, the therapist must work hard to maintain an attitude of detachment in order to continue working in an upbeat, hopeful manner, despite the unpleasant conditions that may exist in the client's life. The recovery process, particularly when it involves changes in relationships, often brings increased conflict, greater emotional distress, and other aversive consequences along with it in the short run. Clients who are not committed to working through such aversive consequences will not be able to sustain new behaviors regardless of the support they might receive from others.

In our view, there are only three areas in which the therapist has a legitimate mandate to interfere with the client's choices: (1) when there is direct intent to kill or harm oneself; (2) when there is direct intent to kill or harm another; and (3) when there is abuse, neglect, or other clear-cut victimization of children. Other than offering the general dictum that the client may be ill-advised to ponder dramatic, major life changes during a period of extreme turbulence (or during the early stages of treatment), the therapist should avoid interfering with the client's decisions outside of the three areas mentioned above.

One of our clients achieved a breakthrough in dealing with her depressed husband when she learned how to distinguish between *supporting* and *controlling*. When she gave up the need to control, she found that she became less angry with her husband. She also found that, when her husband was ready, he solved his own problems in a much more direct, efficient, and powerful manner than any way she might have suggested. Therapists who become caught up in giving advice or otherwise trying to change the client's behavior have probably crossed the line between support and control. In the process, they violate client boundaries and communicate the unintended message that the individual is not competent enough to solve his or her problems. Therapists who become controlling also often ignore the importance of the client's *motivation* to change. People who are truly motivated, and who have removed psychological barriers, will find a way to solve their problems. *The therapist's emphasis ought to be placed on helping individuals remove roadblocks that prevent change not on writing new life scripts for clients.*

SUSTAINING FOCUS ON THE SELF

There are many reasons why a client might find it difficult to use treatment sessions to focus on the self. As we mentioned in an earlier chapter, we seldom achieve substantial progress with clients who habitually externalize all blame for their difficulties. Individuals who experience little or no legitimate dissatisfaction with themselves should probably be encouraged to find settings outside of treatment to ventilate their complaints about others.

On the other hand, many clients who are initially unable to focus productively on themselves can learn to do so if the therapist can find an acceptable starting point for them. Certain individuals, for example, are so obsessed with the thoughts, feelings, and behaviors of others that they are simply unable to identify or articulate inner experiences. They need to learn how to direct attention inward in a sustained manner, without being distracted by external stimuli. Other clients may look inward to some degree, but they may become so preoccupied with certain themes, such as worthlessness or anger, that they fail to process substantial amounts of data. Through the use of overt interventions and embedded messages, the therapist can provide a complex framework that will enable the client to remain focused on the self.

In the example that follows, the therapist kept redirecting the client's attention back toward understanding the factors underlying her involvement in an abusive affair, one that had ultimately caused great harm to her and her family. In keeping the client focused on an area of such intense self-dissatisfaction, the therapist had to help her to avoid being overwhelmed by feelings of worthlessness and guilt. On the other hand, the therapist also needed to validate the client's understandable anger at the abusive partner. He had to provide the client with the opportunity to express her anger in an appropriate manner without permitting her to use up all her time in his office perseverating on themes of hatred and revenge. In the same vein, in order to keep the client focused on herself, the therapist needed to discourage her from acting out her angry feelings or attempting to control others in an inappropriate manner.

Gina was the 40-year-old mother of two daughters, the older of whom was a freshman at a nearby women's college. She entered treatment after her older daughter, Paula, disclosed that a male neighbor had been sexually abusing her from the time she was 12 years old. The abuse had involved forcible rape on many occasions, as well as other acts of brutality. Gina and her husband, Spike, had long recognized that Paula's difficulties with self-esteem and peer relationships were serious problems for her. In fact, they had consulted the therapist when the girl was a freshman in high school. At that time, the therapist had repeatedly questioned Paula regarding possible sexual abuse, but the girl never acknowledged any such difficulties in her life. As it turned out, the neighbor had kept the daughter from disclosing the abuse by threatening to harm Gina and the rest of the family if Paula revealed his actions to anyone.

Gina herself made another alarming disclosure to the therapist. She had carried on a long-term affair with the perpetrator, during the same time period in which he had abused her daughter! She also revealed that she too had been the victim of rape and other violent acts at the hands of the same individual. Gina's secret now had become too big to contain. Soon after her disclosure to the therapist, Gina realized that both Spike and Paula were aware of her extramarital relationship. Now the entire family had to pick up the pieces somehow.

Understandably, Gina was literally exploding with anger at the perpetrator, who now no longer had any contact with the daughter or the rest of the family. She alternated between an all-consuming rage at the neighbor and an overwhelming sense of guilt over her own actions, which had indirectly resulted in her daughter's victimization. During her sessions, Gina would raise her fists and vow through clenched teeth, "I'm gonna get that son of a bitch." Indeed, for nearly a year after her daughter's disclosure, she continued to believe that she would never rise up out of her depression unless she could strike back at the perpetrator. Although she was able to acknowledge that Paula was herself too depressed and confused to make long-range plans or commitments, she still pressured her daughter at times to take legal action against the neighbor. Gina also was obsessed with other plans for revenge against the perpetrator, plans which if realized, could have easily created additional problems for herself and her family. In her individual treatment sessions, Gina preferred to focus on her anger with the perpetrator, her obsessive thoughts of revenge, and her chronic complaints about Spike. The therapist found it hard to redirect Gina's attention to other important issues, such as the current state of her marriage, her ongoing role in Paula's recovery, and the underlying issues that had caused *her* also to remain in an abusive relationship with the perpetrator.

The therapist had a number of goals in mind for Gina and for the family. First of all, he wanted to normalize Gina's affective reactions to the abuse, particularly that which her daughter had experienced, without giving her license to act out in any way against the perpetrator. He wanted to serve as a support to Gina as she struggled to understand and accept what had occurred to her family, while communicating his sense of optimism regarding their chances for recovery. Although the therapist wanted to validate Gina's anger toward the perpetrator and her frustrations with her husband, he also wanted to direct her attention back toward her own issues. The therapist needed to help Gina understand what had made her remain in an abusive relationship for so long. In order to do so, he knew that he needed to learn much more about her family background, her belief systems, and her style of relating.

The therapist, a male of about the same age as the perpetrator, decided that it would be preferable to have Paula see a female therapist individually. He believed it was vital for the time being for him to work with Gina individually and to see various configurations of the family as needed. For the most part, the family sessions involved the parents and Paula, although occasionally the therapist only saw the spouses. The family sessions were primarily organized around enabling the parents to support Paula's recovery without infringing upon her privacy or autonomy. By encouraging the parents to keep Paula's welfare in the foreground at all times, the therapist tried to insure that neither one would pressure her to take any sort of action against the perpetrator. He also wanted to strengthen the boundaries around the family as a whole, for example, by encouraging the parents to keep their recent difficulties private. The therapist had hoped to move Gina's treatment eventually into a couples format, but he was never able to interest Spike in working explicitly on his own issues or the problems in the marriage. Unfortunately, Spike also showed no enthusiasm or aptitude for examining his reactions to his wife's infidelity.

The therapist consistently stressed that he empathized with Gina's rage at the man who had abused both her daughter and her. He defined her anger as a normal response to an abnormal, destructive situation. Although the therapist repeatedly expressed his confidence that Gina would eventually achieve some greater peace of mind, he also told her repeatedly that she could expect continued emotional turbulence in the short term, as she dealt with the implications of all that had happened in her life. He stated again and again that if he were confronted with a similar situation with his own daughter, he could only hope that he could stop himself from doing something rash, since he would certainly entertain many violent and destructive fantasies, just as Gina was doing. Unfortunately, he often reminded her, some of the powerful forms of revenge she contemplated involved actions that could result in her being injured or incarcerated. Whenever she considered the effects of such outcomes on her children, Gina would conclude that she could not afford to act on her fantasies of retribution, regardless of how angry she felt. She also came to recognize that having fantasies was not synonymous with acting them out. Over time, she felt a greater sense of control over her destructive impulses.

Gina was always quick to agree that regardless of how she felt toward the perpetrator, her main concern was the welfare of her daughter. Periodically, particularly when he suspected that she might be putting subtle pressure on her daughter to take legal action against the perpetrator, the therapist would ask Gina to review information regarding Paula's current level of functioning. The therapist would recall how, even after she disclosed the abuse, Paula had expressed the belief that the perpetrator *really cared for her*. Unlike her mother, she had not yet experienced a powerful sense of anger at the man, an indication, according to the therapist, that she had not fully realized the extent of her victimization. Moreover, the daughter still found it extremely difficult to discuss the abuse, even with her own individual therapist. Gina had always found it painful to witness her daughter's passivity and unassertiveness. Even when she could identify clear gains that Paula had made in many areas, she would still readily acknowledge that these passive aspects of her daughter's behavior were still a long way from changing.

Summarizing the data, the therapist would ask Gina whether she thought her daughter was ready to undertake the pressures of a long and bitter legal battle. Was Paula prepared to tell her story again and again, to one stranger after another? Was she self-confident enough to tolerate hours of interrogation at the hands of hostile attorneys? Could Paula sustain her commitment to a process that could take as long as 2 or 3 years? Was she ready to face the accused in court? Invariably, Gina answered "no" to all the therapist's questions. After nearly 10 months of individual treatment, Gina began to accept the fact that legal action against the perpetrator would only take place in the distant future, if it occurred at all. Consequently, she stopped raising the issue with her daughter.

The therapist utilized the same strategy repeatedly to draw the client's attention toward what he considered to be the most crucial issue in her individual treatment, namely, her *own* long-term participation in a highly abusive, degrading affair. Whenever Gina railed against the perpetrator, the therapist at some point would state that he could appreciate how difficult it must be for her to accept the fact that she had to assume the role of a helpless bystander now, since, despite her anger, she herself could not take direct action. After all, she had always considered herself a fighter and had described her behaviors in the family many times as "controlling." The therapist would then briefly review a number of instances in which Gina had demonstrated her willingness to fight, especially on behalf of her children, and her unwillingness to relinquish control, particularly to her husband. Having volunteered all the information the therapist was presenting about her, Gina naturally would agree with him. Then the therapist would move the discussion toward his main treatment agenda. Why, he would ask her, would such a fighter allow herself to be dominated, abused, and *even raped*? Not surprisingly, Gina initially had no coherent answers to this question. The more she discussed the details of the relationship, and the more the therapist reflected her disclosures back to her, the more perplexed Gina grew about her own behavior—and appropriately so. As she described it, the abusive components of the extramarital relationship had occurred with increasing frequency over the last 2 years of the affair. Despite her increasing discomfort over the abusive treatment, Gina had continued on in the affair, finally terminating it only as a result of her daughter's shocking disclosures.

The therapist continued to imply that Gina was unlikely to gain control of other problematic areas of her life, particularly her marriage, until she truly understood the mechanisms that had prevented her from leaving such a destructive relationship. Other than encouraging her to take actions in the family that supported Paula's sense of safety and overall recovery, the therapist had little interest in the details of Gina's relationships, except as they replicated boundary violations, denial, and other mechanisms that seemed to be linked to the abusive affair. At times, he found it necessary to redirect the client's attention in a manner that raised her anxiety over her participation in the destructive relationship. For example, Gina could easily slip into lengthy diatribes against her husband Spike, who despite his bumbling ways, was hardly an abusive presence in her life. The therapist would typically listen attentively for a while to Gina's complaints about Spike, which usually centered on his quiet, but stubborn refusal to be influenced by her. When she paused, or seemed to run out of steam, the therapist would say "I know there's a lot of tension at home. I hope that we can help you find a way to make improvements in your marriage eventually. It doesn't surprise me that you have problems communicating with your husband. After all it was just a few months ago that you were tolerating *being raped* in a relationship." In order to keep Gina focused on the affair, and to block any tendency on her part to deny the severity of her victimization, the therapist made sure to link the experience of having been raped with any reference to the relationship made during the sessions.

In the meantime, the therapist continued to explore the abusive affair and its connections with other relationships in Gina's life, particularly in her family of origin. Based on the information Gina supplied about the extramarital relationship, it was possible for the therapist to sensitize her to the use of denial quite early in treatment. Gina recognized that she had minimized her guilt over the affair by telling herself that it wasn't affecting anything else in her life. Now she found that this extramarital realtionship had in fact resulted in damage to her entire family. Gina also saw how she had coped with the physical abuse and the sexual assaults in the affair by telling herself to forget about them. Moreover, she had continued to maintain an idealized picture of her lover, believing that he truly saw her as the "ultimate woman." As treatment progressed, Gina recognized just how much she had denied the terrible emotional toll of the abusive relationship on her. Despite her continuing anguish over her daughter, Gina reported feeling much better about herself now that she was free of the guilt and degradation associated with her affair.

There seemed to be more than enough stress in the client's family of origin to account for the severe denial, the helplessness, and the poor self-esteem that had enabled her to continue on in such a destructive relationship for so long. The third youngest of four children, Gina had grown up in Albania, under considerably impoverished conditions. The youngest child, a boy 4 years her junior, was quite ill, apparently from a form of leukemia, for much of his life. He eventually died at the age of 12. When Gina was 7, her father had the first of many psychotic breaks, during which he became paranoid and quite violent. He was permanently institutionalized as a result of an episode in which he had held the family hostage and had managed to kill one of the policemen who came to intervene. Unlike her mother and her siblings, Gina had always remained loyal to her father, in spite of the fact that he had nearly killed the entire family. She dutifully made regular visits to the institution where he was held, until his death in her midteens. In her historical accounts Gina idealized her father, describing him as having doted on her, for example, while glossing over the wild, frightening behaviors triggered by his psychotic episodes.

One result of the father's absence from the family was that Gina became the primary caretaker for her sick younger brother, as he slowly deteriorated and died. In the meantime, her academic and social development stopped. Far from being appreciative of Gina's efforts, the mother was consistently critical of her, as well as openly contemptuous of her continued loyalty to the father. At age 17, Gina agreed to an arranged marriage to Spike, an American man whom she had never met. In retrospect, she concluded that she had consented to the marriage because it had offered her an opportunity to leave home.

As treatment progressed, the client remembered more and more material of a traumatic nature, material that rendered her participation in such an abusive relationship much more understandable. When Gina was scarcely 12 years old, her mother sent her off to a series of boarding situations, in which the girl had to function as a child laborer, under incredibly harsh conditions reminiscent of a Dickens' novel. Eventually the client was able to recall numerous incidents of physical and sexual abuse that had occurred while she worked away from home. Over time, Gina was able to recognize the connections between her abusive relationship and her experiences in childhood and adolescence. She began to understand how her poor self-worth, her angry outbursts, and her controlling behaviors originated in her chaotic family life, only to be exacerbated by the abusive experiences she encountered outside the home as a young adolescent.

The therapist consistently underscored instances of denial on the client's part, particularly when she was being mistreated by others. He repeatedly asked her to examine very carefully the motivations of people who crossed her path, especially when it came to the males who seemed to take an inordinate amount of interest in her. The therapist also kept the spotlight on various individuals who habitually violated the privacy of the client and her family. As long as she resisted the tendency to engage in denial, Gina proved increasingly capable of discouraging would-be admirers and/or victimizers. She also began to pull away from a number of exploitative friends and acquaintances and learned to avoid becoming entangled in additional relationships of a similar nature. Such changes in thinking and behavior on Gina's part resulted in stronger boundaries around the family as a whole, which in turn created a safer, more supportive climate for the daughter's recovery.

Gina also began to understand how her controlling behaviors reflected an attempt to cope with the stressful conditions in her family of origin. The therapist was always quite assertive in confronting her whenever she resorted to manipulating or pressuring her family in any way, but he was able to do so in a way that did not threaten the treatment alliance. Gina found that by monitoring her controlling behaviors, she was better able to identify the specific fears that stimulated her actions. As time went on, she was able to correct more and more of the irrational content associated with her fearful thoughts. Although both her husband and her daughter continued to behave passively and somewhat irresponsibly, Gina found that she was more capable of relinquishing control than she had ever imagined. Despite a lack of romantic attraction to her husband, which was certainly understandable given many of her previous experiences, Gina did grow more caring and tolerant in her attitudes toward him as she changed in other ways. She also came to experience considerable gratitude toward him for remaining loyal to her and to Paula, despite all that had happened.

Gina was able to reduce the frequency of her own therapy to one visit per month. She had made significant changes in her thinking and behavior, resulting in improvements in nearly all the important relationships in her life. In the meantime, the therapist continued to hold periodic meetings with the family as an adjunct to the daughter's individual sessions. Paula's treatment, which would no doubt continue on for some time, had resulted in remarkable improvements in the young woman's self-confidence and communication skills. She clearly no longer felt the need to withdraw or dissociate in response to stressful interactions with her parents during the family sessions. Although he suspected that he might see Gina more intensively at some point in the future, perhaps after the departure of the younger daughter from the home, the therapist was confident that she would never subject herself to physical or psychological abuse again.

THE THERAPEUTIC USE OF CRISIS

Time does not stand still while the therapist and client engage in the long-term process of changing dysfunctional schema. Significant life events in the course of treatment, such as marital separation, divorce, deaths, and problems with children, often do not allow us the luxury of contemplating family of origin material from a relatively detached perspective. Moreover, successful treatment of family of origin issues may actually induce a crisis in the client's life, as he or she becomes painfully aware of a spouse's drinking, a child's drug problem, a boss who replicates the actions of an abusive parent, and so on. For the alert therapist, however, crisis can spell opportunity. In many instances, recovery cannot occur without it. We encourage therapists to anticipate likely crises in their client's lives and to plan in advance how to respond to such events within the broader context of the treatment plan. A crisis allows the therapist to widen the scope of the therapy at the same time it deepens the client's sense of involvement in the treatment process.

The therapist must approach each legitimate crisis in the client's life as an opportunity to stimulate or encourage forward movement in recovery. From a cognitive perspective, crisis can reflect the breakdown of the process of assimilation and accommodation through which each person normally adjusts to ongoing life events. When the client reaches out to therapist for help during a period of turmoil, it is a de facto acknowledgment by the individual that existing concepts and/or coping strategies are not sufficient to handle current stressors. By making contact with the clinician, the client is also acknowledging a level of trust in the therapist, despite whatever may have transpired in the treatment process up to that point. Although the client's level of emotional distress may be high, he or she also may be more open than ever before to the therapist's influence. The clinician needs to capitalize on the client's increased reliance on the therapeutic relationship during a period of crisis to promote specific treatment agenda.

Clinicians who specialize in interventions for chemical dependency (Johnson, 1973) utilize significant others to orchestrate a crisis in the substance abuser's life, generally with the goal of facilitating immediate referral to inpatient treatment. The individuals who participate in the intervention process essentially trade on their accumulated good will with the identified patient. They confront the substance abuser strongly, but in a supportive, loving context. In the meantime, the clinician has already made all the necessary arrangements for inpatient treatment, so that an immediate response can occur the moment the substance abuser acknowledges a need for help. The intervention process appears to derive its power from the influence of the assembled group combined with the clinician's quick execution of a carefully planned response to transient changes in the substance abuser's thinking and behavior. The "window of opportunity" for the clinician and the client's significant others will only remain open for so long, however. Unless the substance abuser seeks inpatient treatment immediately or bonds very quickly with a self-help program, he or she will be likely to fall back into denial in a short amount of time.

It frequently behooves the therapist to make contingency plans for crises in the client's life, just as the clinician who conducts interventions does. This type of planning is particularly important when one is working with clients who, for various reasons, currently find it hard to focus productively on issues the therapist deems to be crucial to long-term recovery. Some types of individuals for whom such plans could be helpful include:

1. Substance abusers.
2. Clients who engage in addiction-like compulsive behaviors (e.g., gambling, phone sex) associated with potentially escalating negative consequences.
3. Clients who are currently utilizing denial strategies to minimize potentially serious stressors in their lives.
4. Clients in potentially destructive relationships that are currently at the limerant stage.
5. Clients with emerging, but perhaps poorly recognized, problems with partners, children, or other significant individuals in their lives.
6. Clients who have devoted their sessions exclusively to symptoms and/or obsessions.
7. Clients who have been extremely defensive or resistant to discussing certain issues in treatment.
8. Clients who have insisted on carefully controlling or limiting the content of treatment thus far.
9. Clients who have externalized blame to an extensive degree or have otherwise found it difficult to sustain a focus on the self in treatment.
10. Clients who have refused to comply with treatment norms, homework assignments, or other recommendations from the therapist.
11. Clients who have resisted marital, family, or group therapy,

psychiatric consultations, or other adjuncts to individual treatment.

In planning for crises, the therapist should attempt to answer the following key questions:

1. What are the "real world" consequences that might be associated with the crisis?
2. What potential symptoms might occur, on the part of the client, and/or significant others?
3. What provisions need to be made (e.g., medication, hospitalization, breaking confidentiality) in order to respond to the symptomatic dimensions of the anticipated crisis?
4. What kind of therapeutic posture will be most effective in responding to the client when the crisis occurs?
5. What changes in the therapeutic relationship would the clinician like to see as a result of the crisis?
6. What issues will be important to attempt to highlight during the crisis, and in what order?
7. How will the therapist frame the crisis to the client?
8. What previous gains or experiences in treatment will the therapist draw on in the crisis?
9. What areas of competence or past successful coping experiences on the part of the client can the therapist draw upon in the crisis?
10. Are there cognitive distortions, likely to be present in the crisis, which the client may have worked through successfully on other occasions?
11. In offering his or her help, what increased demands will the clinician want to place on the client?
12. How will the therapist seek to expand the focus of treatment during and/or after the crisis?
13. How might the therapist seek to expand contact with significant others and/or other professionals involved with the client during or after the crisis?
14. What noncompliant, defensive, or otherwise troublesome behaviors on the part of the client would the therapist want to address and reduce as a result of confronting the current crisis?
15. What adjuncts to the current treatment (e.g., group or family therapy, Twelve Step Program) does the therapist wish to promote in response to the crisis?
16. How can the therapist help the client come out of the crisis feeling like a winner?

11

The Use of Affect

AFFECT AS THE INEVITABLE OUTCOME OF ADAPTIVE INFORMATION PROCESSING

The bulk of our clients from dysfunctional family backgrounds have virtually no idea how to integrate the experience of affect into their lives. Some seldom experience strong emotions of any kind. Others may be unable to articulate the emotions they do experience. Certain individuals may have difficulty discriminating among various feeling states. Finally, even when they are able to experience and identify their emotions, our clients often find themselves confused about what to do next. Moreover, the emotional reactions of others may also frighten them—for a variety of reasons.

Early experiences with parents or other significant caretaking figures play a powerful role in the adult's ability to experience, tolerate, and express strong emotions. Certain clients may report having been afraid their whole lives that they would inevitably follow in a disturbed parent's footsteps. Not surprisingly, individuals with a family history of mental illness typically find it quite difficult to believe that feelings of anxiety do not lead to psychotic symptoms. They also may become unduly threatened when others appear to be anxious. In a similar manner, individuals whose parents were incapacitated by depression may be unable to tolerate feelings of sadness or despair, in themselves or others, without experiencing considerable panic or shame. Clients who were raised in physically abusive families may be phobic about experiencing anger in any form, or having to confront similar feelings in others. Likewise, victims of childhood sexual abuse may find it extremely threatening to experience sexual arousal, particularly during a period of trauma revelation.

Even happy feelings can scare some individuals, particularly if they anticipate destructive consequences as a result of letting down their guard in some manner. One of our clients would find herself recalling an oft-repeated line from her abusive mother whenever she began to feel any form of pleasure or happiness. "Laugh on Friday, cry on Sunday," the mother used to say. The same client, who suffered from chronic symptoms of depression, also repeatedly had the thought "If I feel better, I'm going to die."

Given the beliefs about affect expressed in the paragraphs above, it is no wonder that so many clients want simply to turn off their emotions. Such a coping strategy may have been both necessary and appropriate at one time, particularly during stressful periods in childhood and adolescence. The client with a history of impulsive and/or destructive behaviors might be even less inclined to risk the potentially disastrous consequences associated with intense affect.

The basic cognitive model of psychopathology holds that the affective response to any situation is generally a direct consequence of the way in which that situation has been perceived by the individual. Dysfunctional cognitions and disturbances in information processing produce distortions in the individual's affective responses. The cognitive therapist views the client's affect as appropriate or inappropriate solely in light of the associated meaning(s). Events that are intrinsically meaningful and rich with implications will produce an equally rich mixture of affective responses. An event that might be unreservedly positive in its *overall* impact, such as having one's child accepted at Harvard, might still evoke various painful emotions, for example, sadness in response to having a youngster leaving home.

Typical cognitive therapy strategies, having been developed primarily in order to treat depression and anxiety, aim to reduce emotional excesses through modification of the underlying ideation. *Therapists from other theoretical orientations often mistakenly assume that cognitive treatment aims solely for the reduction of affect in all situations.* Our model of treatment calls for a *variety* of therapeutic responses to emotions depending on the needs of the client. At times in the treatment process, the therapist will utilize interventions that *intensify* the client's affect, particularly when dealing with significant areas of denial. In other situations, during work on traumatic material for example, the therapist may encourage the client to learn strategies to control or *contain* intense emotions. Moreover, throughout treatment the therapist will generally make ongoing efforts to *normalize* many of the client's affective reactions.

In any given case, the therapeutic process will consist of *repeated cycles* in which periods of content *exploration* and emotional *intensification* alternate with intervals of affective *containment* and *normalization*. Such cycles can also occur on a small scale many times in the course of a typical treatment session, particularly if the material discussed is threatening or otherwise highly meaningful to the client. At times the therapist may be driving the cycles of exploration and containment, establishing a sense of rhythm, within and across sessions, that seems to suit the client's pace. Such circumstances are exhilarating and immensely gratifying for the clinician involved, since they produce such positive results for the client. In other instances, particularly when the case involves childhood trauma, neither the therapist nor the client feel in command of the exploration–containment cycle. Under these conditions, the therapist may need support from peers and supervisors, particularly if his or her caseload contains several individuals undergoing similar difficulties.

Our work with adults who were raised in dysfunctional families indicates that many such individuals suffer in equal measure from emotional *deficits* as well as excesses. Such individuals habitually underreact emotionally to situations most persons would find extremely distressing. The absence of affect can be as dysfunctional as the presence of inappropriate affect, if it is based on distortions in meaning. Often the emergence of intense affect on the part of the client is an important indicator of therapeutic progress, not because it reflects catharsis or abreaction, but because it reflects a more adaptive level of information processing. As we discuss in a subsequent section in this chapter, the therapist may need to examine his or her own affective reactions in order to determine whether the client's emotional responses are appropriate in a particular situation.

INTENSIFICATION STRATEGIES

It is entirely appropriate for our clients to experience emotional discomfort if that discomfort is based on a realistic appraisal of a particular situation. There *are* problems which are worth losing a night's sleep over. Full recognition of a major difficulty in one's life, a spouse's alcoholism for example, cannot take place without inducing considerable distress. The client who views his or her life through a detached perspective, as if another person were involved, is in all likelihood still screening out vital data. Sustained worry or anxiety over a particular issue often reflects expanded information processing, and in many instances, it indicates that for the first time the client has truly recognized the full magnitude of the problem. In many instances, the individual will remain stuck in a hopeless, helpless position unless and until he or she can begin to define the situation as a crisis. Once the client does recognize the true significance of a real life issue, then he or she can dedicate the time and energy necessary to address the problems involved.

The therapist may carefully attack the client's denial regarding a particular matter, such as a spouse's drinking, for months or even years during treatment. In these instances, the therapist actually wants the client to become more upset, because of the significance of the issues involved. When the client begins to show distress over the matter, the therapist will often end up amplifying those dysphoric feelings, by encouraging the client to process as much of the associated data as possible. This part of the treatment process can be taxing, both for therapists and clients.

Therapists who lack experience in breaking down denial processes, or who may identify too closely with a particular client, may worry about the potential effects of inducing "productive anxiety." They may worry that clients will fall apart when they come face to face with painful truths about their lives. Although the authors have had a substantial number of clients who decompensated in response to trauma-revelation material, we find that individuals rarely show similar reactions to current day realities, even when severe stressors are involved. On the other hand, we can recall numerous instances in which all sorts of traumatic outcomes occurred because clients were unwilling or unable to recognize threatening situations in their lives.

As long as the client is sober, nonpsychotic, and free of any biologically based mental disorder, we see no reason to shield him or her from reality, however painful the recognition process may be. The client who has forged a strong collaboration with the therapist does not have to undergo the recognition process alone. Even while working to enhance processing of disturbing material, the therapist continues to be supportive and empathic toward the client. In fact, once the client has switched into a more realistic appraisal of a particular situation, the therapist is now free to assume an even more supportive role in the treatment, even to the point of encouraging the client not to panic, to slow down, and to allow ample time for reflection before taking action.

Intensification strategies attack denial by keeping the client in contact with affectively charged information. There are various ways in which the therapist may attempt to accomplish such a task. Suppose, for example, a client has minimized signs of a potentially serious substance abuse problem on the part of her son. The therapist decides to return to the subject during the subsequent interview, so that the client can have another opportunity to review the data about her son. The therapist has many choices as to how to proceed, each one emphasizing a slightly different aspect of the content or a more intense confrontation of the client:

1. *Do you mind if I ask you some more questions about it?* Here the therapist implies an interest in the topic but draws the client's attention back to the content in a neutral manner.

2. *Did you feel we discussed all the facts about your son adequately? Were you more worried about your son at the end of that discussion?* Here the therapist suggests a direction the client could have (and perhaps should have) taken. The clinician's questions also provide the potential foundation for a discussion about denial if the client did not think about the subject. Embedded in the therapist's inquiries is the assumption that there is more to worry about and more to talk about.

3. *After our last session, I found myself thinking about the concerns you expressed about your son. Let's go back over the facts again for a moment.* These remarks may stimulate the listener's curiosity about the therapist's reactions, but they also move the spotlight quickly back to the client. The therapist raises the client's discomfort level, but then stands back and reviews the known data on the subject, allowing the facts to speak for themselves if possible.

4. *I became very concerned for your son's safety after the last session. It bothered me so much I almost called you a couple of times during the week. I want you to know that I'm not usually a "worry wart" about these things, so I think it's significant when a situation troubles me like this. Let's review the reasons why you were upset first, and then I'll explain why the implications were so frightening to me.* This strategy invites close attention to the therapist's affect and cognitions, before moving the client to an examination of the objective data and the personal implications thereof. As in the previous example, the therapist forestalls elaboration of his or her reactions in favor of an interactive review with the client.

5. *I want you to know that I became very frightened for your son's safety after we talked. Let me tell you what ran through my mind and why. If I sound all wet to you, please tell me, and I'll be happy to back off.* This strategy is useful with instances of severe denial, particularly if the therapist works directly from raw data supplied by the client. The therapist moves forcefully into the foreground, and remains on center stage for some time. In fact the therapist may stand, pace, or otherwise change positions frequently during the discussion which follows, in order to provide dramatic punctuation, and perhaps more importantly, to keep the client's attention riveted on a "moving target." The success of this type of intervention rests on the strength of the therapeutic bond and on the ability of the therapist to create and maintain a commanding presence

without provoking negative reactions on the client's part. The therapist should probably avoid such a provocative approach in the earlier phases of treatment, unless he or she has achieved both a remarkable rapport with the client, and a strong grasp of the individual's response tendencies.

Use of the Therapist's Affect

The affect the client evokes from the therapist is a crucial variable, not only with respect to diagnostic concerns but also as an aid to analyzing the therapeutic process itself. It is often useful for the clinical supervisor to understand the dynamics involved in a "stuck" case by examining the therapist's affective experience first, then working backward to the issues of the client. The therapist's affective reactions to the client can be an integral part of supervision, just as the client's feelings about the therapist can serve as an important focus in treatment. As the following case vignettes illustrate, even when the therapist's own issues are involved in his or her reactions to a specific case, it is typical in our experience to find on further analysis that the client's issues are *also* exerting strong influence in the situation.

A therapist was late in getting to the office one morning, as she was occasionally wont to do. Consequently, her supervisor peeked into the waiting room to inform the therapist's female client that she would be a few minutes late. During the interaction, which lasted all of 10 seconds, the supervisor maintained steady eye contact with the client, without allowing his gaze to stray to other features of her anatomy. Afterwards, he could not remember what the client had been wearing, nor could he even recall the general shape of her body. Nonetheless, as a result of a 10-second interaction, the supervisor found himself curiously turned on, hoping for an excuse to go back into the waiting room to speak to the client. At first, the supervisor felt somewhat ashamed and embarrassed, as if by feeling the attraction to the client he had done something wrong. However, as he reflected upon the incident he realized that the client *had* communicated some kind of sexual invitation to him, albeit nonverbally, during the brief interchange. This had not been his imagination, nor had it been some sort of distortion based on wish fulfillment on his part. Having worked through his embarrassment, the supervisor discussed his reactions with the treating therapist. As it turned out, the client in question disclosed a long and rather frightening history of sexual promiscuity, involving many liaisons with men who were nearly total strangers to her. Interestingly, she also complained of many unwanted sexual advances, wondering how it was that *she* was the focus of so much unwelcome interest from men.

Although she had intelligence, education, attractive looks, and a cheerful, friendly demeanor, Kimberly was stuck in a terrible marriage. Her husband, a police officer, was a hostile, demanding alcoholic, who thought nothing of spending hundreds of dollars each month buying marijuana and drinking in bars with his cronies. In the meantime, Kimberly worked two jobs to keep the family afloat financially. At times she would return home from work to find that her husband had passed out while caring for their two preschool-aged daughters. Kimberly rarely confronted her husband, or anyone else for that matter, in a direct way. She viewed herself as a helpless victim, without options. She experienced bouts of depression as well as bulimic symptoms. During the past few years, she had initiated affairs with two men she met at work, both of whom, predictably, had significant substance abuse problems of their own.

Kimberly ended up seeing two different individual therapists, because the first clinician who treated her moved out of the area. The two therapists, both females, had very similar affective responses to the client. They found themselves becoming anxious about the client's husband, whom they viewed as highly impaired, unmotivated to change, and unlikely to tolerate a divorce without making life miserable for the client. Both therapists felt a strong urge to protect Kimberly and both experienced a corresponding sense of helplessness when they realized that they could not directly affect her situation. Both came to believe at some time while treating Kimberly that, because of an array of logistical barriers, she *was* hopelessly trapped in her marriage.

The supervisor, who worked in turn with each therapist, played the role of devil's advocate when discussing the case. He reminded each therapist of women they had treated who had surmounted more severe obstacles to leave their husbands. He also exhorted the therapists to remain mindful of the client's denial processes and her compulsive behaviors. The supervisor reasoned that if Kimberly truly recognized the potential jeopardy to her children, she would treat her situation as an emergency. *Then* the client might view the complications of divorce as obstacles that she was ready to overcome. Moreover, the supervisor encouraged the therapists to consider the meaning of the client's affairs. Those relationships, which were clearly self-defeating in nearly every respect, indicated that the client was still committed to acting out rather than to confronting her problems directly. Further, her choice of partners also indicated that she was still gravitating to the same type of men.

When confronted with the data, both therapists could recognize that despite *their* affective reactions, the *client* still did not have a full appreciation of the negative features of her home situation. Furthermore, she was still not taking full responsibility for her choices. Both therapists realized that their protective urges reflected not only the client's pain but also her *abdication of responsibility*. Kimberly was not yet ready to confront the problems in her marriage directly. The supervisor suggested strategies for raising Kimberly's anxiety about her children and her sense of self-dissatisfaction over the affairs. Over time, dismay over the marriage grew, aided in no small part by her husband's escalating substance abuse. Eventually the client did terminate the marriage, primarily in order to protect her children.

Therapists commonly have difficulty working with some of the intense emotions they may experience in the course of treating certain cases. It may not be easy for clinicians to admit to supervisors that they feel enraged, intimidated, or erotically stimulated by particular clients. Many therapists expect a great deal from themselves. They may view each occurrence of "unwanted" emotional reaction to clients as a personal failure, rather than as a source of data to be utilized. The supervisor needs to create the kind of supportive atmosphere that encourages self-disclosure of potentially shameful feelings on the part of the therapist. In our opinion, it is helpful for the supervisor to normalize the therapist's affective reactions by disclosing his or her own feelings of anger, frustration, overresponsibility, intimidation, sexual attraction, and so on, as they have arisen in the treatment of certain cases.

The therapist should always take note when he or she seems to have a stronger emotional reaction to a situation in the client's life than the individual does. The client may recount an incident in a fairly detached tone, while implicitly and/or explicitly minimizing the significance of the situation in question. The therapist, meanwhile, may experience fear, anger, sadness, or other emotions. At times the therapist's affective response may continue on for hours after the session is over. Why the disparity in the reactions of therapist and client to the same material? From a cognitive perspective, we would suspect that the client's relatively unemotional response indicates denial mechanisms at work, so that he or she fails to process fully the ramifications of the situation in question. On the other hand, the therapist's affective response generally stems from a more complete appraisal of the data at hand. Unlike the client, the therapist is able to recognize potentially upsetting elements in the individual's life. Consequently, the therapist "carries" the client's affect. The therapist's task is to restore the affect to its rightful owner, in a manner of speaking, by stimulating more adaptive information processing on the part of the client.

For example, the highly promiscuous client mentioned in a pre-

vious paragraph would relate tales of casual, high-risk sexual encounters in an airy, singsong tone of voice, revealing not the slightest hint of
distress with herself or her behaviors. The therapist found the client's
stories distasteful and disconcerting. She became fearful when she
heard how the client continued to risk being raped, assaulted, or in-
fected by her sexual partners. As treatment progressed, the therapist
also became quite angry with the client, who continued on in her promiscuity, blissfully unaware of the potential consequences and implications. The therapist's anger and frustration reflected the strength of the
client's continuing denial mechanisms. Initially, the client was almost
totally incapable of sustaining a focus on the dangerous and degrading
aspects of her compulsive sexual behavior. Over time, however, the
therapist was able to identify elements of the promiscuity the client
found upsetting, *which she then sought to amplify at every opportunity.*
Eventually, the client reached the point where she herself labeled the
sexual behavior as a dangerous compulsion, although she continued to
deny the degrading aspects of her experiences.

In order to be able to tolerate the frustration of working with such
powerful denial mechanisms, the therapist had to divest herself of any
hopes of producing immediate changes in the sexual behavior. The
therapist could only assume that the self-destructive patterns would
continue until the client could begin to look at them more realistically.
On the other hand, the therapist also did not hesitate to voice her anger
and disgust with the client during supervision sessions. The supervisor
tried to help the therapist bring her negative feelings back into the
treatment sessions, not by bludgeoning the client into submission, but
by continually highlighting relevant data in a powerful, confident, but
noncoercive manner.

The therapist should be circumspect about *directly* expressing his or
her emotional reactions to a situation that the client has denied or
minimized. Remember that the goal of treatment is to change thinking
patterns by orchestrating *learning experiences* for our clients. We want to
enable them to process data that challenge their long-accepted ways of
conducting business. *Our interventions should direct the client's attention
back toward the data, not toward ourselves.* Disclosing one's affective reactions to the client's material can perform such a function admirably at
times, but there are pitfalls involved. Before disclosing his or her emotional reaction regarding a particular situation to the client, the therapist
needs to ponder several important questions:

- Will the client be distracted by the therapist's emotions, so that
  the therapeutic relationship, not the precipitating situation,
  moves to the perceptual foreground?

- Will the client feel ashamed or responsible for having upset the therapist?
- Will the client want to protect the therapist in some way subsequently, perhaps by failing to disclose similar information in the future?
- Will the therapist's affect stimulate a loyalty conflict for the client, thereby distracting him or her from the data?
- Will the client feel ashamed about having minimized the situation, thereby promoting greater self-disparagement?

Facilitating Productive Self-Dissatisfaction

Most of us would never change without a profound sense of dissatisfaction with ourselves and our actions. Guilt can be a constructive influence in a client's life, in that it can provide the individual with the motivation to break chronic patterns of self-defeating behaviors. The therapist needs to learn the delicate art of stimulating and/or perpetuating appropriate self-dissatisfaction, without punishing clients on the one hand, or rescuing them on the other. The following case example illustrates a successful exchange with a client, who became more distressed about her behavior as the dialogue with the therapist proceeded.

Although she had stopped drinking several weeks earlier, Valerie still had not attended an AA meeting and was beginning to minimize the extent of her alcohol problems, as evidenced by statements such as "I can take it or leave it." As he listened to Valerie slip back into denial, the therapist felt temporary annoyance with her and, more significantly, enduring anxiety about the continuation of her sobriety. The therapist's feelings at this point were diagnostic of the client's difficulties. It was a significant index of Valerie's denial regarding alcohol that the *therapist's* affect was beginning to boil over, not hers.

The therapist used his mounting concern as a signal to provide direction in the session with Valerie, but he did not share his feelings with her. Although the therapist wanted to transfer his dysphoric affect to the client so that she would take care of the problem, he did not want her to be distracted by *his* responses to her alcohol abuse. He suspected that the client would immediately react defensively if she experienced him as controlling or disapproving. Any approach that deflected Valerie away from her own reactions to the issue of alcohol would only facilitate the client's already substantial denial on the subject. Consequently, the therapist assumed a concerned, supportive posture, while he initiated a lengthy Socratic dialogue with the client.

The therapist asked Valerie's indulgence while he asked her to describe her feelings toward her two young children. The client acknowledged that her children were her first priority in life and that she would unhesitatingly make any sacrifice necessary to protect them. She agreed that she would not knowingly expose them to the possibility of physical or psychological abuse. The therapist emphasized that, although he had asked Valerie to articulate her feelings about parenthood, he had always assumed that she was a loving, competent mother who would unhesitatingly put her children's welfare ahead of her own.

Through the use of questioning, the therapist then conducted an interactive review with Valerie, using data already known to both of them, regarding the previous behavioral consequences of her drinking. By her own admission, the client had interacted with her children many times when intoxicated or suffering from a hangover. She described how she would behave in an ill-tempered manner on such occasions. Valerie also recalled having driven while intoxicated many times, since the bulk of her drinking occurred outside of the house. The client acknowledged that she even had the children in the car in several instances while driving under the influence of alcohol. She shuddered as she considered the degree to which she had endangered her children. The therapist also encouraged Valerie to imagine what the consequences would be for the children if she were imprisoned, badly injured, or killed as a result of drunken driving. She readily envisioned negative results for her children, especially in the event of her death.

The therapist then returned to the main issue, which was alcohol. He summarized the data that had illustrated so graphically that alcohol had caused the client to violate her most sacred values by inducing irresponsibility as a parent. By affirming Valerie's competence as a mother, the therapist was able to raise her anxiety about drinking and the denial process, without flooding her with feelings of worthlessness. In addition to underscoring her worth as a parent, he repeatedly pointed out that *alcohol* was the villain, not Valerie. He encouraged her to ponder with him the insidious power of the denial process, as evidenced by her current statements minimizing the previous impact of her alcohol abuse. Again, *denial* was the culprit in the therapist's presentation, not Valerie. Alcohol had threatened what she held most dear, and with the resurgence of denial, it was beginning to threaten her once again. One of the advantages of AA, the therapist explained, was that it assisted the individual in the daily war with denial.

As this discussion unfolded, the therapist's dysphoric feelings diminished and eventually disappeared, while Valerie's anxiety rose steadily. The therapist maintained a concerned, but nonjudgmental, posture and stopped short of making any concrete recommendations to her about alcohol or AA, since the client was already well aware of his views on those topics. At the next session, Valerie announced that she approached a colleague who was active in AA and had already attended several meetings with her.

CONTAINMENT STRATEGIES

Containment strategies aim to reduce affect and/or mitigate the effects of strong emotions. The literature on cognitive therapy (see McMullin, 1986 for a review of techniques), behavior therapy (Goldfried & Davison, 1976), and hypnotherapy (Brown & Fromm, 1986) all contain many examples of techniques that foster a greater sense of affective self-control on the part of the client. As we shall discuss in a subsequent section, containment-oriented interventions are extremely important when working with trauma survivors.

The therapist can promote containment by:

Supporting activities that will lower arousal level, for example, relaxation, meditation, aerobic exercise.

Encouraging appropriate self-care on the part of the client, particularly in the areas of nutrition, physical rest, and proper medical attention.

Confronting ongoing factors that may undermine self-control, for example, substance abuse.

Supporting the use of prayer, participation in confession, attendance at church or synagogue, or other adaptive religious activities, if the client is so inclined.

Promoting the development and maintenance of more secure boundaries in the client's life.

Recommending temporary restrictions in the client's sexual involvement if flashbacks or other strong affective reactions have been associated with such activities.

Encouraging the use of Twelve-Step or other self-help group resources during crisis periods.

Facilitating the use of appropriate medications.

Mobilizing the client's support system if possible, or if necessary, hospitalizing the individual.

Helping the client learn imagery techniques, rational responses, and other methods for coping with unpleasant emotions.

Assisting the client to test out the validity of fearful cognitions.

Encouraging the development of adaptive distraction techniques by the client.

Encouraging the client to implement containment strategies when experiencing intense affective responses during treatment sessions.

Utilizing a stress inoculation approach, for example, by rehearsing strategies for handling flashbacks or other symptomatic periods.

Providing the client with a comprehensible framework for understanding why particular affective reactions occur.

Helping the client to recognize normal, appropriate affective reactions to significant life events.

Highlighting data that indicate that the client *is* capable of exercising appropriate self-control even during periods of discomfort.

Helping the client to identify and confront any legitimate sources of threat that may exist in the environment.

Providing the client with a consistent, stable therapeutic relationship, involving continuous feedback, well-articulated expectations, and a clear treatment contract.

Addressing factors in the therapeutic relationship that might cause the client to feel unsafe or otherwise uncomfortable.

Allowing the client to retain near-absolute control over the content of treatment sessions.

Postponing discussion of affectively charged material to later sessions should the client feel unprepared for such dialogue.

Confronting acting out episodes, particularly those which occur in response to the clinician.

Coping strategies already in the client's repertoire may give the therapist some clues as to the type of containment techniques that might succeed best with the individual. For example, a client who maintains a regimen of strenuous exercise has probably learned distraction techniques to cope with monotony and/or exhaustion. The therapist may explore whether the client can transfer such skills to manage symptomatic periods. Similarly, a female client who has borne children via natural childbirth may have developed effective breathing and imagery techniques that could be readily adapted for containment purposes. Unfortunately, the therapist may not always be able to find coping strategies in the client's repertoire that can be appropriated for containment purposes. In such instances, it can helpful to expose the client to a *menu* of potential containment strategies so that the therapist can build on those techniques that seem to provoke interest or enthusiasm. The therapist should studiously avoid promoting strategies that appear superficial, gimmicky, or otherwise ineffectual to the client, regardless of how well such interventions might have succeeded with other individuals.

The therapist should encourage the client to examine carefully any instances of successful containment. We find that enormous benefits result whenever clients can attribute improvements in self-control to their *own* efforts. Indeed, in many instances when clients control themselves successfully, they will assign credit elsewhere unless the therapist intervenes. Clients do need to recognize, however, that containment strategies will not magically eradicate dysphoric affect. The therapist should emphasize repeatedly that the goal of treatment is to enable the client to *tolerate* negative emotions, without resorting to acting out, severe dissociation, or other self-defeating coping strategies.

NORMALIZING STRATEGIES

Treatment generally involves *ongoing, repeated* efforts to help the client develop new norms regarding the experience and the expression of affect. Normalizing strategies can involve the full range of techniques for promoting awareness (e.g., orienting, Socratic dialogue, and so on) described in Chapter 9. The therapist will also use embedded messages to promote normalization of affect. The therapist can utilize adjunctive resources such as self-help books and support groups to help the client develop a clear picture of what constitutes appropriate affective responses to various situations. Such "objective" sources of data are often far more successful in changing the client's attitudes than any reassurances offered by the clinician.

Throughout the course of treatment, the therapist promotes the normalization of affect by repeatedly obtaining and underscoring data from the client's own experiences that support the following points:

1. Strong emotions are expected to accompany all of the important experiences of life.

2. Most if not all important events and relationships in life stimulate a rich *blend* of emotions, some which may contradict one another. Ambivalent feelings are normal and appropriate in a wide range of situations.

3. It is normal for an individual to go through repeated affective *cycles* in response to a highly meaningful event. It takes time to appreciate all the ramifications of important life situations. Consequently, the individual's emotional responses will change and diminish over time, only to recur at various junctures. Sometimes the recurrence of affect will follow a predictable pattern (e.g., anniversary reactions, missing someone over the holidays), and sometimes it will appear to be random in nature. Both circumstances are entirely normal.

4. No one can prescribe the *right* emotions to feel in response to a

particular experience. Although there are common themes that seem to recur, each individual reacts in a unique way. Similarly, no one can prescribe the right *sequence* of emotions one should experience in response to a significant event. Again, people react to important situations in their lives with idiosyncratic affective patterns. Finally, no one can prescribe the optimum time it will take an individual to "recover" from an upsetting event such as a death of a loved one.

5. *Lack* of affect in response to a particular situation is not necessarily indicative of more competent functioning. Indeed, it can reflect a potentially crippling inability to confront reality. Stoic detachment often inhibits the development of more effective problem-solving skills and coping strategies.

6. The suppression of intense affect is not nearly as successful as it may appear. In an intimate relationship, for example, an acting job is probably much less effective than the would-be Thespian realizes. A husband who works hard to suppress angry feelings toward his wife ultimately behaves differently with her anyway, by withdrawing, by reacting more irritably to minor matters, by acting in a passive–aggressive manner, and so on. Similarly, the woman who "decides" not to experience any more grief about the loss of her mother will still find herself in tears unexpectedly.

7. Denial strategies can create new problems for people. Individuals who habitually suppress intense affect invariably "throw out the baby with the bath water," in that they also steer themselves away from vital information in the process. Ultimately, the loss of data compromises the individual's ability to make well-informed decisions, particularly about relationships.

8. Attempting to suppress intense affect is very *costly* in terms of time, energy, and aggravation. It takes more time and effort trying *not* to cry than it does to tolerate a few moments of sobbing or tears. Moreover, the suppression of affect can assume the status of a full-time job in the client's life, as is true in so many cases of anxiety and panic. On the other hand, once an affective response occurs, the individual *can* utilize *containment strategies* to modulate the intensity, the duration, and the aftereffects of his or her emotional reactions.

9. Strong emotions, experienced either by oneself or by significant others, need not produce grave consequences. The individual who *experiences* powerful feelings will not necessarily feel compelled to act them out.

10. People do not *choose* their emotions, or the thoughts that may stimulate their feelings, the way they choose their actions. Affect is a spontaneous reaction to the perception of meaning. Emotions, unlike actions, are morally neutral.

11. Habitually withholding reports on one's affective state can sabotage efforts to establish and maintain intimacy in a relationship. Persistent failure to communicate about inner experiences with one's partner actually constitutes a potentially destructive form of withdrawl.

12. *Sharing* one's emotions in a constructive, nonblaming manner can build intimacy with a supportive partner.

13. Invalidating the feelings or perceptions of others can be a destructive interpersonal strategy. Attempts to support, reassure, or comfort others should generally not include efforts to restructure cognitions or change emotions. Empathizing with an individual's feelings can occur without necessarily endorsing, or even addressing the perceptions that may be involved.

14. Progress in therapy will not remove negative emotions from one's existence, since loss, disappointments, rejections, failures, conflicts, and a host of other unpleasant experiences are all a part of life. Indeed, if treatment is successful in attacking denial strategies, it will probably *increase* the frequency and intensity of the individual's emotional responses to certain life situations.

15. Negative emotions, particularly anxiety, are likely to intensify whenever an individual begins to confront a phobia or any other area of avoidance. Increased exposure to feared situations, particularly if it occurs in a graded manner, will in the long-run almost inevitably result in reduced affect and a greater sense of self-control.

16. Affective responses may serve as *cues*, signaling the need for self-exploration. Individuals can increase self-awareness by tracing emotions back to their sources. Persistently exaggerated affective responses to certain situations or classes of situations may reflect the operation of external stressors and/or inner mechanisms that are not apparent without reflection. There generally is an explanation for why a particular emotional response has occurred. Knowing why we feel as we do will not necessarily suppress or even dampen our emotions, but it does enhance control over the disruptive secondary consequences associated with intense affective reactions.

In order to facilitate more adaptive expression of affect on the client's part, the therapist first needs to understand how caretaking figures responded to the individual's emotional reactions in childhood and adolescence. Did anyone listen? Were the child's emotions minimized? Was the child punished or rejected for experiencing certain emotions? Was the child labeled in some manner as a result of verbalizing certain emotions (e.g, "You're the emotional one," "You get angry just like your father does," and so on)? Was the client encouraged to use denial strategies to deal with painful situations (e.g., "Just put it out of your mind," "We will never speak of this again," and so on)? Did the child make a *decision* at some point about not expressing (or even experiencing) certain feelings?

CONFRONTING ACTING OUT

The process of psychotherapy is always influenced by the personal and professional values of the therapist. We suspect that mental health professionals who are committed in their own lives to what Twelve-Step Programs call "fearless self-examination" will probably be most effective in recognizing and confronting acting out patterns in their clients. Although clinicians need not be apologetic about their values, they certainly must remain acutely aware of them. Without self-awareness and self-discipline, the therapist can turn the treatment process into a personal crusade. Clinicians need to respect the diversity of individuals from different backgrounds. Consequently, therapists ought to have some objective criteria, so that they can easily identify acting out on the part of their clients without having to draw *solely* on their own idiosyncratic values or reactions. We find that the following elements consistently characterize acting out behavior:

1. Acting out behavior is pressured, *compulsive* behavior. The individual may feel uncontrollably drawn to certain individuals and situations or pushed to behave in a particular fashion. The fact that compulsive behaviors may lead again and again to the same negative consequences does not generally stimulate the client to utilize better self-control. The individual will usually fight anyone tooth and nail in order to be able to continue the acting out behaviors.
2. Acting out involves the abdication of personal responsibility on the part of the individual. When asked later to account for their actions, individuals typically externalize blame and/or describe themselves as having had no other choices or options in the situations involved.
3. Acting out behaviors reflect the direct operation of dysfunctional basic schemas and coping strategies, generally without the client's explicit acknowledgement.
4. Acting out behaviors are usually *fear-driven coping strategies*— attempts by the individual to avoid various aversive consequences. Many cute, peace-loving animals can become threatening to humans if cornered. Similarly, individuals who are strongly motivated by fears of various kinds can easily behave

destructively toward others, often without recognizing it. Readers should review relevant sections in Chapter 3 on "Solomon's Dogs," and "Compulsive Behaviors."

5. Acting out behaviors are usually accompanied and/or supported by substantial denial on the part of the individual. Individuals consistently minimize the impact of their actions, offer rationalizations, and otherwise resist sustained analysis of their behaviors.

6. Acting out behaviors produce long-term negative consequences for the client and/or significant others. Regardless of the short-term benefits that may result, acting out extracts its toll in the long-run, often on innocent parties.

7. Acting out behaviors involve departures from the client's baseline levels of social, interpersonal, ethical, spiritual, intellectual, and/or vocational functioning. The majority of our clients feel quite displeased with themselves once they examine their acting out behaviors in a realistic manner.

The therapist must take note whenever the client engages in acting out episodes, particularly those which result in the victimization of others. Many clients have the capacity to be victimizers, as well as victims. Even clients who would not knowingly exploit or abuse others are capable of behaving in a manner that produces destructive interpersonal consequences. Enabling and/or controlling behaviors, although they may be prompted by the best of intentions on the part of the client, can be toxic to others. For example, the parent who subsidizes a drug user, ignoring evidence that the funds are going directly to the purchase of illegal substances, is unwittingly or not, promoting death just as strongly as any dealer. When the effects of such behavioral patterns are being examined, the question of the enabler's motivation is absolutely irrelevant. Similarly, anxious individuals with strong controlling tendencies can create a tense, punitive atmosphere for everyone around them, particularly their young children. In the process of managing their own fears about parenting, some of which may be realistic, certain controlling clients may inadvertently scapegoat the children they seek to protect.

Any time the therapist fails to confront a clear episode of acting out, he or she has made a concession of sorts to the less competent side of the client. In effect, the therapist who bypasses such a confrontation is saying that the individual is unable to change or even talk about the behaviors in question. Indeed, the client may *not* yet be ready either to change the behaviors or to address the issues involved. The clinician may need to wait until a later point in the recovery process to address the relevant material, for example, when the therapeutic relationship has developed, when a period of crisis occurs, and so on. However, the therapist's *first* instinct should be to move *toward* acting out material whenever it surfaces in treatment. If it is clinically advisable to wait, let the therapist do so *reluctantly* and perhaps somewhat impatiently. In the meantime, the clinician can remain vigilant for any opportunities to steer the client's attention toward the material in question.

There are two favorable characteristics, at least from a therapist's point of view, associated with acting out behaviors. Acting out behaviors tend to recur, and they tend to produce crises in the client's life. Consequently, in the course of treatment the therapist ought to have multiple opportunities to address similar behaviors on the part of the client. These "second and third chances" allow the therapist to learn from previous errors and to formulate a more effective posture for confronting acting out episodes in the future. Once the therapist has developed a model of the client's behavioral cycles, it should be possible to anticipate certain types of crises in the individual's life. As we discuss in our section on crisis, the therapist can utilize such occasions to confront material that the client had been unwilling or unable to examine previously.

The following case involved a client, Laura, whose defensive, controlling style led to many interpersonal conflicts. The therapist found it difficult to confront the client's hostile behavior toward others until she directed an angry outburst at him. The clinician was then able to utilize the acting out episode as a pathway to much more profitable therapeutic work on the client's interpersonal style and the chronic sense of worthlessness that served as the foundation for much of her self-defeating behavior.

Laura grew up in a large family of French-Canadian immigrants that had been plagued by alcoholism for many generations. When the client was 10, her stepfather initiated an incestuous relationship with her that continued until just after she reached puberty. After Laura finally resisted the abuse, and disclosed it to her mother, the entire family scapegoated her. The mother even went to the point of demanding that Laura confess her sin of "lying" to the parish priest. Laura was a fighter, however. She acted out in every way she could, until she was placed in a foster home. At 17, she became pregnant by a young soldier from a nearby army base, whom she eventually married when the infant was 6 months old. The husband, himself a product of an extremely chaotic home, was unable to cope with the demands of his new family. He began to drink heavily and spent most of his time in seedy bars.

Volunteering for duty at a remote overseas base, he eventually broke off all contact with the family.

Left alone with a toddler to support, Laura refused to be defeated by her discouraging circumstances. Making use of grants, food stamps, and every available resource she could find, the client was able to put herself through a part-time nursing program. Her energy, tenacity, and strong work ethic enabled her to rise through the professional ranks fairly quickly, so that she found herself in a high-level administrative position at a comparatively young age.

Work had always been an oasis of sorts for Laura. The client's daughter, who suffered from attentional problems and learning disabilities, had been a handful almost from the beginning. Now an eighth grader, the girl was approaching what Laura knew from her own experience was a very dangerous age. The client complained that her daughter was lazy and manipulative, noting that the girl's father had behaved in a similar fashion. There were constant battles between the mother and the daughter over trivial matters, usually housekeeping chores.

Laura's relationships with men had not improved much from the early days. Along the way, there had been a second failed marriage to another alcoholic, albeit one with a medical degree. Except for a brief affair with a recently separated man who ultimately returned to his wife, Laura had pretty much given up on dating in recent years. Committed to a stoic, basically anhedonic lifestyle, she kept herself narrowly focused on her responsibilities, as a professional and as a mother.

Laura entered therapy because she had begun to experience increased friction with two key subordinates at work. They accused her of being rigid, prejudicial, and verbally abusive. Although Laura acknowledged somewhat grudgingly that she had engaged in public shouting matches with the subordinates on a few occasions, she did not believe that her actions had contributed significantly to the continuing interpersonal friction. In her view, the subordinates had engaged in a vendetta against *her* over minor issues, for purely personal motives. Threatening legal action, they had met privately with Laura's manager. Subsequently, the manager had issued an official memo to Laura, censuring her and admonishing her to avoid similar behavior in the future. For the first time in her career, Laura had a dark cloud hovering over her head. Despite the friction that had occurred, the supervisor clearly expected her to deal with the two hostile subordinates in a more effective manner, ideally without antagonizing them further. The fact that the subordinates had won a public victory over her only made Laura more angry with them. She found herself experiencing considerable anxiety, which interfered with her ability to concentrate and stimulated powerful feelings of embarrassment.

Laura considered herself knowledgeable about the mental health field and had not been impressed by the therapists who worked at the hospital. Curiously, however, she persisted in addressing her therapist as "Doctor," although he had used his first name when he introduced himself. Although a tear or two managed to slip out while she discussed the work conflicts, the client generally behaved in a controlled, somewhat formal manner during treatment sessions. Laura found the therapist's suggestions for containing anxiety to be quite helpful, but she did not seem responsive when he attempted to underline the broader issues that seemed to be involved in her current distress. Although the client recognized superficial similarities between the current work problems and the scapegoating that had followed her disclosure of sexual abuse, she was not able to identify any common cognitive elements, particularly those that involved worthlessness. Even when questioned directly by the therapist, Laura tended to deny any significant difficulties with self-esteem. Likewise, she claimed to have left the problems in her family of origin, and the stormy, degrading experiences of adolescence, far behind her.

The therapist was reasonably sure that Laura often created problems for herself interpersonally, both at home and at work. He saw her as a compulsive, highly driven individual who probably lost sight of her interpersonal impact once she became anxious to any significant degree. Although Laura was never less than polite and respectful in his office, the therapist suspected that she could behave in an extremely controlling, abrasive, and perhaps even manipulative manner, particularly when threatened. He assumed that such behavior was based on dysfunctional thinking patterns, but he had great difficulty finding tangible evidence of cognitive distortions in the client's externally focused accounts of her interpersonal conflicts. Laura always seemed to present herself as the reasonable party, victimized by the jealousy of her subordinates, or the irresponsibility of her daughter. Moreover, both the subordinates and the daughter *did* behave outrageously at times.

During the 12th treatment session, Laura showed a different side of herself to the therapist. She arrived at the office in a tense mood, fresh from another annoying encounter with the hostile subordinates. Almost from the moment she walked in the door, Laura launched into an angry diatribe against her adversaries. The therapist wanted to make more constructive use of the interpersonal material than he had been able to do during previous discussions. Consequently, he remained quite active while Laura told her story, interrupting her frequently with questions and interpretive comments. In retrospect, the clinician's intrusive approach may have been ill-advised. The therapist was trying too hard, perhaps because he was afraid that Laura would be critical of him for not being more helpful to her.

Operating under the assumption that part of the subordinates' power over Laura stemmed from their ability to induce feelings of worthlessness and self-doubt, the therapist again tried to integrate information about her abusive family background with the current work conflicts. Laura seemed to have more and more difficulty answering the therapist's questions as the discussion proceeded. Although the client never stated directly that she was uncomfortable with the therapist's input, her responses seemed to become increasingly terse and uninformative. Suddenly, at least from the therapist's point of view, Laura became livid with him. Her face turned a crimson hue, and the pitch of her voice seemed to rise several octaves. "I know what you're driving at, and I won't put up with it," she shouted. "That's all everyone does is blame *me* for everything that goes on." The client grew more upset as she continued to berate the therapist. "What do you know about problems anyway, with your nice little middle-class life? No one knows the kinds of things *I've* had to put up with. What do people really care about *me*? I'm sick of them, and I'm sick of therapy, and I'm sick of *you*." Much to the therapist's surprise, Laura punctuated the final sentence by flinging her purse across the room.

The remainder of the session was unproductive. The therapist calmly told Laura that she would need to refrain from throwing anything else during the session. Taking a moment to compose herself after the outburst, Laura quickly lowered her voice to a more reasonable volume. From her intonation and other nonverbal indicators, it was clear to the therapist that Laura was still quite angry with him. She continued to appear somewhat cold and distant, despite the clinician's attempts to smooth over the incident.

The therapist decided to postpone discussion of the incident until the next session. Although the therapist certainly wondered whether Laura might terminate treatment at this point, he acted as if he fully expected her to schedule another appointment. Somewhat to his surprise, the client did so quite readily. As Laura left the office, the therapist shook hands with her, just as he always did. As he did so, he told the client, "I just want you to know that I continue to be committed to working with you and that I'm just as optimistic as I've ever been about your ability to get something valuable for yourself from treatment." Since his words were spoken as Laura walked out of the office, the therapist knew that she would not have the opportunity to reply. He hoped that the client would recall his closing comments when she reflected on the session later.

Laura's angry outburst certainly left its imprint on the therapist.
Initially, he felt quite responsible for her behavior. The clinician spent
some time berating himself for not allowing the client to tell her story
unimpeded. There were factors in the therapist's own family of origin
that precipitated him to blame himself whenever he was the target of
hostile, guilt-inducing behavior from a depressed female client. Gradually, the clinician realized that although he had behaved in a more
intrusive manner than usual during Laura's narration, he certainly had
not treated her with disrespect during the discussion in question, or at
any other time for that matter. No, the therapist concluded, nothing *he*
did had warranted the client's destructive response. Somehow, he had
inadvertently communicated blaming messages to Laura regarding her
problems at work. It was the client's *perception* of being blamed that had
triggered the angry outburst.

The therapist's own family of origin experiences could have easily
led him to sweep angry outbursts from hostile, dependent clients, especially females, under the carpet, partly out of fear and partly out of a
misplaced sense of responsibility. As a result of his own therapy, the
therapist had found he could confront clients who behaved in such a
manner much more successfully than he had in the past. Moreover, the
clinician knew that the incident could provide him with an effective
entry point into the issues that were creating difficulties for the client in
several important relationships. Consequently, the therapist was determined to process all the implications of the outburst with Laura during
the next interview. The therapist made a list of the things he hoped to
accomplish in the discussion of the incident, and tried to picture the
most effective sequence for raising certain related issues with the client.

The therapist began the next session by asking Laura what her
reactions had been to the previous interview and how she had felt about
coming for today's appointment. Making far less eye contact than was
customary for her, the client said she was surprised that she had become
so angry, so quickly. Laura stated that she still could not believe she had
reached the point of flinging her purse across the room. Many times
during the past week she had worried that the therapist would now
think she was crazy. Laura had also wondered whether the clinician
would even continue to work with her after the angry outburst. However, the therapist's reassuring remarks at the close of the previous
appointment had continued to echo in the client's thoughts, thereby
comforting her somewhat. Having experienced considerable guilt over
her actions, Laura reported feeling quite embarrassed about returning
for her next session. Although she had invented many plausible excuses
for canceling the appointment, the client said she knew she needed to
see the therapist, since her anxiety level had been quite high all week.

Before questioning Laura more specifically regarding her phenomenology of the incident, the therapist needed to underline a few points. With clients who were less contrite about their behavior, he normally would have spent time defining very clearly the limits of acceptable behavior in psychotherapy sessions, as well as the potential costs of transgressing such limits in the future. However, now that Laura *herself* had identified her behavior as symptomatic and contrary to her values, the therapist could afford to take a somewhat magnanimous posture, while still calling for a full examination of the incident. The clinician now wanted to redirect the client's attention away from her behavior and his reactions to it toward the underlying cognitive mechanisms. He said, "I had thought you might be embarrassed about coming back here today. That's why I specifically told you I still wanted to work with you just before you left the last time. I'm glad you remembered those words of mine during the week. I know it wasn't easy to come back here. I think it took some courage. I know that what you did last time wasn't like you at all. Your guilt and embarrassment are proof of that. Something pretty powerful must have been happening inside you to lead you to behave in a way that was so clearly contrary to your own personal values. I'd like to talk some more about your inner experiences during that session but only to see if we can learn something from it. Is that okay with you? I don't want to make you feel as if we're "rubbing your nose in it." Do you think you can tell me if the discussion starts to feel that way?"

Laura agreed that she would alert the therapist if she began to feel significant discomfort during the forthcoming discussion. She told the therapist that she remembered experiencing a blinding rage with him just prior to the outburst. She remembered thinking "He's going to blame me too." The client recalled feeling a sense of *absolute desperation* as she began to suspect that the therapist was siding against her. The therapist asked the client to articulate what it was about the situation that made her feel *desperate* (as opposed to disappointed, annoyed, uncomfortable, and so on). Laura seemed to draw a blank in response to the question.

Before probing further, the therapist decided to underscore a few key points that he hoped would reduce the client's defensiveness during subsequent discussion of her angry behavior. Since Laura had previously shown many signs of denial, including a tendency to quibble with him over the precise usage of certain affectively oriented terms, the therapist was careful to incorporate a great deal of her *exact* language into his remarks. He said, "I think I have some ideas as to why you felt so desperate, but before we discuss that issue, I just wanted to underline a very important point. Most of the people I've worked with don't get any particular pleasure out of getting angry or hurting others in any way. You're no exception to the rule either. Notice that before you became angry you felt *desperate*. I believe that the angry behavior you and most other people engage in is only a way *to cope with something else that is very threatening*, something like *absolute desperation*. Consequently, you're going to find that I'm a lot more interested in the issues that stimulate anger rather than the angry behavior itself."

Now the therapist was ready to assist Laura to explore the sense of desperation that had given rise to her angry outburst during the last session. In doing so, he employed the formulation that had guided him the previous week, namely, that many of her interpersonal problems occurred when her basic sense of self-worth was being threatened in some manner. Having laid the groundwork described in the previous paragraphs, the clinician was now free to facilitate Laura's self-exploration through the use of Socratic dialogue without fear of provoking another defensive response from her. The conversation proceeded as follows:

Th: Let's explore why you became upset to the point of desperation when you thought I held you responsible for your problems at work. This may seem like a digression, but how well do you think I know you at this point?

Laura: I think you know a lot about me. You know things about me even my close friends don't know, especially about my past.

Th: Are you referring to the incest and the things that happened after you blew the whistle on your stepfather?

Laura: Yeah, and some of the crazy things I did when I was a teenager. I don't discuss those days with anyone now.

Th: How much do you value my opinion? When it comes to feedback about you, your attitudes, your behavior, how much credibility do I have?

Laura: I would say a lot. You knew that I came here in the beginning a nonbeliever as far as therapy was concerned. Your feedback has been practical, down-to-earth. You've taught me how to deal with these anxiety attacks much more effectively. At least now I know that I won't go crazy just because I have one. I think you've been a straight shooter with me. Believe it or not, even last week's incident made me respect you more. I know how hard it can be to keep your cool when someone attacks your credibility as a professional.

Th: So unlike your two subordinates, and your supervisor, neither of whom you particularly respect, I am someone whose opinions you value?

Laura: Yes, that's right.

Th: How do you think it would affect you, then, to be criticized by someone whose judgment and competence you respected, someone who knew things about you few others did? How do you think you would begin to feel about yourself, in the face of real or perceived criticism from someone like that?

Laura: On a good day, I might tell myself that you really didn't understand the particular situation, or that you were being unfair. Maybe I'd get mad at you and show it. On a bad day, or maybe even just an average day, I think I'd probably feel devastated if I thought you had a low opinion of me. I'm sure I'd start to feel pretty lousy about myself. But isn't it just human nature to want a person you respect to like you in return?

Th: I think you're absolutely right. It would be pretty bizarre if you, or anyone else, *didn't* want someone you respected to like you. But remember now that we're talking about how you begin to feel about yourself once you perceive that someone in my position *does* have a negative opinion about you. For the most part, you seem to think that it would be a pretty devastating experience for you, causing you to feel badly about yourself as a person. Do you think you would begin to ruminate about other faults or misdeeds of yours, beyond whatever I might have chosen to criticize?

Laura: Yeah, I think I could start beating up on myself pretty badly, especially if I had to be alone without any distractions for long periods of time. (Sighs) I guess there are a lot of things I don't really like about myself that I try not to think about most of the time. Maybe those things could start crashing down on me anytime if I let them.

Th: Has there ever been a time when you've let that happen, or when maybe you couldn't do anything to keep it from happening?

Laura: Well, I felt pretty close to that the first couple of days after our last session. I was sure you were down on me, and I thought you had a good reason to be. I felt rotten about myself in every way, not just because I had gotten so mad at you. All the old standbys, you know, working double shifts, cleaning like a madwoman, just didn't seem to make any difference. I still felt like a total failure in every way.

Th: Let me remind you that the point of this discussion was to find out how it affected you when you thought I was blaming you for the

difficulties you were experiencing at work. Remember that initially
you couldn't tell me too much about your reactions, except that
before you became angry you felt desperate. Thanks to your willingness to persevere though, I think we've been able get a clearer
picture of the *source* of your desperation. Actually, we've probably
learned a great deal of valuable information during this discussion,
which I will share with you in a few minutes. Listen to what you've
just told me: By giving you negative feedback, I would have the
ability to make you feel terrible about yourself, so terrible that you
would begin to ruminate about faults and misdeeds totally unrelated to the current situation. As you just indicated, despite your
efforts to distract yourself, the sense of worthlessness could easily
torment you for days afterwards, just as it did last week. I think
anyone might come out fighting if they thought they were being
backed into that kind of corner, don't you?

This particular discussion with Laura far surpassed any of the therapist's expectations in that it yielded a wealth of new material about her
self-image and her coping strategies. Through the Socratic dialogue, the
client was able to identify thinking patterns that she had not been able
to access previously. She indicated that feelings of worthlessness affected her, and motivated her actions, much more significantly than she
had recognized previously. The client also began to see how her compulsive work behaviors helped her to cope with feelings of worthlessness by serving as a distraction and by providing a sense of self-esteem,
however transient. Moreover, Laura was starting to understand how
feelings of worthlessness also affected her interpersonal relationships.
The client realized that although her behavior during the previous
session had been based on distorted perceptions, her anger was actually
a response to an enormous, but unacknowledged threat, namely, the
therapist's ability to make her feel very badly about herself.

As the therapist continued the discussion, he explored the broader
implications of Laura's angry outburst. He asked the client to describe
other times when she had struggled with feelings of worthlessness,
encouraging her to identify consistent situations and recurring themes
associated with her self-deprecating thoughts. He began to underscore
how the events of the client's adolescence might have affected her
self-image, initially by asking Laura to imagine how her teenage daughter might have reacted to similar childhood experiences. The therapist
also explained how the success of Laura's preferred coping strategies,
a powerful combination of denial and hard work, made it appear not
only to the outside world, but even to *her*, that worthlessness was not
a problem. He described how a snake phobic might restrict many of his

or her activities in an attempt to avoid the feared reptiles, *all the while experiencing very little of the actual anxiety that had produced the problem in the first place.* Laura seemed to understand that whether or not she experienced feelings of poor self-esteem at any given time, every day was for her a struggle against worthlessness.

The therapist had now set the stage for a major change in the focus of treatment—away from Laura's complaints about others, back toward the real problems, her attitudes about herself and the over-driven coping strategies she employed to ward off feelings of worthlessness. However, the client's difficulties at work and with her daughter continued to produce considerable distress in her life. Understandably then, she would still want to spend time in her sessions discussing those difficult relationships. The therapist needed to develop a format for discussing Laura's interpersonal problems that would continually underscore *her* issues, without eliciting the kind of defensiveness that had occurred previously. He also wanted to prepare the client for other distorted perceptions of the therapeutic relationship that might occur in the future, so that she would view such reactions as a valuable source of data and continue to disclose them.

During a later session, the therapist asked Laura's permission to review again both the angry outburst and the discussion that had followed it. He reminded the client that the issue of her own worthlessness was the basis of her hostile response, emphasizing once again how uncharacteristic of her the angry behavior had been. The therapist also described the historical antecedents of Laura's defensiveness, recalling how she had been scapegoated and falsely accused by her family at a time when she had desperately needed support and validation. What basis would Laura have in her experience to trust *anyone* with her most vulnerable side, the therapist asked, particularly a male authority figure? He added that although he was sure that there would not be any additional angry outbursts on her part, he did suspect Laura would have difficulties trusting him at times in the future. Stressing the importance of the therapeutic relationship as a source of vital data about *all* his clients, the therapist expressed his hope that Laura would continue to share all such reactions with him, even those she might consider foolish or unacceptable. He emphasized that it was particularly important for the client to let him know if she were to feel blamed by him again at any time in the future. While on the subject of the treatment relationship, the therapist also took an opportunity to point out another instance of denial on Laura's part by recalling how, during the initial interview, she had been quite confident in her belief that the therapist's warnings about possible reactions to him could not possibly apply to *her.*

Using the therapeutic relationship as a conceptual anchor, the therapist now redirected Laura's attention to the other interpersonal problems she experienced. He told her he had been thinking about some additional implications of her reactions to the therapeutic relationship. If she had experienced such a powerful sense of threat dealing with him, he wondered, what must it be like for her when she had to interact with people who really *were* blaming and hostile toward her? Joining strongly with Laura, the therapist summarized the various destructive behaviors of her daughter and her subordinates at work. The therapist told the client that he could now understand much more clearly how threatening and devastating conflicts with the individuals in question could be for her. He reminded Laura that all of us develop "tunnel vision" when anxious, just as she had probably done when she became angry with him a few weeks previously.

The therapist said that he could visualize the client becoming equally defensive when threatened at work or at home, perhaps committing tactical errors which hurt her in the long run, or worse, behaving in a way that hurt her self-image, particularly as a mother. He told her "I know how much you love your daughter. I'm sure it's a terrible blow to your self-esteem every time you lose control of yourself with her. But I think if we continue to take care of business in here the way we have been, you're going to see some improvements in the way that you handle her." Laura's eyes filled to the brim with tears as the therapist discussed her feelings about herself as a mother. The therapist closed the discussion by emphasizing that in no way was he saying that Laura had *deserved* the abusive treatment she received from others. She was not responsible for the actions or choices of others. Although the therapist would be addressing Laura's defensiveness and self-defeating behavior in interpersonal situations in the future, he said he wanted her to know that he was not interested in assigning blame to her for things she could not control.

As Laura began to open up with the therapist, it became clear that angry outbursts occurred on a fairly regular basis in her life. She and the therapist were able to forge and sustain a strong alliance, so that eventually she was able to share her most upsetting behaviors with him without fear of recrimination or rejection. For Laura, having a relationship in which she could share her deepest fears and her greatest failings was a completely new experience and undoubtedly a healing one as well. At times it was very upsetting for the client to consider the effects of her angry actions on others, particularly her daughter. Although the therapist never excused Laura's behavior or minimized its destructive impact on the daughter, he consistently encouraged the client to remain mindful of her strong points as a parent, even as she analyzed her past errors. Laura found that the more she confronted her acting out behaviors and the underlying issues that triggered them, the more she was able to exercise self-control. Fortunately, the client was also able to avoid creating additional difficulties for herself at work.

With the therapist's assistance, Laura gradually recognized the role worthlessness played in motivating many of her day-to-day behaviors. As she did so, she began to work in a less driven, compulsive manner and found herself becoming less perfectionistic as a housekeeper. Not surprisingly, the degree of conflict between mother and daughter began to diminish as a direct result, thereby providing Laura with an opportunity to play a more supportive parental role. Although it was clear that the daughter needed more structure and parental involvement than most teenagers, Laura learned to exercise constructive leadership without being so critical and controling. Despite being able to acknowledge the need for more pleasure and recreation in her life, Laura never seemed to find the time to pursue such interests in any consistent way. Likewise, the client continued to believe that it was safer for her to avoid intimate relationships completely. She repeatedly stated a desire to keep her life relatively calm and uncluttered while she finished the task of raising her daughter. During the 3 years Laura spent in treatment, she showed little or no enthusiasm whenever the clinician attempted to broach the subject of her relationships with men. Although he probed the matter from time to time, the therapist found it easy to support the client's sense of priorities. When Laura terminated, however, both she and the therapist agreed that sometime down the road the issue of intimacy would probably motivate her to return to treatment.

To summarize, when clients act out either during or between sessions, they can provide the therapist with an opportunity to propel treatment forward. The thoughts, feelings, and behaviors of clients during such incidents should yield insights into how they function during their most difficult moments. Angry outbursts or other gross departures from treatment norms should never pass without comment from the therapist. Even a magnanimous verbal dismissal of an episode by the clinician (e.g., "I don't think there's a need to go into any detail about last week's session. You were clearly in an extremely agitated state of mind by the time you got here") is preferable to colluding with the client to maintain silence. *The therapist provides security for the client, not only by being empathic and caring but also by remaining in charge during a behavioral crisis and its aftermath.* Below are a number of additional recommendations regarding the therapeutic response to acting out episodes, particularly those which involve the clinician:

1. Allow sufficient time for your initial emotional responses to subside. Take note of them and the associated cognitions for later reference. Answer your own cognitive distortions if you can, especially those which concern your worth as a therapist or as a person. Ventilate with a colleague if one is available. Do something pleasurable for yourself after work if you have the opportunity. You've probably earned it!

2. Process the entire incident later, either on your own or with another professional. See how the client's current behavior fits in with current hypotheses about the sources of his or her distress and consider revising formulations where appropriate. *Most acting out episodes in nonpsychotic, nonchemically dependent clients are fear-based.* Make sure you have a clear understanding of the nature and source of the client's fearfulness or devise a plan to investigate the matter during a session as soon as is appropriate. Spell out the implications for the therapeutic relationship suggested by the individual's behavior and your responses to it. Consider how your own issues might be involved in either the interaction with the client or your subsequent responses to it. Formulate a multifaceted plan for addressing the episode during subsequent sessions. Think in terms of a *sequence* of issues that you would like to see unfold in your dialogue with the client.

3. Approach the individual when he or she appears to be in a more reasonable frame of mind. Explore the client's inner experience of the incident in question as thoroughly as possible, including his or her reactions afterwards.

4. Determine if the client is truly dissatisfied with his or her actions. Strive to amplify productive self-dissatisfaction if it seems necessary and appropriate. Consider sharing your own affective reactions, particularly fear, if it will help the client develop a more realistic picture of the effects of his or her behavior on others.

5. Define the limits of appropriate behavior in the therapeutic relationship, if you think the individual needs to have the matter spelled out explicitly, or if you are concerned that the acting out behavior will recur. If necessary, don't hesitate to indicate the costs of any destructive or threatening behavior directed at you in the future. Remember that you are not obliged to continue working with an individual who has a destructive or otherwise toxic effect on you. If you seek to terminate with the client, make sure you do so in a manner that satisfies prevailing ethical and legal guidelines.

6. Find a worthwhile, competent part of the individual, which is clearly separate from the acting out behavior, and use it as the foundation of your alliance. Keep the worthwhile part of the client in the foreground of the discussion, even as you address the acting out episode. Look for opportunities to affirm the individual's worth. Define

guilt as a positive factor, a manifestation of the client's *true* character or values. Attempt to block or restructure ideas of worthlessness. Relabel the individual's worthless feelings as an impediment to developing greater self-knowledge and preventing future occurrences of undesirable behavior. Repeatedly reaffirm your continued willingness to work with the client (if this is indeed the case).

7. Take full ownership of any behaviors on your part that may have contributed to the client's distress. Validate any of the individual's perceptions that may have been accurate (e.g., if you were angry, didn't listen, asked intimidating questions, and so on). Do not allow the client to protect you or otherwise minimize the negative impact of your behaviors. Draw appropriate parallels to other pertinent relationships in the client's life if he or she attempts to excuse or minimize the significance of your actions.

8. If you truly believe that the individual is not capable of working constructively on the issues involved, deliver some sort of *official dismissal* of the incident. Strive in your remarks to separate the *appropriateness* of a behavior from questions of its *causation*. Resist any pull from the client to downplay the negative aspects of his or her behavior.

9. Help the individual become aware of the issues that have triggered the acting out. Look for opportunities to break new ground or highlight material that has been difficult to discuss with the client in the past. Repeatedly underscore the fear-driven nature of the acting out behavior. Likewise, help the client to reframe the acting out behavior as a *coping strategy*, an attempt to solve a problem. Identify the specific cognitive and behavioral mechanisms involved and integrate them with relevant data from the individual's family of origin. Underscore similarities between the current incident and other pertinent situations in the client's life. Encourage the client to develop containment strategies to use in the event he or she begins to respond in a similar manner in the future.

10. Help the client understand the acting out behavior in the context of the therapeutic relationship. Carefully examine the individual's reactions to the therapist and his or her expectations regarding treatment. Prepare the client for the possibility that some of the threatening elements in the therapeutic interaction that stimulated the acting out episode may recur in the future. Utilize a stress inoculation approach with regard to future distortions in the therapeutic relationship. Sensitize the client to the "early warning signs" associated with the previous episode. Encourage the individual to find an alternative means for signaling his or her distress to you. Elicit the client's help in determining the most effective way for you to respond to analogous situations in the future.

11. Review the discussion about the episode during the next session. Strive to keep the issues and mechanisms associated with the acting out behavior in the therapeutic foreground during subsequent sessions. Refer the client back to what he or she learned during the discussions at every available opportunity in the future.

ACCESSING THE "INNER CHILD": FOR WHAT PURPOSES?

Much has been written of late regarding the so-called "Inner Child" (see Whitfield [1987] for a review of the concept), particularly in the self-help literature. Many of the authors who use the concept of the Inner Child seem to subsume a number of phenomena under one all-encompassing umbrella: (1) childhood memories, particularly those of a traumatic nature, and the associated emotional responses; (2) the state of psychological immaturity, emotional vulnerability (particularly to caretaking adults), and interpersonal dependency that is associated with childhood; and (3) enduring schemas, information-processing mechanisms, emotional reactions, coping strategies, and relationship patterns associated with childhood experiences. Clearly, our treatment model also demands that the therapist and client explore such phenomena.

Somewhere in the course of treatment we nearly always search for ways to induce the *experience of oneself as a child*, particularly when working with clients who are survivors of childhood physical or sexual abuse. We suspect that the motives behind our induction of such experiences, and the ways in which we utilize them in subsequent treatment, may be somewhat different from practitioners who do not have a cognitive orientation. Let us review then, the main reasons for asking a client to recreate the phenomenology of a child:

1. To stimulate recollection of specific factual childhood experiences, particularly of an abusive or otherwise traumatic nature, for assessment purposes.
2. To bolster the client's belief in the accuracy of certain childhood recollections and, by extension, in the validity of formulations that link historical events with current distress.
3. To enhance the client's appreciation of his or her physical, and/or psychological vulnerability to abuse, threat, manipulation, coercion, rejection, or other stressors at a particular age.
4. To enhance the client's appreciation of his or her physical, intellectual, and/or behavioral limitations at a particular age.
5. To correct distorted attributions of causation and assignments

of responsibility for behaviors and experiences in childhood, particularly in connection with parents or other caretaking figures.

6. To promote and sustain awareness of victimization in childhood and its effects.
7. To promote self-forgiveness and self-acceptance.
8. To foster awareness of effects of losses in childhood through death, desertion, separation, neglect, chronic rejection, or other manifestations of impaired parenting.
9. To enable the client to recognize thoughts, feelings, behaviors, and/or relationship patterns from childhood that have been replicated in areas of current functioning, or that otherwise play a causal role in his or her present difficulties.
10. To identify specific images or key phrases that the therapist can use subsequently to reorient the client's attention to particular childhood experiences which may be relevant to some area of current distress.

Perhaps the reader has already noticed that there are several goals that we do *not* pursue when we assist our clients to access the "Inner Child." We wish to spell out concretely, however, some approaches to childhood imagery used by other practitioners that we deliberately avoid:

1. We do not seek to flood the client with childhood imagery for the purpose of producing "affective discharge," catharsis, or abreaction. Of course, we find that for many clients, guided exploration of childhood material reduces any fearful or phobic reactions that may be connected with the specific recollections. Moreover, as we have indicated earlier in the section, the client's affective response to any recollection has a number of important therapeutic implications. However, the therapist must remember that affect is generally the product of thinking. Asking the client to reexperience painful or traumatic childhood events over and over again will never make a silk purse out of a sow's ear. *Events that are intrinsically unpleasant will always remain distressing to some degree or another, no matter how many times the individual reexperiences them.* For example, there is no way to feel good about having been the victim of sexual abuse as a child, even if all vestiges of self-blame were to disappear. In some instances, when treatment has been successful in changing the way in which the client processes information, it may no longer be possible for the individual to think about childhood events in a highly detached manner, as if they had all happened to another person. Consequently, as a by-product of recov-

ery, the client actually begins to experience *more* pain associated with childhood recollections. Why ask the client to experience the same unalterable realities again and again, when the associated meanings continue to evoke the same healthy but inevitably painful emotional responses? Our final objection to the cathartic or abreactive approaches is that they tend to neglect the most important part of our treatment model, the explicit integration of childhood experience and current difficulties in the client's life.

2. We do not attribute a special curative power to the fabrication of an alternative historical reality for the client. Although some clients, perhaps a small minority, derive some positive results from creating alternative childhood scenarios for themselves, we do not think such a technique is uniformly powerful or useful.

3. *Clients never cease to be adults, even while working on historical material, and should continue to be treated as such by their therapists.* Some therapists apparently believe that clients who have been abused or neglected actually need to be parented all over again, *in literal terms.* We have heard anecdotal evidence of clients who have been physically held and stroked by their therapists under the guise of "reparenting." We believe firmly in the power of the therapeutic relationship to create a "corrective emotional experience" for the client, particularly by providing a positive parental figure on a temporary basis. However, we anticipate a range of harmful effects associated with allowing clients to regress to a childish or even infantile state, let alone with violating their physical boundaries, particularly if they have already suffered physical or sexual abuse.

4. Although specific themes and emotions seem to recur across individuals, people do not go through an invariant sequence or combination of reactions to childhood material. Each client will utilize historical data in an idiosyncratic manner. There may be no particular virtue to having the client experience an emotional state for its own sake, particularly if the individual has processed the essential meaning of the content in question. For example, many of our clients experience great sadness and a sense of loss over the cruelty or injustice they suffered, over the support and nurturance they missed, over the personal limitations they have struggled with, and so on. Other clients acknowledge the same information fully, but experience affective responses of much lower intensity. For them, the recovery process leads them to other content and other issues. We do not think it is necessary, intrinsically helpful, or perhaps even possible for these individuals to grieve the losses of childhood as one would a contemporary loss. Moreover, they may find it to be highly demoralizing or otherwise toxic to flood themselves with unpleasant affect. In most instances, we are far more interested in assisting clients to identify current feelings of worth-

lessness, habits of self-blame, and recurring relationship patterns that are related to losses and parenting deficits in childhood than in encouraging them to perseverate on depressing themes that fail to teach any additional lessons.

5. The quality and extent of the client's memories do not necessarily influence the outcome of treatment, particularly if the historical material that is known already provides a good fit with current distress.

6. We generally do not want to have the client internalize the concept of an Inner Child, if it involves a belief in an actual intrapsychic structure that carves out some sort of independent existence outside of the individual's control. Metaphors facilitate learning in treatment, but they can begin to stimulate helplessness and pessimism if they become *reified*. Moreover, the identification of powerful tendencies toward certain types of thinking and behavior never absolves the individual of responsibility or accountability for the choices he or she makes in life. We believe that most of our clients find it less overwhelming and consequently more hopeful, to work on discrete, readily identifiable attitudes and information-processing deficits rather than try to modify an amorphous, demanding, and seemingly unchangeable entity such as the Inner Child.

THE TRAUMA REVELATION PROCESS

A full examination of the complexities of trauma work is clearly beyond the scope of this volume. Nonetheless, the reader will note that many earlier sections, particularly those that addressed boundaries in the therapeutic relationship, directly apply to survivors of childhood trauma. We urge readers to consult various resources on trauma work, both in the professional (e.g., Courtois, 1988; Herman, 1992; Ochberg, 1988) and the self-help (Bass & Davis, 1988; Black, 1985) literature. We also recommend that clinicians familiarize themselves with multiple personality disorders (e.g., Putnam, 1989; Ross, 1989), since such difficulties appear to be associated with severe childhood trauma.

Courtois (1988) cites research that places the prevalence of reported incest among outpatient therapy clients at 25% to 44%. She emphasizes, however, that most victims do not divulge their incest experiences during intake or early in treatment. Rather, the majority of victims manifest the effects of their abuse in disguised fashion. Consequently, Courtois emphasizes the need for therapists to become skilled at detecting and exploring clues suggestive of incest. We refer the reader to the excellent volume by Courtois (1988) for a detailed description of the common ways in which incest victims present in treatment.

We have worked with many clients who experienced a process of trauma revelation in the course of treatment, usually involving child-hood sexual abuse. Although most of these clients were well aware that they were raised in dysfunctional family circumstances, they had not viewed themselves as victims of physical abuse, sexual abuse, or any other traumatic experiences in childhood. After a period of treatment, such clients begin to report disturbing dreams or intrusive waking imagery, often with violent or sexual content. In some instances, the trauma revelation process may begin not with "flashbacks," but with a simple thought on the client's part, for example, "I'm beginning to wonder if I've been sexually abused." In our experience, once the client begins to voice such speculations, traumatic imagery, recollections, and other material are likely to follow. Moreover, the majority of our clients who experienced trauma revelation eventually reported multiple, var-ied episodes of abuse, by more than one perpetrator.

Flashback phenomena and other types of recollections will often reflect encoding limitations present at the time the traumatic events in question occurred, in that the intrusive recollections may involve little more than bodily sensations and/or affective states. Many of our clients experience the powerful emotions associated with traumatic experien-ces without any other associated cognitions. Clients find flashback ex-periences doubly frightening if they are not associated with clear, con-crete recollections. We assume this occurs because the client's affective response to the trauma was preserved somehow as an *intact memory,* having been encoded more successfully than other aspects of the ex-perience.

As discussed earlier in this chapter, the therapeutic process with any client will consist of repeated cycles in which periods of content *exploration* and emotional *intensification* alternate with intervals of affec-tive *containment* and *normalization.* With trauma cases, the client tends be the one who drives the exploration process, although often enough new material simply seems to *appear,* in the form of intrusive imagery, spontaneous recollections, and vivid dreams. Instead of utilizing active exploratory methods such as Socratic dialogue, the therapist will gen-erally assume a more supportive, integrative role. Under such circum-stances, the clinician will typically spend a proportionally greater amount of time supporting the containment and normalization of affect, and helping the client to *organize* and *integrate* traumatic material.

Postural Considerations

Coming to treatment sessions can be a tortuous experience for a client during a period of trauma revelation. The consulting room, once a safe haven from difficulties and uncertainties in the outside world, may now begin to feel like a chamber of horrors for the client. Since clients may dread coming to sessions, problems with cancellations and missed appointments may occur. If significant others are aware of the client's affective or symptomatic reactions to trauma revelation, they may begin to scapegoat the therapist or the treatment process. Because of the powerful negative feelings associated with sessions that focus on the traumatic content, the client may now experience the therapist more as a tormentor than as a helper. The client may feel angry at the therapist for "causing" the unpleasant emotions without offering any relief in the short-term. The client may feel the pull of a profound loyalty conflict, torn between the therapist on the one hand and the family members who may have perpetrated the traumatic experiences on the other. The client may fear that he or she is being brainwashed by the therapist into renouncing family ties. The client's reactions to the therapist also may begin to mirror the content of the traumatic material itself. The victim of sexual abuse may begin to wonder whether the therapist is a potential seducer. He or she may fear that the therapist has a voyeuristic interest in hearing the details of erotic images or experiences. The client may also feel as if the therapist has manipulated him or her to disclose sensitive information unwillingly. Some clients may report sexual dreams or fantasies involving the therapist as the perpetrator. Clients who have been physically abused may find themselves afraid of the therapist's anger, even to the point of worrying that they may be physically assaulted.

Because of both strong feelings of worthlessness and a sense of responsibility associated with the events in question, many clients also experience heightened concerns about being rejected by the therapist during the process of trauma revelation. They may suspect that the therapist is becoming disgusted by the experiences they disclose or annoyed at their inability to recall the historical events more quickly or accurately. Courtois (1988), who has written extensively and eloquently on the complexities of the therapeutic relationship with survivors of childhood sexual abuse, notes that victims of incest might well try to protect themselves from such anticipated harm by provoking rejection from others. Courtois recommends that therapists must constantly attend to their countertransference reactions to the incest survivor, bearing in mind at all times that they are working with a frightened individual whose best line of defense might involve engaging in such self-defeating actions. The therapist continually walks a tightrope with such clients. Should the therapist react in an overly supportive manner, the client may become suspicious and frightened, expecting something bad to follow on the heels of an offer of comfort or nurturance. On the

other hand, should the therapist be too distant, the survivor may feel
rejected and, of course, believe that he or she is to blame.

The client with a history of physical or sexual abuse needs a therapeutic relationship with clear limits and expectations in which his or her
boundaries are consistently and carefully respected. Consequently, the
therapist should be even more *collaborative* than usual with such individuals and most particularly so during a period of trauma revelation.
The clinician's first priority should be to monitor and to sustain the
client's sense of *safety* in the therapeutic relationship. We encourage
readers to go back and reexamine the postural issues discussed in
Chapters 7 and 8, particularly in the sections covering the maintenance
of appropriate boundaries in the therapeutic relationship. The client
needs to know that he or she is fully in command of the process of
disclosing and exploring traumatic material during sessions. Whenever
possible, the therapist should explain *why* it is so important for the client
to be in charge of the process, emphasizing the need to avoid replicating
past boundary violations in the therapeutic relationship. The therapist
should also emphasize that for most victims of childhood trauma, the
use of denial, or "shutting down" was a sound survival strategy. The
client, even now, does not necessarily *decide* to produce material or not
to produce material. In essence the therapist is saying, "There are times
when you'll need to shut down, for any number of reasons, and that's
okay. *Your* pace is the best pace."

*The therapist needs to act as a guide for the client, by providing informa-
tion about the nature of the trauma-revelation process itself.* The therapist
should forewarn the client about some of the potential side effects
associated with the process, including increased dysphoric affect, intrusive imagery of a distressing nature, sleep disturbances, feelings of
disloyalty to family members, sexual dysfunction, difficulties in relationships, and of course, resistance to treatment. The therapist needs to
normalize the client's intense affective responses to traumatic material
through a number of methods. It is often helpful for the therapist to
share examples of other clients who have undergone similar affective
responses to trauma disclosure. Likewise, bibliotherapy resources, such
as *The Courage to Heal* (Bass & Davis, 1988), also enable clients to realize
that they are experiencing "normal reactions to abnormal situations."
The therapist should underline his or her availability during the trauma
revelation process, by scheduling more frequent sessions or by emphasizing a willingness to meet or talk on the phone with the client on an
as-needed basis during stressful periods. In stressing availability, however, it is important for the therapist to avoid communicating an expectation that the client cannot handle the intense reactions stimulated

by the trauma-disclosure process. Instead, the therapist should emphasize the *desirability* (as opposed to the *necessity*) of offering support to the client and of assisting him or her to understand the significance of new images or recollections, as they come up.

The therapist should also forewarn the client regarding potential difficulties in the therapeutic relationship that may arise during the trauma revelation process, offering if possible some hypotheses as to the types of distortions that might take place. Again and again, the therapist needs to give the client explicit *permission* to experience and to share reactions to the treatment relationship that are connected to the traumatic material, no matter how bizarre and seemingly inappropriate they may be. The therapist should take pains to normalize such reactions whenever they are disclosed by the client, while stressing that he or she does not take anything personally. The therapist should also laud the client's courage in dealing with the traumatic material, while disavowing the need to speed up the process in any way.

Trauma-revelation material may begin to implicate family members as potential perpetrators of physical or sexual abuse, albeit sometimes incorrectly so. It may be quite distressing for the client to think that a loved parent or grandparent may have been a victimizer. Predictably, some clients feel incredibly guilty even considering such a possibility. They may wonder if they are conveniently transferring blame for their own personal problems to other family members by fabricating tales of abuse or trauma. It may be helpful for the clinician to emphasize to the client that the identity of the perpetrator has not yet been established. Likewise, the therapist also needs to remind the client that although dreams and images may provide the basis for *hypotheses* about traumatic childhood experiences, they are not necessarily *literal* depictions of real events. On the other hand, the therapist should look for opportunities to highlight instances of irrational, self-defeating family loyalty on the client's part, especially in situations which are somewhat removed from the traumatic material. If the client has already worked through feelings of disloyalty in connection to other family of origin material, so much the better. In such instances, the therapist may well be able to demonstrate to the individual how family loyalty is again impeding the acknowledgment of important early influences in the client's life.

The trauma-revelation process seems to occur in fits and starts, even with highly insightful, motivated clients. Understandably, many clients want to know how they can accelerate the process, not realizing that the process involves *integration* of information, not just the disclosure of facts. However, we often observe that clients may show considerable progress in their day-to-day functioning long before all the relevant traumatic experiences have been discussed. For clients who have struggled with a strong sense of worthlessness and culpability their entire lives, the mere recognition of having been victimized stimulates changes in long-standing patterns of thinking and behavior. The therapist should continue to provide the client with realistic expectations about the nature of the revelation process, while underscoring the data that indicate that recovery is still proceeding despite the absence of all the "hard facts" about the abuse itself. The therapist should also emphasize that although the client may never know the *absolute* truth, he or she can expect to learn enough to produce significant improvements in current life difficulties.

The perpetrators of childhood physical and sexual abuse are predominantly male. As a consequence, we assume that there will be clients of both sexes who cannot work effectively with a male therapist, particularly on trauma-related issues. Clients who initially had no preference for the gender of their therapists, or even those who had specifically chosen a male therapist, may begin to feel extremely uncomfortable working with a man once the trauma-revelation process begins. When working with victims of childhood trauma, male therapists need to monitor the client's gender-specific reactions throughout the treatment process. Even when there has been a long-term relationship established with the individual, the male clinician must remain open to the possibility that the client may feel safer working on certain issues with a female. The clinician who suspects that gender issues might be retarding therapeutic progress must find a nonthreatening way to explore the problem and the potential solutions with the individual. Feelings of disloyalty and fears of antagonizing the therapist may prevent clients from expressing their true preferences under such circumstances. These individuals may need *permission* from the clinician before they are able to discuss their reactions in a comfortable, open manner. On the other hand, as the therapist raises the issue of alternative treatment arrangements, he or she also must avoid sending rejecting messages to the client. It will probably be necessary for the clinician to reaffirm a desire to continue working with the client repeatedly in the course of such discussions, so that the individual can examine the options without feeling pushed away. Further, the client should be told that choosing to work with a female therapist need not result in a *permanent, irreversible* break with the male clinician. The individual needs to know that there are opportunities to make various *flexible* arrangements, which may involve returning to the male clinician for treatment at some point in the future if the client so desires.

Containment

The process of trauma revelation is quite taxing for clients on an affective level. The dreams or imagery may be terrifying and/or disgusting, producing ripples across previously untroubled waters in the client's life. Clients may begin to experience unwanted affective or symptomatic reactions in situations where no difficulties had occurred previously. Some clients report intense feelings of anger or panic, whereas others experience a powerful sense of shame associated with revelations of abuse. Some clients with no prior history of self-destructive behavior may experience suicidal or self-mutilative urges connected to the disclosure of traumatic material. Other compulsive behaviors or obsessive thoughts may increase in frequency and severity. The client may experience difficulties in intimate relationships, particularly in sexual contacts. The client's distress during sexual relations often signals the need for a moratorium on such activities. The client also may become enraged again and again at a relatively supportive partner, with minimal or no provocation.

Not surprisingly, fears of losing emotional or behavioral control are likely to intensify during the trauma-revelation process, sometimes with good reason. Indeed, the therapist may well need to consider the use of medication and/or hospitalization with certain clients for whom such interventions had never been indicated previously. During trauma work, the therapist should help the client select and develop a *range* of containment strategies directed at the associated symptomatology. The therapist will need to watch the client carefully for signs of distress, withdrawl, or dissociation during any discussions of traumatic material. It may be necessary to interrupt such discussions immediately in order to allow the individual to reestablish contact with the therapist or achieve a greater sense of self-control. Although the clinician will want to process symptomatic reactions and/or episodes of acting out on the client's part, especially if these events occur during treatment sessions, such discussions will require particularly delicate timing with trauma cases. Likewise, the therapist will even need to be cautious when presenting formulations or capsule summaries, since any references to traumatic material may have the capacity to stimulate flashbacks, dissociation, or other symptoms on the client's part.

Negative interactions with partners or other family members can easily undermine the client's self-control. *Along with individual treatment, the majority of our trauma clients need to be involved in some form of couples work.* At the very least, concerned partners need *information* about the trauma revelation process so that they can respond in a constructive way to the client's distress. Unfortunately, however, many victims of childhood trauma are also involved in destructive ongoing relationships that only serve to replicate earlier episodes of abuse. Their partners may well be unwilling or unable to participate constructively in treatment efforts of any kind.

Integration

In processing traumatic material with the client, the therapist will have a number of cognitive goals in mind:

1. Establishing the validity of traumatic recollections.
2. Normalizing the affective reactions associated with traumatic memories and/or the recognition of victimization.
3. Challenging the individual's sense of responsibility for having been victimized.
4. Identifying the impact of trauma on the client's development in childhood and adolescence.
5. Underscoring how the effects of trauma may have been exacerbated by other negative influences in the family of origin.
6. Linking the traumatic experiences to symptoms, specific beliefs, cognitive distortions, information-processing biases, coping strategies, recurring relationship patterns, and other mechanisms observed in the client's current life.

Needless to say, it will be necessary for the therapist to process the same trauma-related material and themes repeatedly with the client using a variety of strategies (e.g., Socratic dialogue, interpretation of dreams, discussion of assigned readings, and so on).

Clients often react to the initial stages of trauma revelation with a sense of disbelief, particularly if they had not experienced previously any evidence of physical or sexual abuse in childhood. The fragmented, sometimes illogical nature of the dreams and imagery also makes it hard for clients to experience a sense of reality or certainty about traumatic incidents. Statements such as "This can't be true," or "I must be making this up" are familiar refrains during the early stages of trauma revelation. Clients who have learned to distrust their own perceptions, who harbor fears of being crazy, and/or have been labeled as "overly sensitive" or "too emotional" by their families of origin will find it particularly hard to attach any credibility to their initial sensations and recollections.

The clinician has an ongoing responsibility to help the client organize and integrate all the diverse material related to childhood trauma. The therapist also needs to help the client evaluate evidence that bears on the potential validity of childhood memories. With the clinician's assistance, the client should continually try to determine whether emerging traumatic recollections provide a good "fit" with the following: (1) known information regarding the individual's family of origin (e.g., other evidence of neglectful or abusive parenting); (2) adjustment problems experienced by the individual in childhood or adolescence; (3) psychological difficulties in adulthood, particularly boundary and/or sexual problems; (4) the individual's characteristic cognitive distortions and coping strategies in adulthood; (5) the existing body of traumatic material already revealed in treatment, including dreams and intrusive imagery.

Gradually, a more detailed, comprehensible picture of the client's traumatic experiences may begin to emerge. Along with the continued dreams or imagery, the client may report new childhood memories that seem related somehow to the disturbing content. Sometimes the client may not be able to articulate why a particular piece of information seems relevant to the issue of childhood trauma, other than to say that the material in question seems to spark powerful affect. The therapist will then need to help the client generate hypotheses as to the significance of the material. At times, the therapist may need to keep the particular content in mind for a while, hoping that its meaning will become clearer as subsequent memories emerge. Recollections of other family members may also help to provide the client with missing details and a greater sense of confidence in the reality of his or her perceptions.

The clinician should try to keep the client aware of any themes that seem to recur in the trauma material, particularly those that run through apparently unrelated content. Some clients are quite surprised when the therapist reminds them that last week's nightmare, despite a slightly different script or cast of characters, has essentially the same thematic elements as an upsetting dream reported a month earlier. As they recognize the thematic consistencies, some clients do begin to think, "I can't be making all of this up. I'm not that good a storyteller."

After she had been in treatment for a year and a half, Leona began to report fragments of her dreams. Two dreams were particularly terrifying for her. In one, she was standing in a moving subway car. From behind her, she could hear the sound of a man's heavy breathing. Although she was frightened to the point of wanting to run, Leona found herself unable to move. She was frozen in her spot on the train, forced to listen while the ominous heavy breathing behind her continued. In the other dream, Leona could only remember the sensation of a large forearm across her chest, immobilizing her. She also reported

CHAPTER 11

other imagery of a sexual nature, which she connected to the house she grew up in, but not to any specific family members. Interestingly, she also mentioned an extreme aversion to flannel material, the kind used in shirts and bathrobes. At the mere mention of flannel, she would become visibly anxious and agitated, often rubbing her fingertips along her thighs in a very stereotyped, nearly involuntary motion. As a means of stimulating recollections, the therapist suggested that Leona go to a fabric store and purchase some flannel. She first reported that she completely forgot the homework then flatly refused to complete the assignment.

One day, Leona received a phone call from an older sister that put the dream material into clearer perspective. While reading a magazine article on incest, the sister recalled having been sexually abused as a youngster by the paternal grandfather, who had lived with Leona's family for many years. The sister remembered that the grandfather would ask her to sit on his lap while they watched television together in a darkened room. Holding her across the chest with one forearm, the grandfather would reach into her panties with the opposite hand and insert his finger into her vagina. The sister also remembered that the grandfather would rub his erect penis through his clothes against her backside, while he manipulated her. Presumably he was breathing more heavily than normal while engaging in such behavior. Both Leona and her sister identified that the grandfather typically wore flannel pajamas around the house.

The client at first strongly resisted the idea that she might have been sexually abused by her grandfather. "It can't be. It's gotta be *me* who has the problem," she would insist. Nonetheless, the therapist continued to highlight the consistent elements reflected in the material presented by both Leona and her sister. Although she still struggled with a sense of disbelief, Leona found herself increasingly less inclined to dismiss the consistencies the therapist noted. In the meantime, she continued to provide new data that also fit well with previously disclosed material, further buttressing the notion that she had been the victim of sexual abuse in childhood.

In our experience, the newly revealed traumatic material invariably helps to shed new light on the client's adult adjustment. *The therapist should highlight repeatedly the aftereffects of abuse manifested in the client's current functioning, particularly those that involve symptoms or other presenting complaints.* Unless the client's contemporary material is totally trivial, the therapist should be able to make connections on an ongoing basis between current content and what is already known about traumatic events in childhood.

The therapist also needs to help the client reexamine his or her history in light of emerging disclosures of traumatic material. Many of our clients still feel ashamed and stigmatized by developmental difficulties they experienced in childhood and adolescence. Indeed, they may have been actively scapegoated by parents or other family members for such difficulties. With the therapist's help, these clients may now be able to relabel various shameful episodes in their lives as *understandable reactions to victimization*. Wherever possible, the clinician should underscore the connections between specific features of the client's traumatic experiences and problems the individual may have manifested while growing up. Courtois (1988) presents a number of behavioral and physical symptoms that characterize incest survivors at various ages. Common indicators emerging in early and middle childhood include: symptoms of anxiety and/or depression (e.g., regressive behaviors such as enuresis, thumb-sucking, and clinging behaviors; fretfulness; withdrawal; insomnia; nightmares); compulsive and inappropriate sex play; sexual precociousness; physical trauma to the mouth, genitals, or rectum; gastrointestinal disturbances; and conduct disturbances. Symptoms emerging during adolescence typically involve angry, impulsive, and rebellious behaviors, although persistent withdrawal and other depressive features may also suggest abuse. Other difficulties experienced by teenage victims of sexual abuse include: sexual promiscuity; substance abuse; self-mutilating behaviors; suicidal ideation and gestures; eating disorders; dissociative experiences; and runaway behaviors. The therapist also should provide the client with a framework for understanding how the destructive effects of traumatic experiences may have been *amplified* by other negative influences in childhood and adolescence, for example, chronic rejection by a nonabusing parent, ongoing substance abuse in the home, peer or sibling violence, and so on.

During the trauma-revelation process, the actual content of treatment sessions will tend to be more diverse and less uniform, simply because the therapist is allowing the client to be in control to a much greater extent than at other times. Because the content may shift frequently, the therapist needs to invest considerable effort in maintaining the client's sense of continuity in treatment by offering formulations and capsule summaries more frequently than usual. The high levels of discomfort associated with trauma cases will certainly interfere with the client's ability to recall the content of treatment sessions, particularly if the individual has a tendency to dissociate under pressure. Consequently, the therapist needs to be willing to review the same points again and again, until the client is able to retain information more consistently.

One of the hallmarks of traumatic material, in our experience, is *the incorporation of a child's perspective* into the dreams or imagery. That is, the material the client presents will contain events or phrases that directly reflect a *child's experience* rather than an adult's perspective on a child's experience. We remind the reader that children, particularly those who have not yet reached the stage of formal operations, tend to be limited and egocentric in their perceptions of the world around them, particularly when dealing with questions of causation. Moreover, young children may not even have the words or the concepts to describe traumatic experiences, especially if sexual contact is involved. Consequently, we assume that the quality of the client's traumatic recollections will reflect the cognitive limitations of the child who experienced them in the first place.

The clinician needs to be alert to any features of the client's dreams or images that seem to reflect a child's perspective. It is invariably useful to point out such details to the client, as a means of strengthening his or her belief that something traumatic *did* indeed happen, despite the haziness and confusion that accompanies the historical material. Perhaps a number of examples will give the reader an appreciation for various elements in clients' dreams and images that reveal the perspective of a child:

Teresa described a series of sexually degrading dreams in which she noticed the same kind of tile on the floor. She recalled that this tile pattern was on the floor of the house she lived in before age 9. She recalled that her alcoholic grandfather, whom she later suspected of having abused her sexually, had the same kind of tile at his house. Teresa also reported a dream in which the tops of tables and dressers in the house were *at eye level*. On another occasion, the client dreamt she was the mistress of a gangster. She went to great lengths to conceal from him the fact that she had spilled juice on her dress. Eventually she had sex with him, to prevent him from noticing the soiled garment.

On an episodic basis, Betsy would experience severe panic attacks while alone in her room at night. During these periods of anxiety, she would report an extreme, unreasoning fear of the dark. She also reported being terrified of shadows in the darkened room, particularly if she thought she detected movement out of the corner of her eye. At times even lumps or large wrinkles in the covering on her bed itself made her feel panicky. She was unable to identify a specific stimulus (for example, intruder, fire) that might cause an *adult* to be afraid in such situations. The therapist noted that during a period of heightened anxiety at bedtime, his 5-year-old daughter had reported identical perceptions.

12

Building Coping Strategies

Clients must understand that changing long-standing beliefs and coping strategies takes time and effort. On the other hand, the therapist needs to give clients the clear message that, if they are motivated to change and willing to put in the time, they will experience gradual progress. In our model, we try to educate clients early on as to what the change process requires in the way of effort. Without additional thought and/or practice by the client between appointments, the comparatively brief time spent in therapy sessions may not be effective in promoting change. We recommend that therapists invest considerable time throughout the treatment process assisting clients to make realistic assessments of past therapeutic accomplishments and to formulate reasonable expectations of future psychological growth. The authors are strong advocates of homework and practice. Later in this chapter, we discuss the use of homework assignments as a means of achieving a variety of treatment goals.

CLARIFYING EXPECTATIONS OF THE CHANGE PROCESS

Successful psychotherapy, insofar as the authors know it, is a process of *evolution*. Moments of epiphany occur rarely and are far less influential in the long run than some of our clients might suppose. Meaningful, lasting changes in our clients' lives seem to occur very gradually, in fits and starts, with lengthy periods during which nothing much in the way of progress seems to be happening. Although there is ultimately something miraculous about the recovery process, it does not occur by magic but through hard work and determination on the part of the client. Insight can transform lives, but only when it is *integrated* into daily living. Such a task demands extensive self-observation, practice, repetition, and attention to detail.

Movies and television do as poorly at depicting what goes on in psychotherapy as they do at reflecting other aspects of real life. Other than Woody Allen movies, in which *nothing* happens in therapy, media depictions of treatment sessions invariably involve powerful revelations and intensely cathartic experiences. In a dramatic moment, the client usually achieves some sort of breakthrough and is never the same again. If only we therapists could achieve the dramatic results our celluloid counterparts seems to produce! Even the nonfictional media presentations of psychotherapy and other recovery-oriented topics (for example, shows by Oprah Winfrey or John Bradshaw) tend to emphasize the cathartic or abreactive elements of treatment, not the long periods of dirty work. Of course, clients who expect to achieve the same results in "real life" are destined to become quite disappointed. The therapist has the responsibility to provide an accurate picture of the typical recovery process and to help the client maintain realistic expectations throughout treatment. Without such ongoing leadership from the clinician, the client may reach the wrong set of conclusions about the therapist's competence and/or the value of treatment, as well as his or her ability to change.

The recovery process we discuss in this volume is comparable to the task of learning a foreign language in adulthood. An adult student literally has to *unlearn* habits associated with his or her mother tongue in order to acquire fluency in the new language. He or she must learn a complete set of concepts and behaviors associated with different rules of pronunciation, grammar, and syntax, as well as a whole new vocabulary. The beginning student may master written exercises, or rote responses to drills in the classroom or on tape but may still be unable for some time to use the new language spontaneously in real life situations. Background noise, vagaries of voice quality, inflection, and dialect, and of course, anxiety, all will prevent the student from transferring classroom learning to faster-paced interactions. Only through repeated "in vivo experimentation" will the student acquire survival skills in the new language. Despite having made considerable progress in mastering the new language, the more advanced student may still "think" in the mother tongue when it comes to expressing new or more complex ideas. The student may never reach a true colloquial or idiomatic usage of the new tongue however, so that he or she will remain unable to understand the true meaning of puns or humorous remarks made in the language. Moreover, although the student may become fluent enough in the new language to live and work successfully in a foreign country, he or she will always have an accent that is recognizable to a native speaker.

The therapist may want to offer the metaphor outlined in the previous paragraph to the client at the beginning of treatment. Many of our clients can grasp the similarities between psychotherapy and learning a foreign language, particularly if they have had some experience in trying to master another tongue. Needless to say, however, some of our clients could not conceive of mastering *anything* having to do with academics or intellectual functioning. A variety of other skill areas, such as athletics, handicrafts, and music also can illustrate similar processes of rote practice, repetition, and subsequent spontaneous performance. Even the client who claims to be totally unskilled in *every* area has probably learned to drive a car. In a pinch, the therapist can use the acquisition of driving skills (after ruling out the presence of phobias of course) as an illustration of the learning process associated with successful treatment. Unfortunately, however, not all of the alternative metaphors parallel psychotherapy as closely as the linguistic one, since acquiring a new language demands the *unlearning* of previously ingrained habits.

Like the student of a foreign language, the client in cognitive therapy must learn new beliefs that will compete with older, more well-established schemas and cognitive distortions. Similarly, the client will identify new information-processing priorities, which will in time begin to supplant more *reflexive* habits of overvigilance and denial. In the early stages of treatment, the client will be able to identify information-processing errors, cognitive distortions, and the influence of basic schema on thoughts, feelings, and behavior—*but only after the fact, and with considerable assistance from the therapist*. During this period, the client may find it extremely difficult to generalize cognitive or behavioral changes from treatment sessions to "real life." In fact, some clients with extremely strong denial systems may report being unable even to *remember* the discussions from previous sessions, let alone utilize the content from them. Once the client leaves the therapist's presence, old belief systems may begin to reassert themselves with a vengeance. Moreover, although the client may begin to understand some new concepts such as "denial" or "poor boundaries," he or she may be largely unable to recognize manifestations of these problems that occur on a daily basis.

The therapist should provide the client with a framework to understand why it is difficult to keep new insights associated with treatment in focus between sessions. By offering examples that illustrate the fluidity of belief systems across situations, the therapist will help the client appreciate the profound changes in thinking that accompany certain stressful or threatening events. Clients who ordinarily might be resistant to examining potential distortions in thought content may find it fascinating to observe the inconsistencies in their cognitions across situations. By underlining the inconsistencies, the therapist paves the way for subsequent examination of both specific content and the operation of overvigilance and denial. Likewise, the therapist should be sure to label as significant any difficulties the client has in recalling meaningful material from previous sessions, particularly if the individual demonstrates a good memory in other areas. Clients who are resistant or lack insight may require an approach that appeals to intellectual curiosity. Without providing the answers, the therapist may repeatedly pose questions to the client such as "Why would a bright person like you, who has demonstrated an ability to recall all sorts of obscure details, be unable to recall a conversation that was so personally significant?"

The therapist should encourage clients to use various strategies that will enhance recall and integration of the content discussed during treatment sessions. As with all types of therapeutic assignments, it is vital for the clinician to propose a strategy that is compatible with the client's learning style and overall level of intellectual functioning. As we mentioned earlier in this volume, many our clients find it helpful to make audiotapes of their sessions. Since most cars today are equipped with tape players, clients often find it convenient to play back their sessions while driving. Unfortunately, some clients who struggle with powerful feelings of worthlessness are not able to listen to themselves without considerable discomfort. Such individuals should be willing, however, to bring a small notebook to the therapist's office in order to jot down the major points of each session. When clients have persistent difficulties with recall and integration, the therapist should also be even more diligent than normal about beginning each treatment hour with a summary of the main points from the previous session.

As we emphasize elsewhere, during the early stages of treatment, the therapist tries to keep the client focused primarily on the task of building awareness. Any expectations on the client's part of being able to use therapeutic insights as a foundation for major life changes would be somewhat unrealistic during this period. Some of our more parentified, control-oriented clients are prone to think that they know all there is to know about the operation of a particular issue in their lives after just one or two discussions with the therapist on the topic. They may want to move into the implementation of some sort of action plan before they (or the therapist for that matter) really understand the *day-to-day ramifications* of the issues in question. These clients may need to be slowed down and even humbled a bit, *not by the therapist but by the data*. With a literal or figurative shrug of the shoulders, the therapist may indicate that, at this point, he or she simply does not know enough about the client to be able to conceptualize how personal issues might affect future plans or decisions. Working from a relatively nonthreatening posture that communicates "*I* don't know enough about you yet to help you implement an action plan," the therapist will seek to highlight data that underscore significant gaps in the client's self-knowledge. The therapist must assume a highly supportive stance as he or she helps the client to recognize that issues such as worthlessness produce effects that are complicated, wide-ranging, and deeply embedded in everyday life. Avoiding the slightest hint of an "I told you so" attitude, the therapist will remind the client what a complex procedure it is to recognize and to change ingrained patterns of thinking and behavior. Later in recovery, these same clients may acknowledge having been in a hurry to move from awareness to implementation because, for a variety of reasons, they were terrified by the prospect of sustained examination of certain threatening personal issues.

As recovery progresses, the client may begin to internalize the treatment techniques, to the point of being able to conduct post-hoc analyses on his or her own, without the therapist's assistance. The client may now grasp the pervasiveness of certain issues and cognitive distortions, but may be quite frustrated at his or her inability to break old habits. In fact, the more threatening the situation, the less likely the client will be to achieve a more rational, detached perspective without the therapist's assistance, even after the fact. The client may experiment with new behaviors during this period, particularly in relationships, but long-term changes in interaction patterns may be quite hard to sustain without more robust cognitive changes to support them. The client may feel embarrassed or ashamed that old relationship patterns continue to occur. He or she may also project feelings of discouragement or self-disgust onto the therapist. The client may say to the clinician "You must be getting sick of me coming in here and talking about the same things over and over again." Again, the therapist should remind the client what a complex task it is to change long-standing patterns of thinking and behavior, particularly in intimate relationships. Moreover, the clinician should reframe the repetition of themes across sessions as a *positive* development in treatment. "It's *good* that we're discussing the same topics again and again. That indicates we're staying focused on the most meaningful issues in your life. I always hope to be doing that more and more as I get to know someone better. In fact, I'd start to become concerned if we *weren't* repeating ourselves at this point," the therapist might say.

During the course of recovery, the client should become more oriented to underlying issues or mechanisms than to symptoms. Consequently, the focus of treatment sessions will become broader, as it begins to reflect the changes in self-awareness. Moreover, the client will eventually internalize enough of the treatment experience so that even when away from the therapist, he or she will be increasingly able to divert attention away from more peripheral considerations, such as symptoms, back toward larger, personally significant themes. For example, as we illustrate in the case of Carol presented later in this chapter, the client may learn to dismiss the content of obsessive thoughts in favor of trying to identify the reasons why he or she may have become anxious. More and more of the client's treatment time, as well as his or her personal reflection between sessions, will be devoted to examining recurring themes underlying the symptomatic periods.

ANALYZING INSTANCES OF SUCCESSFUL COPING

Every victory the client achieves over his or her personal demons deserves acknowledgment and review by the clinician, regardless of the magnitude of the actual gains involved. Instances of more effective coping, particularly those the client spontaneously reports, provide the therapist with an excellent opportunity to underscore previous insights and to stimulate new habits of thinking and behavior. Often our clients will want to gloss over their successes, becoming uncomfortable if such experiences receive much more than a cursory examination in treatment. Nonetheless, the therapist should approach each instance of successful coping as if it were a meal in an expensive restaurant, to be savored and digested slowly. The clinician should "massage" the data the client provides, in order to promote multiple treatment goals simultaneously, as the following case example illustrates. Since a particularly meaningful incident might involve many significant thematic elements, it may take the therapist more than one session to review a success experience adequately.

Once reviewed, each instance of successful coping should become part of the common data bank utilized by the therapist and the client during the rest of the treatment process. Throughout treatment, the therapist will continually orient the client back to episodes of successful coping until the individual truly begins to internalize the concepts and the sense of competence associated with them. Moreover, by encouraging recall of past successes and the coping strategies involved in them, the therapist can help the client to feel more hopeful and confident during periods of crisis.

The case of Kathleen provides an interesting example how the therapist might approach an instance of successful coping. As a child, Kathleen experienced the dual stressors of poverty and family disorganization. Since both her parents were "underfunctioning" alcoholics, the bulk of the parenting obligations in the family fell to Kathleen, who was the eldest child. Meanwhile, the parents consistently scapegoated Kathleen, while they tended to enable several of the other siblings.

Kathleen's father was prone to be physically abusive toward his wife and the children. He became especially punitive when the client, as a college student, began to differentiate from the family. Kathleen remembered that when she was 20 years old, her father came charging into a Homecoming party, and eventually slapped her in front of her date. At that point, Kathleen moved out of the house. She never re-turned—but not without an enormous cost. Kathleen always felt as if she had abandoned her siblings, particularly her "baby" sister, who had only been a toddler at the time of separation. For many years, she held herself responsible for that sister's descent into drug addiction and prostitution in young adulthood.

Kathleen opened a session by telling the therapist that she had finally confronted Howard, her hostile boss. Instead of dissolving into tears or listening impassively when he became enraged with her over a minor matter, as she usually had done, Kathleen stood up to him this time, demanding in no uncertain terms to be treated with respect. To her surprise, Howard immediately backed off after her impassioned state-ments. Subsequently, he seemed to have taken a somewhat more re-spectful attitude toward her.

"What was it that made you able to stand up to Howard *now*, given the long history of this kind of behavior on his part?" the therapist asked. Kathleen cited two reasons. One, Howard had attacked her *character* this time, not merely her professional performance. Conse-quently, his comments had enraged her. Secondly, during the exchange with her boss, she kept recreating in her mind's eye a powerful image she had experienced in a previous treatment session. Attempting to underscore the abusive nature of Kathleen's relationship with her boss, the therapist had asked her *to visualize what her body would look like if Howard had left a bruise every time he had verbally attacked her.* Evidently the image of her bruised, discolored body had stuck with Kathleen, serving to remind her of the destructive impact of the relationship with Howard and the urgent need to defend herself against his attacks.

The therapist reminded Kathleen of other instances in which she had attempted to stand up for herself, with Howard and with other people in her life, only to be flooded afterwards with a terrible fear of retaliation, and in some cases, a sense of guilt for having been angry. Had she experienced any similar feelings this time, he asked, and if not, why not? Kathleen reported that she had felt no guilt whatsoever about her actions, since she remained firmly convinced that her supervisor's actions had been totally inappropriate. On several occasions after the incident, however, she had begun to feel afraid of what Howard might do to her in retaliation for her assertive behavior. The client had found it reassuring to review the matter with her husband, who was knowledgable enough about the past conflicts with Howard, and personnel practices in general, to underscore her rights as an employee in the situation. Moreover, Kathleen was also able to remind herself that given the history of her relationship with Howard, she would continue to be unsafe *unless* she began to defend herself. When she began to feel fearful about a retaliation from Howard, Kathleen also reported that she found it helpful to recall once again the image of her bruised body.

The therapist asked Kathleen about the future of her relationship with Howard. She replied that she had no intention of returning to the abusive conditions of the past. She stated that she would even quit her job now to prevent being abused by him. She would either find a way to replace the lost income, or if necessary, settle for a lower standard of living in order to escape Howard's cruel treatment. She was also willing to fight him through the legal system to insure fair treatment as an employee. Kathleen's husband was fully supportive of her position, she said. Looking back now from her current perspective, she could identify the tremendous toll the job had taken on her physical and psychological well-being. The therapist reminded her that she had tended at times in the past to downplay the stressful impact of the job, particularly when Howard was in the midst of one of his occasional periods of good behavior.

The therapist then systematically reviewed previous discussions with Kathleen about Howard, paying particular attention to the components of the relationship that mirrored her family of origin issues. He recalled how trapped and hopeless the client had felt about her job, particularly because of the relationship with Howard. She had believed it was impossible to assert herself with such a cruel and abusive individual. The clinician emphasized that the sense of competence Kathleen experienced in her confrontation with Howard came as the direct result of tremendous dedication and hard work on her part. The therapist stated his hope that Kathleen's success in confronting her supervisor would give her a greater sense of optimism about her ability to solve the other significant problems in her life. He suggested that she try to recall the eventual outcome of the relationship with Howard whenever she began to feel hopeless or helpless in similar situations. The therapist also stated that he intended to refer back to this episode as well whenever the client became discouraged by comparable circumstances in the future.

The therapist reminded Kathleen of the similarities she had identified between Howard, an abusive male authority figure, and her alcoholic father. He recalled how the client had reported often feeling small, powerless, and overwhelmed by fear in Howard's presence, just as she had with her father. Kathleen also had disclosed similar experiences in the therapeutic relationship and in her marriage. At times, she had mistakenly perceived the therapist as overpowering, hostile, and even potentially physically abusive. Although she had wanted to dismiss the importance of Howard's opinion of her, Kathleen found herself earnestly working to achieve his respect, as a professional and as a person, despite his consistently rejecting style. In the same way, she had vainly struggled for her father's love and approval. When Howard attacked her, Kathleen typically had questioned her own professional competence and felt responsible for the problems in the relationship, just as she had blamed herself when her father had abused her. At times, she had even wondered whether Howard was somehow aware of shameful personal issues that had impelled her to seek treatment. Finally, Kathleen utilized denial strategies in her relationship with Howard, much as she had with her father. She was likely to "forgive and forget" past transgressions on Howard's part if he began to show her even a minimal amount of courtesy or respect. Several times, she had convinced herself that she had turned some kind of a corner with him, only to be hit with another devastating verbal attack when she had her guard down. Somehow she was never able to sustain a view of Howard as an *enemy* who demanded continued wariness and self-protection on her part.

The therapist spelled out how the confrontation with Howard underscored a number of gains Kathleen had achieved for herself. Above all, she had acknowledged the victimization by her boss and all its implications for the present and for the future. This time, neither denial nor self-blame had prevented the client from remaining focused on his abusive treatment of her. Kathleen had not felt responsible in the least for her supervisor's actions. She had disengaged herself from concerns about his perceptions of her competence. Despite her fear of the supervisor, the client had recognized that she did not need to act like a helpless victim in his presence. The therapist noted that Kathleen had found a way to defend herself in an effective, yet dignified, manner. She did not become enraged to the point of losing all self-control, as she had once feared. Moreover, the clinician pointed out that by recognizing that the supervisor's treatment of her constituted a real *emergency* in her life, the client had achieved a major victory over denial. She began to be more fearful about continuing the ongoing pattern of abuse that already existed than about any potential future retaliation from Howard. Unlike previously, Kathleen did not make the mistake this time of assuming that a quiescent period on Howard's part signaled some sort of permanent change in the way he related to her. She now operated on the

assumption that he would *continue* to be a threat to her as long as she
had contact with him. The therapist pointed out to Kathleen that Howard might indeed respond more destructively when she attempted to
defend herself in the future. He also praised the client's efforts to develop a contingency plan with her husband in preparation for a time
when she might need to leave her job.

The therapist again reviewed the confrontation with Howard in a
similar manner during the following session. Kathleen continued to
have distressing interactions with her supervisor for some time, but she
never retreated to the helpless position she had assumed in the past.
Eventually she successfully filed grievances against her boss on a number of key issues. The therapist referred to various aspects of the episode
with Howard innumerable times during Kathleen's subsequent treatment, particularly when the client found herself intimidated by another
person.

As the vignette above illustrates, the therapist should utilize an
instance of successful coping to promote a number of treatment goals:

1. Affirming the client's worth by underscoring the success experiences with as much fanfare as the individual will comfortably tolerate.
2. Insuring that the client credits the *self* for any legitimate
   changes that have occurred rather than attributing them to
   chance or other external factors.
3. Challenging hopelessness and helplessness by utilizing the instance as an example of what the client might also be able to
   accomplish at some point in other areas of life.
4. Linking the incident in question explicitly to specific events or
   interactions in the client's family of origin.
5. Enumerating other manifestations in the client's current life
   that also reflect the operation of the same family of origin
   mechanisms, including relevant events which may have occurred in the therapeutic relationship.
6. Identifying the specific cognitive distortions and information-
   processing difficulties that have prevented the client from responding more effectively to similar situations in the past.
7. Identifying the specific changes in thinking, information processing, and behavior that accompanied the episode of successful coping.
8. Underscoring any negative consequences the client may have
   anticipated that did *not* occur, such as loss of emotional or
   behavioral self-control, retaliation from others, and so on.
9. Outlining specific implications for the client's future, either

with the particular person or situation involved, or with analogous situations in the individual's life.

10. Encouraging the client to rehearse specific cognitive and behavioral responses to comparable situations that might occur in the future.

We have presented the vignette from Kathleen's treatment because it illustrates how the therapist's analysis of an instance of successful coping can effectively integrate many aspects of the treatment plan. However, at the time the incident occurred, she had been in treatment for some time with clearly positive results. In fact, the confrontation with her boss only occurred after she had spent considerable time and energy working on the relevant issues in treatment. Various problems will arise, however, when the therapist attempts to review the successes of clients who have not yet advanced as far in the recovery process.

Many clients are unable to identify instances of more successful coping, particularly when the situations reflect more modest, *incremental* changes. Clients who do not perceive themselves as making progress may only disclose information that suggests positive changes in an incidental manner during the course of discussing other issues with the therapist. With such individuals, the therapist must remain alert to explore any data that may reflect changes from baseline functioning, however modest these may be. Using Socratic dialogue, the therapist may need to walk the client carefully through the relevant data in the hope of facilitating recognition of progress. Such recognition from the individual may be grudging at best, at least for the present, and may come only after the therapist has grappled with a host of potential disclaimers and disqualifications raised by the client.

RESISTING VICTIMIZATION

Like Kathleen, who was discussed in the previous section, many of our clients learn during the course of treatment how to resist various forms of victimization. In order to resist victimization, the client must develop a complex set of cognitive and behavioral skills. Below are a number of issues that we seek to bring to the attention of any client who is being victimized in an ongoing relationship. In our experience, integration of a number of points regarding victimization and self-defense must occur before the client will be ready to resist mistreatment in an effective and consistent manner.

Recognition of victimization is often long overdue, having been delayed by cognitive distortions and information-processing errors, particularly denial strategies. Therefore, it behooves one to analyze in some detail the various factors (e.g., self-blame for the perpetrator's actions) that had obscured the victimization previously. In similar fashion, one should also examine closely the potential connections between such factors and one's family of origin experiences. Regardless of what perpetrators might think or say, verbal abuse and/or harassment of various kinds can be just as destructive as physical assaults. Similarly, one can also be victimized by those who make relentless, unnecessary demands on one's time and energy, even when such behaviors occur under the ostensibly benign rubric of "friendship" or "love."

The recognition of victimization of oneself and/or one's children is accompanied by powerful affective reactions. Anger and fear are appropriate responses, and these may intensify over time. Situations that were once endured will now become more and more intolerable, until one can achieve a greater measure of safety. One can learn to *contain* one's emotions in a reasonably successful manner without having to suppress information processing as a result. Moreover, one's affect can serve as a cue for *reflection* and/or *action*.

Once identified, threats to personal safety (and/or the safety of one's children) must take precedence over other concerns. Until one is safe, habitual distractions, such as obsessing over one's shortcomings, must be pushed to the background again and again.

It will be necessary to mount a campaign of resistance against victimization. One confrontation, however dramatic it may be, will not suffice. In all likelihood, there will be a succession of battles to fight, some with upsetting consequences. The victimizer, after all, has no reason to think that things are going to be any different than they have been in the past. Only *consistency* and *repetition* will convey the strength of one's resolve to the victimizer. Consequently, it is vital to prepare for an *extended* period of conflict whenever one attempts to reverse a pattern of victimization in a relationship. Likewise, one should assume that the other person will respond with his or her full repertoire of aversive behaviors, not once, but on multiple occasions, and perhaps with even greater intensity than in the past.

The nature and magnitude of ongoing threats to personal safety (and/or the safety of one's children), not the abstract principles of philosophy or theology, must dictate the nature of one's response to victimization. There is no one right or appropriate way to defend oneself. The ethics of self-protective strategies must be evaluated in light of the safety issues involved. Behaviors which are deemed impolite, aggressive or otherwise inappropriate in most social contexts might be quite adaptive and *necessary* when one is attempting to resist various forms of victimization. One must remember that even rigid prescriptions such as "Thou shalt not kill," are waived in society when an individual is threatened with danger to life and limb.

In order to plan a campaign, it is necessary to assess very carefully one's resources including existing assertiveness skills, potential allies, institutional supports, and so on. Assessment of resources is often complicated by negative beliefs about the self, and distorted perceptions of the victimizer. Superior firepower does not necessarily dictate victory. Effective self-defense or self-assertion need not involve either overt anger or aggressive behavior. Gandhi brought the mighty British Empire to its knees without ever firing a shot. In many situations, a whisper may have greater impact than a scream, depending in part on the strength of the resolve behind it. In planning a campaign of resistance, one should never overlook the importance of factors such as cleverness or surprise. Likewise, even the most fearsome adversary always has weaknesses that one can exploit to some degree. *Any assessment of the victimizer that does not include reference to such weaknesses is incomplete, and probably reflects distorted perceptions of the individual in question.* One also needs to evaluate thoroughly any previous attempts to set limits on either the victimizer in question or the perpetrators of past abuse in order both to identify potentially successful strategies and to highlight any problems in implementation that may have occurred.

In order to sustain a successful campaign of resistance, it is necessary to monitor and counter the following cognitive mechanisms on an ongoing basis: (1) any type of denial regarding the perceptions of past harm and future threat that have necessitated the self-protective actions; (2) self-blame for the perpetrator's actions; (3) any type of denial regarding the perpetrator, including excuses for his or her behavior, attributions of overly favorable motives, and so on; (4) irrational expectations that the perpetrator will change, particularly as a result of the self-protective actions taken in response to victimization; (5) protective urges toward the perpetrator, particularly ones that surface before one has achieved a greater sense of safety; (6) unrealistic fears regarding the perpetrator's ability to retaliate or otherwise control subsequent situations; (7) a sense of helplessness or an unrealistically low assessment of one's potential power and competence; (8) irrational fears regarding the intensity of one's own affect and its potential impact on self or others.

Practice does indeed make perfect. In the course of a campaign of resistance, one will develop a growing repertoire of self-defense skills. These skills will increasingly reflect one's personality, communicational style, and moral values. Likewise, one can become more successful at communicating in a clear and consistent manner, thereby avoiding the mixed messages that often sabotage efforts to set limits in relationships. Finally, repeated experiences with conflict can help one to develop a

greater degree of confidence "under fire." One should always attempt
to savor those moments in which it was possible to stand up to mistreatment, since such reviews build wisdom and confidence.

*Resisting victimization does not necessarily result in the end of relation-
ships.* Setting limits can at times be the first step in repairing a relationship. By asserting oneself effectively, one may be able to gain a new
level of respect from others. Since many bullies are cowards at heart,
they often back off dramatically once they know that a victim will resist
mistreatment in a consistent manner. Once empowered, one may finally
be able to confront underlying issues, such as a partner's substance
abuse, which have been responsible for ongoing relationship problems.
Nonetheless, positive changes in the behavior of a victimizer may well
be transient in nature, particularly if they have occurred because one
has threatened to end the relationship. *Until such changes are solidly
established, one should resist any tendency to suspend vigilance or to assume
a less assertive posture.* Moreover, unless the victimizer fully acknowledges his or her destructive impact, he or she will probably remain a
threat indefinitely, regardless of any behavioral changes which may
have occurred.

*One must prepare for the possibility that the victimizer will be unable or
unwilling to change in any manner.* In some instances, the most assertive
posture imaginable may not provide a greater sense of safety, as long as
one remains within arm's length of a potential victimizer. Under such
circumstances, the only effective line of defense will be to terminate
contact with the victimizer. When terminating a relationship, one must
attempt to communicate in a clear, consistent manner, avoiding mixed
messages as much as possible. "Surgical" terminations (i.e., involving
quick and complete severing of contact) are vastly preferable to other
alternatives, particularly since the perpetrator may well seize on any
opportunity to sustain some form of contact with the victim. One cannot
end a relationship and at the same time help the other person deal with
the emotional ramifications of the termination. There may well be a
series of false starts before one is able to sever the connection with a
victimizer, but with support, one can learn how to achieve a definitive
end point in the relationship.

*One will continue to encounter potential victimizers throughout life's
journey.* Moreover, abusers, manipulators, and others of their ilk are
always "trolling" for new victims to hook. Consequently, one must
attempt to integrate as much data as possible from one's experiences,
particularly those which involve successful resistance to victimization.
It is necessary to develop "early warning mechanisms," in order to
eliminate or minimize contact with such individuals as quickly as possible. It is also useful to develop a profile of the types of individuals

to whom one is most susceptible (for example, hostile dependent males) and their characteristic "hooking" behaviors (e.g., threatening suicide, complaining of not being loved enough, and so on). Similarly, one should review carefully the assertiveness strategies that have worked in the past and the cognitive distortions that might interfere with implementing similar tactics in the future. The net result of all this reflection will probably be a semi-irreversible change in one's pattern of vigilance, particularly in relationships. Such an attentional change need not result in one becoming paranoid, defensive, or overly aggressive, however. Instead one can attempt to implement the words attributed to Jesus in Matthew 10:16—"Behold I send you forth as sheep in the midst of wolves: be ye therefore wise as serpents and harmless as doves."

CHARACTERISTICS OF EFFECTIVE HOMEWORK ASSIGNMENTS

The following characteristics help to promote the effectiveness of homework assignments:

1. Homework flows smoothly from the content of treatment. The assignment should clearly reflect the actual material of the session.

2. There should be a rationale for the homework assignment that the client readily comprehends. Our preference is to avoid assignments with strong paradoxical overtones, since they usually involve an implicit rationale that the therapist declines to share with the client. As we have discussed in earlier chapters, we prefer to establish and maintain a highly collaborative relationship with the client, with an emphasis on clear boundaries and expectations. Paradoxical assignments, in our opinion, would only engender confusion and mistrust in clients who may have already been extensively victimized by other authority figures in their lives. Even when the therapist has carefully explained why he or she has made a particular assignment, the client may still believe that there is another, hidden agenda. Such reactions may reflect the client's issues around trust, worthlessness, rejection, and so on. As one client said "Whenever you asked me to do any homework about incest, I thought that your real agenda was to show that it was *my* fault it happened."

3. The client should understand on a concrete level what is involved in the assignment, so that he or she knows how to succeed at it. As a check on comprehension, the therapist may ask the client to repeat back the instructions for the assignment in verbatim terms. It is impor-

tant that the therapist avoid belittling the client in doing so, however. The therapist may say: "I find that I'm not always clear when I give my clients homework. Would you do me a favor and just repeat back to me what you understand the assignment to be?" When assigning written homework, the therapist should emphasize, perhaps repeatedly with some clients, that he or she has no interest in spelling, punctuation, grammar, syntax, or handwriting.

4. The format of the assignment should resonate with the client's personal style. A familiarity with the client's history (particularly in academic areas) and current lifestyle should help the therapist match the format of the assignment to the client's unique characteristics. Without such knowledge, the therapist may assign the wrong kind of homework. For example, a client with a history of learning disabilities and school failure may be so mortified to have the therapist see his bad spelling and handwriting that he continually fails to produce any written homework. Similarly, it may be counterproductive to expect a client who seldom even glances at a newspaper to read an entire book, even if it is a very down-to-earth volume on a recovery-related subject. On the more positive side, the therapist who knows that a particular client has a very strong religious involvement may obtain far more information by asking her to think about a particular guilt-related topic when she is in church on Sunday.

5. The assignment is most effective when it orchestrates a learning experience for the client, regardless of the outcome. As discussed elsewhere (Beck et al., 1979; Bedrosian & Beck, 1980), the therapist should try to set up a homework assignment as a "no-lose situation," so that even if the client is unable to complete it, his or her failure will provide an opportunity to learn something. Behavioral assignments, particularly those that generate binary outcomes (e.g., "Go to an AA meeting this week"), may set up clients for failure and therapists for frustration unless they are accompanied by the appropriate instructions. For example, the therapist may ask the client with the AA assignment to note the cognitions that keep him or her from attending the agreed-upon meeting.

6. The therapist always reviews the homework assignment in a deliberate manner. As Haley (1976) points out, the therapist undermines the seriousness of his or her future recommendations by failing to discuss previously assigned homework. Failure to discuss a homework assignment without a compelling reason (e.g., an immediate crisis in the client's life) discourages the client from taking the therapist and the treatment seriously. It is much better in our opinion, for example, for the therapist to declare an assignment as having been ill-conceived or poorly timed, rather than to fail to mention it at all. The therapist should

always reward whatever time or effort the client has invested in the assignment by attending carefully to the results produced by the assignment. Some individuals (and not only obsessive-compulsives!) will produce more content in response to a homework assignment than the therapist can comfortably review in the session, particularly if he or she also needs to attend to other matters during the hour. The therapist should note the time allocation problem and allow the client to decide which portions of the homework he or she wants to discuss first. The therapist should also inquire as to how the client feels about not having the time to cover all the issues raised by a homework assignment, particularly if the problems keep occurring. By taking care to discuss such matters explicitly, the therapist communicates strong respect for the client's work and the effort it took to produce it.

7. The homework assignment, and the way it is discussed, should resonate with the therapist's posture. For example, when treating an incest survivor, the therapist will want to continue to convey the utmost respect for his or her boundaries while discussing homework. If there is written homework, the clinician may not ask to see it, but might request the client either to read it aloud or to comment on it instead. The therapist may emphasize that the client does not need to share all that he or she has written.

MENU OF HOMEWORK ASSIGNMENTS

The cognitive-behavioral literature (for example, Barlow, 1988; Beck & Emery, 1985; Beck & Freeman, 1990; Beck et al., 1979; Bedrosian, 1988; Burns, 1980; McMullin, 1986) contains a plethora of self-help tasks that can be assigned to clients between sessions. The homework we assign typically involves a mixture of established techniques (e.g., readings, tapes, thought recording tasks) and exercises that have developed spontaneously in response to the immediate issues of the client. As many of the following tasks illustrate, the therapist may design assignments that will promote several different treatment goals simultaneously.

Practicing Containment Strategies

Practice deep muscle relaxation, meditation, or related techniques on a daily basis.

Write down reassuring statements regarding anxiety on a small file card, for example, "I'm not going to go crazy." Carry the card with you at all times and read it over any time you begin to feel tense.

Prepare a list of the coping strategies you need to utilize during episodes of anxiety. Keep it in your purse or your wallet.

Fill out a weekly activity schedule. Identify changes that would afford you greater control over your time. Modify your schedule to include more social contact and less stressful activities.

Set up barriers (e.g., an answering machine) to reduce your availability to others.

Ask one or two trusted friends or family membesr if they can be available for support, if necessary, during symptomatic periods.

Set up regular calls to your Twelve-Step sponsor and/or increase attendance at meetings.

Tell your partner about the difficulties you've been experiencing during sexual relations.

Normalization Experiences

Ask your best friend how she responded when her eldest child left home for college.

Ask friends or family members how they felt returning to work after the birth of their children.

Ask your sponsor to recount his thoughts, feelings, and behaviors during the first six months of sobriety.

Ask a friend to describe her experiences with unwanted sexual advances, particularly those which occurred at work.

Read a book about grief, incest, or other significant experiences in your past or current life.

Attend a workshop on the experiences of adult children of alcoholics or an ongoing ACOA support group.

Investigating Specific Perceptions or Interpretations

List the differences between your own child's family experiences and those to which you were exposed.

List the differences between your parenting style and that of your parents.

Ask your wife if she was afraid of you when you became angry last week. Request that she specify which of your statements or behaviors frightened her.

Ask your husband whether he noticed how depressed you felt on Thanksgiving. If he did, see if he can describe in detail the changes he observed in your mood and/or behaviors.

Ask your son if he felt responsible for the fight you had with your husband last week and, if so, offer him emphatic reassurances to the contrary.

Meet with a sympathetic member of the clergy in order to determine the validity of your views on religious matters, particularly involving issues such as sin.

Observing Recurrent Themes, Coping Strategies, and/or Relationship Mechanisms

Keep track of the situations in which you begin to "space out."

Note events happening in your daily life that might make *someone else* angry.

Keep a log of the subjects you dismiss as too trivial or unimportant to discuss with your wife.

Make a list of the most important qualities you would like to see in a partner. Rate your long-term partners on those qualities.

Log the things you do to avoid criticism from your partner or others.

Log how much time and energy you spend obsessing about your partner.

Monitor the thoughts you have about your partner as you drive home.

Monitor your thoughts, feelings, and behaviors during instances in which you feel protective toward your partner.

Record the excuses you make for the negative behaviors of your partner and other significant people in your life.

List the things you do to try to get your partner to take care of you (for example, feign illness, complain of tiredness, and so on).

Keep a log situations in which you begin to feel worthless.

Log situations in which you think you overreacted to problems with your children.

Identifying and/or Countering Cognitive Distortions

Make a list of the fears that kept you from confronting your boss (partner, parent, and so on) in the past. Write down the reasons why each of the fears were unrealistic.

Chart how often you anticipate being criticized, disliked, or rejected by others. Monitor your thoughts, feelings, and behavior when you begin to expect such treatment. Attempt to counter your negative predictions with more realistic cognitions.

Copy and/or recite a prepared list of self-affirmatory statements. Try to do this daily if possible.

Make a list of valued personal attributes that you typically minimize.

Make a list of your partner's positive attributes that you tend to downplay or ignore.

Identify instances in which you exhibit an irrational fear of another person's anger. Answer these fearful thoughts with some of the conclusions we reached during today's session.

List the negative consequences of participating in unwanted sexual experiences.

Write down the reasons why you deserve or have the right to say no to unwanted sexual advances.

Make a list of your rights or minimum expectations in a relationship.

List the negative consequences associated with not asking for what you want from your partner.

Exploring Historical Material (Refer to Section on "Ways of Stimulating Recollections" in Chapter 9, p. 224)

Prepare a three-generational family history.

Look over childhood pictures, school yearbooks, and other historical mementos.

Read and highlight selected passages in workbooks or other self-help texts.

Walk through your old neighborhood, noting carefully the thoughts and feelings you experience.

Ask an elderly relative to share his or her reminiscences of the family.

Read a story, or watch a movie, about a young boy or girl who coped with family problems or other traumatic circumstances.

Integrating Therapeutic Insights and/or Improvements in Functioning

Write a summary of today's session and your reactions to it.

Listen to the tape of todays session and write about the responses you have.

List the changes in your thoughts, feelings, and behaviors that have occurred since you became sober.

Write down the things you think have changed in your life since you began treatment. Make sure to allow more than one sitting for the task, spread over a period of several days.

Think of the reasons why you and your wife were able to handle the recent crisis with your son so much better than in the past.

Write down the warning signs you now associate with potentially abusive or victimizing relationships.

Write on a topic that you brought up at the end of the session today, which we did not have time to discuss.

CAROL: BUILDING COPING STRATEGIES ON MULTIPLE LEVELS

The following case involved a number of highly successful homework assignments and symptom-based interventions. As a result of these interventions, the client was able to turn her attention to the larger issues that were connected to her presenting complaints. Through internalizing the process she experienced with the therapist, the client learned not only to control her symptoms but also to utilize them as a *cue* to examine other life concerns. The client identified the traumatic foundation for her obsessive worries and was able to lower her anxiety level markedly as a result. Moreover, the client began to reverse a long-standing pattern of over-involvement with her family of origin. The client's progress in treatment seemed to spur positive changes on her husband's part and in the marriage as well. The client and her husband strengthened the boundaries between their own family unit and their respective extended families. The couple also began to exert more effective leadership in parenting their own children. The case also illustrates how individual and systems interventions can intertwine successfully, supporting the personal growth of one or more individuals *and* the evolution of more effective family functioning.

Carol was the second oldest child in a highly enmeshed Lebanese-American family, headed by her immigrant grandmother. Her family was characterized by overprotective parenting and blurred personal boundaries. When Carol was 10, her older sister found their father dead, the victim of a heart attack while still in his 30s. Thereafter, Carol began to assume a strong caretaking role, toward her mother, grandmother, sister, and younger brother.

Carol entered treatment when she was in her mid-30s, the married mother of two young children. She had begun to experience a spectrum of anxiety symptoms, including palpitations, feelings of panic, and obsessive imagery. The symptoms had started shortly after the client had undergone surgery for a disabling neck injury. Despite having had the surgery, Carol still experienced chronic pain, for which she refused to take medication. Like many individuals who suffer from chronic pain, Carol found that others, including family members and her physicians, were beginning to intimate that her discomfort was "in her head." Consequently, she generally preferred to suffer in silence rather than

risk censure by discussing her pain with others. Carol's physical problems had forced her to quit her job, and they now prevented her from
doing many routine household tasks, such as running the vacuum
cleaner. Since she had more time on her hands, she spent several hours
each day either visiting with her mother and elderly grandmother, or
doing errands for them.

After Carol's father had died, her mother's brother, George, had
served as a surrogate parent in the family. He remained very involved
with Carol and her siblings, even after they had married and left home.
When Carol was in her 20s, George began to experience bouts of severe
depressive episodes, marked by delusional thinking, aggressive behaviors, and chronic suicidal ideation. True to her caretaking role, Carol
wound up "babysitting" for her uncle much of the day when he was
depressed, despite the fact that he had a wife, grown children, and a
number of siblings who were eligible for the job. When he ultimately
shot himself, not only did she hold herself responsible, she was also
blamed by a number of other family members. Although 4 years had
passed since her uncle's suicide, Carol still had not visited his grave. She
also continued to avoid many other places that she had associated with
him.

George's depressive episodes and eventual death figured promin-
ently in some of the symptoms Carol reported. She reported intrusive
images of holding a gun to her own head, of jumping out of a moving
car (as George had often threatened to do), and of the spoken words,
"I'm gonna kill myself." These repetitive images made the client fearful
that she would follow in her uncle's ill-fated footsteps. Consequently,
Carol experienced an overwhelming sense of panic every time the imagery occurred. The more out of control the client felt, the more she
would believe that she indeed *was* going crazy and would need to be
hospitalized, just as her uncle had been.

Carol worried obsessively about the safety of her family. Her fearful orientation was understandable given the sudden deaths of both her
father and George, his surrogate. Moreover, the belief system of the
entire family seemed to revolve around issues of danger. For example,
the client's mother and grandmother habitually invoked fatalistic Middle Eastern superstitions (e.g., if you dream of a wedding, then someone
close to you is going to die), all of which seemed to involve bad omens
and catastrophic events. Wherever Carol happened to be, if she heard
a siren, she immediately visualized something happening to her mother
or grandmother. Likewise the client often expected to hear bad news
about someone when the phone rang. She would call her sister and
mother several times a day with no specific agenda in mind other than
to relieve nagging fearful thoughts about a family member. Carol sel-

dom traveled out of town overnight, but when she did she never allowed a full day to go by without initiating phone contact with the family members back home.

Carol and her husband, Eli, lived in a two-family house owned by his widowed mother, who lived downstairs. Like Carol's mother and grandmother, the mother-in-law was not reticent to offer her strong opinions on every aspect of the couple's life. All three of the maternal figures were quite vocal in demanding time and attention from Carol and her children. Carol's anxiety would skyrocket when she would be unable to reconcile conflicting demands from both sides, particularly during holidays. The enmeshed pattern of relating existed in the spouses' extended families as well. On both sides of the family, it seemed as if there were legions of uncles, aunts, and cousins offering advice or demanding attention. Neither Carol nor Eli seemed skillful at maintaining boundaries around their own marriage. Carol repeatedly became overly involved in the problems of extended family members, much as she had been with her uncle. She often found herself fatigued and overwhelmed as a result of being unable to refuse requests for help from various relatives.

For nearly a year, Carol's treatment was primarily focused on symptom reduction. The therapist's first priority was to help the client feel a greater sense of control over the panic attacks and the intrusive imagery. Carol worked hard at lowering her level of autonomic arousal, by regularly practicing relaxation and visualization procedures. Despite the lingering physical problems the client experienced, she was able to begin swimming regularly, a practice the therapist enthusiastically supported. Her aerobic regimen promoted relaxation and boosted her morale considerably.

Using Socratic dialogue, the therapist repeatedly walked the client through the data that indicated that her panic attacks would not induce psychosis, loss of control, or any other difficulties similar to those her uncle had experienced. Likewise, the therapist regularly attacked the fears about suicide by asking Carol a series of questions aimed at assessing depression, hopelessness, and other correlates of self-destructive wishes. Other than occasional sad moods primarily related to her chronic pain and physical disability, the client experienced none of the severe symptoms of depression she associated with her uncle. She could not recall wanting to die or feeling as if she had no hope for a better life in the future. Moreover, the mere thought of suicide was repellent to Carol, because of the potential destructive impact on her young children. Having lived through the loss of her uncle, she was well acquainted with the terrible aftermath of a completed suicide.

Again and again in the sessions, Carol reached the conclusion that other than the recurrent suicidal imagery, her attitudes, feelings, and behavior bore no resemblance to those of her uncle or any other individual at risk for self-destructive behavior. The therapist asked her to write down the conclusions they reached during their discussions about suicide and to review the list repeatedly between appointments. Carol's list included rational responses to her fearful thoughts, such as "People who are depressed and hopeless commit suicide. I'm not depressed and I'm not hopeless," and "The imagery doesn't mean I want to kill myself." The therapist also suggested that the client try substituting an image of her two children, who were symbolic of her strong wish to live, whenever she experienced the intrusive suicidal imagery. During the session, Carol practiced inducing the suicidal imagery and replacing it as the therapist had recommended. Through diligent practice and repetition, the client was able to use both the imagery and the rational responses to reduce her anxiety about losing control and harming herself.

Once some measure of symptom relief appeared to have occurred, the therapist began to explore the painful memories associated with George's death. Carol continued to avoid a number of locations she had associated with her uncle's depressive episodes, such as the hospital in which he had died. Borrowing a technique from systematic desensitization, the therapist asked Carol to construct a hierarchy of places she currently avoided because of the unpleasant associations with her uncle. Over a period of approximately 2 months, Carol made multiple visits to the sites associated with her uncle, gradually ascending up the hierarchy to the final item, which involved a visit to his house and the room in which he had died. She also complied with the therapist's request that she make regular trips to the cemetery where both her father and uncle were buried. For 2 or 3 months, Carol found it oddly comforting to visit the graves of the two men. Not long after she completed the hierarchy, the client found that she had no further need for regular trips to the cemetery. All these interventions gave the client many opportunities to discuss her relationships with her father and her uncle. She recognized how the obsession with suicide, her fears of losing control, and other recent symptoms all connected to her uncle's death a few years previously. Through dialogue with the therapist, Carol was able to free herself of a sense of responsibility for her uncle's suicide. With the therapist's assistance, the client also began to reflect on the traumatic impact of her father's death on the family and the way in which that event had primed her to assume a parentified role in the household.

Carol would become so obsessed with her symptoms that she would consistently fail to recognize the precipitating factors involved.

It became clear to the therapist that the client's obsessive thoughts and feelings of anxiety increased directly in response to certain key stressors. Whenever the client's symptoms intensified, the therapist encouraged her to search for potential precipitants, by reviewing the status of all the major issues and relationships in her life. Carol internalized the process she learned in treatment, so that when she became symptomatic between sessions, she regularly began to ask herself "What else is bothering me?" Over time, she was able to redirect her attention during symptomatic periods back toward the issues that had originally triggered the discomfort. As a result, the client experienced a greater sense of control over her symptoms, which in turn began to occur with less frequency and intensity.

As she observed the connections between her symptoms and the ongoing stressors in her life, Carol discovered a great deal about herself. First of all, the client recognized that her physical disability and her chronic pain had affected her moods, her self-confidence, and her lifestyle far more than she had acknowledged. On several occasions, she observed that anxious periods would arrive on the heels of increased physical pain or decreased mobility. Carol realized that because she tended minimize her pain and the degree of her disability, she was prone to push herself too hard, or to ignore the signs of overexertion, thereby exacerbating her physical problems. The therapist helped the client acknowledge some of the painful losses she had incurred as a result of her disability. As will be discussed below, the client also recognized the need to explore alternative methods for coping with her pain. Second, Carol began to view her constant involvement in family conflicts as a major and unnecessary source of psychological stress in her life. She gradually learned to resist induction into many of the battles that took place in her extended family. The client continued to be overly involved with her mother and her grandmother, however. Finally, Carol also learned that even in the absence of symptoms, her typical day was filled with worry and fear, primarily centering on the health and safety of her immediate family. The client was able to grasp how her ongoing rumination served as a breeding ground for more serious symptoms of anxiety. As Carol's presenting complaints became less severe and therefore less compelling, she began to address the obsessive fears about her family. With the therapist's help, the client experimented with resisting the urge to call family members when she was worried, in favor of distracting herself or countering the fearful thoughts with rational responses. Carol also grew to understand more clearly how her worries reflected the traumatic events in her past and the fearful world view prevalent in her family.

The therapist believed that it was vital to provide the client with a constructive framework for understanding the impact of her pain and her physical disability. Since Carol was sensitized to any statement that scapegoated her for the chronic pain, the therapist always validated her feelings of discomfort during any discussion of her physical problems. In an effort to normalize some of the client's experiences, the therapist frequently approached the problem of chronic pain in educational terms. For example, the therapist stated that in his experience, other persons often have difficulty accepting an individual's pain as valid, particularly in the absence of a visible injury, lesion, or disease. He often would ask Carol questions such as "Who knows more about your pain than you do?" or "How can someone else tell you what you're feeling?" When she would report that someone had again intimated that the pain might be psychological, or that she wasn't fighting it hard enough, the therapist's standard response was to ask in a light-hearted manner, "Where did he or she get her medical training?" He constantly underlined incidents that indicated that Carol *already* showed a high level of pain tolerance just by engaging in her normal activities each day. Unfortunately, her "everyday" level of pain was invisible to others, since she rarely if ever complained about it. The client began to view herself as a stronger individual, someone who had proven long ago that she could tolerate discomfort. As a result, she found it easier to resist blaming messages from others in response to her pain or her physical problems.

Carol's success at using relaxation exercises and imagery techniques to combat the anxiety symptoms made the therapist wonder if she might be a good hypnotic subject. Ultimately the therapist referred her to a psychologist colleague who was skilled in the use of hypnosis for pain control. Even in making the referral for hypnotherapy, the therapist took care not to give Carol the unintended message that the pain was really only in her head. He began by listing hypnosis as one of several alternatives to traditional medical approaches to pain, such as acupuncture and chiropractic treatment. When she began to express some interest in hypnosis, the therapist discussed its usage primarily as an alternative to anesthesia for surgical procedures and as a pain-control aid for terminally ill patients. Implicitly then, the therapist's discussion of hypnosis grouped Carol's pain with other clearly defined, legitimate medical conditions. As the therapist had hoped, the client did consult his colleague, who taught her how to use self-hypnosis to reduce pain.

Not all the symptom-oriented interventions were successful with Carol. In the initial interview, the therapist had asked her to obtain a book by Claire Weekes between sessions, as was his standard practice at the time with clients who suffered from anxiety symptoms. Naturally, he hoped that the bibliotherapy assignment would help Carol normalize some of her experiences, as it seemed to do for so many other clients. Unfortunately, the client found herself a copy of *Peace from Nervous Suffering,* and never progressed in her reading of it beyond the first chapter. From the moment Carol picked up the book, the word "nervous" seemed to overshadow everything else she read. Everyone in the family had referred to her uncle George's psychological problems with terms such as "bad nerves" and "nervous breakdown." The Weekes book, which normally had such a soothing effect on clients, only raised Carol's anxiety further, since, in her view, it pointed out the parallels between her symptoms and those of her uncle. Although Carol's interpretation of the statements she encountered in the book were clearly distorted, the therapist realized it would be unproductive to challenge such strongly held beliefs without getting to know both the client and her situation better. He told her he wasn't sure if Dr. Weekes was speaking of the same kind of difficulties her uncle had and apologized for having assigned such upsetting reading. Thereafter the therapist avoided bibliotherapy assignments altogether.

Medication also proved to be a mixed blessing for the client. Although Carol's family physician had prescribed a minor tranquilizer for her, she generally resisted using the medication, even during a severe bout of anxiety. In a quietly confident tone of voice, she told the therapist "I'd rather do it on my own if I can." The therapist praised the client for her self-reliant attitude, but he also emphasized that he would not be distressed if she had to use the medication occasionally. The therapist carefully explained the difference between her as-needed medication and the psychotropic drugs her uncle had taken during his psychotic depressions. Although she rarely did take the medication, Carol did draw some solace from knowing that it was available should the need arise. On the other hand, the fact that she did not *need* the medication, enabled the client to view herself as different from her uncle.

During the first year of her treatment, the intensity of Carol's anxiety led to phone calls to the therapist on six or seven occasions. These phone calls were to provide the therapist with a pathway into some of the client's most significant relationship issues. In the therapist's opinion, the calls were all legitimate and appropriate. In each case, a very brief review of some of the issues already covered in treatment was sufficient to lower the patient's anxiety to tolerable levels. The therapist was distressed however, by the fact that the first few calls were initiated not by the client, but by her husband, Eli. In the therapist's view, Eli's behavior reflected the enmeshed, overprotective style of relating so characteristic of both partners' families of origin. Since Carol found it hard to call the therapist, Eli was more than happy to do the job for her. The therapist was concerned that the husband's willingness to take over for his wife perpetuated a family structure in which she was defined as helpless, incompetent, and, God forbid, crazy. Moreover, the husband's enabling behavior only perpetuated Carol's lack of assertiveness.

After one of the crisis calls, the therapist asked Carol to bring Eli along to her next appointment. The therapist was able to sell both spouses on the need for the client to initiate contact with him on her own in the future. The clinician also utilized a number of additional interventions aimed at strengthening the boundaries between the spouses, such as recommending that the husband stop trying to restructure his wife's fearful thoughts. The therapist consistently emphasized the need for Carol to resolve her difficulties in her own way, at her own pace. The therapist held five or six more conjoint sessions with Carol and Eli over the next 2 years. During each couples session, the therapist consistently encouraged greater psychological differentiation between the spouses. The therapist also supported the couple's efforts to separate from both of their extended families. The spouses learned quickly to stay out of one another's business and to assert themselves appropriately whenever invasions of psychological space took place within the marriage. Eli seemed relieved that he no longer needed to take so much responsibility for his wife's thoughts and feelings. He was also able to step back completely and let his wife fight her own battles with her extended family.

The episode of Eli's phone calls provided the foundation for the therapist to address a number of issues in subsequent sessions. First of all, as Carol began to open up a bit more about her marriage, it became clear that the husband engaged in a range of additional overprotective behaviors, generally with his wife's tacit encouragement. Carol's abdication of responsibility, and the sense of helplessness which supported it, were now issues that could be directly addressed in treatment. As a consequence, the therapist was able to shift more of the focus of the sessions away from the client's symptoms toward broader issues such as her inordinate fear of conflict. Similarly, the therapist was able to keep the spotlight on the issues of enmeshment and overresponsibility as they manifested themselves in the client's close relationships, particularly with her husband and her relatives. Carol increasingly resisted being inducted into extended family conflicts. She also learned how to turn down requests for help from various family members without experiencing excessive guilt as a result. The therapist fully expected that decreases in symptomatology, increased insight, and improvements in self-esteem, combined with the emerging needs of the client's own children, would all continue to make Carol's overinvolvement with her relatives a problem for her.

Once she had achieved a significant reduction in the frequency and intensity of her anxiety symptoms, Carol began to prefer intervals of 2 or 3 weeks between appointments. The client found a part-time job that matched both her skills and her physical limitations. Once Carol was able to work again, she became much less involved with her extended family. After approximately 45 treatment sessions spread over 2 years, Carol began scheduling appointments 3 months apart.

About 3 years after Carol had started individual treatment, her 6-year-old son, fittingly enough, began to experience separation problems. The boy seldom slept alone through the entire night, and worse, was starting to show signs of school refusal. The therapist referred the family to a colleague who specialized in childhood adjustment problems. The child clinician helped the family implement a rather straightforward approach to the son's separation difficulties. She tried to affirm the parent's authority, while emphasizing the need for both children to learn greater self-reliance. She also provided a supportive forum for Carol and Eli to work through the guilt feelings they experienced when they were forced to set limits on their children.

Both therapists, whose ethnic and cultural background were quite similar to that of Carol and Eli, also came from enmeshed families in which guilt induction was a common procedure. The clinicians understood and empathized with the family's values, and adapted almost immediately to their client's patterns of speaking and behavior in the sessions. The therapists knew what it was like to be part of an extended family and a tightly knit community, but they also knew, from their own experiences, the importance of differentiation within such a strongly bonded relational context. Consequently, they were always able to convey an underlying message of hope to the couple, even as they highlighted threatening issues, such as enmeshment in the extended family.

The son's problems led to the development of stronger boundaries in the family, particularly between the spouse subsystem and the children. The parents had to work together more closely than ever before in order to resist their son's inappropriate attempts to elicit sympathy. Once the boy started to sleep in his own room for the entire night, the spouses had much more private time available, which in turn enabled them to strengthen their relationship. Moreover, as they encouraged more self-reliance on the part of their son, both Carol and Eli seemed to aim for more independence for themselves. As the family therapy came to a close, the couple decided to move out of Eli's mother's house and purchase a home of their own.

Although she felt somewhat guilty leaving her mother-in-law, Carol moved to her new home without experiencing significant symptoms of any kind. Once she settled in her own house, the client began to guard her own boundaries much more carefully. For example, she quickly identified a potentially intrusive neighbor and carefully limited her contact with the woman. Because of the move, Carol no longer had as much time available for various family members. She was able to tolerate the inevitable guilt-inducing messages she received from her family without becoming bogged down in feelings of worthlessness. More than ever before, the client had a sense of independence. In the meantime, Carol felt a greater sense of safety in her daily life. During one of the client's last treatment sessions, the therapist asked her about one of the superstitions she had discussed when she first entered therapy. Her reply was music to the ears of any cognitive therapist. Folding her arms decisively across her chest, Carol exclaimed, "I don't believe in that shit any more."

13

Utilizing Relationship Material

WORKING ON PATTERNS THAT SHOW UP IN CURRENT RELATIONSHIPS

What are the implications of therapeutic work on family of origin issues for the client's *current* relationships with spouses and family members? Although some authors apparently insist that confrontations with parents or caretakers *must* occur as a part of the recovery process (Forward, 1989), we emphasize that the answer to the question varies with the circumstances of each client. Just so we are certain that separation or divorce is *not* the answer for every spouse of an alcoholic, a compulsive gambler, or any other impaired individual. We do urge our clients to examine the *true motives* behind whatever relationship decisions they do make. We also urge clients to develop realistic expectations of relationships, unfettered by wishful thinking or other forms of denial. We also encourage our clients to think through *in detail* all the consequences associated with continuing, ending, or attempting to modify relationships with significant others. Finally, we want to help our clients live more comfortably with the difficult decisions they have made.

Other writers (e.g., Boszormenyi-Nagy & Spark, 1973) have noted that the client may well experience the relationship with the therapist as a threatening alliance *against* significant others. The therapist needs to elicit the client's reactions to the act of discussing family or marital relationships in treatment. As mentioned in Chapter 7, many clients find it quite threatening to consider the mere *possibility* that their parents had a destructive impact on them in childhood. A sense of disloyalty, and the feelings of guilt which result, may prevent clients from processing sufficient information to connect family of origin difficulties with current distress. Moreover, some clients, particularly those who are phobic about experiencing strong emotions, may become fearful that the examination of childhood circumstances itself will lead to disruptions in their current relationships with parents or other family members. In a similar manner, some clients may fear that therapeutic scrutiny of their marital relationships will lead to intense anger and destructive conflict with their spouses. Other individuals may worry about how the therapist will react if they discuss negative aspects of their current relationships with spouses or family. Often they may be afraid that the therapist will think that they should terminate the relationships in question. On the other hand, clients who find it too threatening to have any contact at all with various family members may imagine, with considerable trepidation, that the therapist will encourage some sort of dialogue with the family members in question.

Needless to say, all of the client concerns described above will complicate any discussions of current relationships that may occur in treatment. Clients who struggle with loyalty issues may feel quite worthless and may even become depressed when they discuss spouses or family members. Consequently, they might clam up, change the subject, or otherwise resist participating in such discussions. Moreover, as we mentioned in our earlier discussion of psychological reactance, both belief systems and the client's willingness to examine them can be strongly influenced by the interpersonal context. The client who fears that the therapist is siding against a spouse or other family members will feel caught in a loyalty bind, as will the individual who perceives that he or she is being led by the clinician into some type of destructive confrontation with a significant other. As a result, the client will reflexively oppose any attempts by the therapist to examine the relationships involved, clinging even more strongly to distorted beliefs in the process. Consequently, the therapist will only be able to explore the relevant material to the extent that he or she can assume a posture which creates a less threatening context for the client.

The therapist should remain alert for signs of discomfort on the client's part during discussions involving current relationships with significant others, and he or she should also take note whenever the discussion about a relationship takes an adversarial tone, particularly if the client begins to defend the other individual in any way. If this occurs, the therapist should immediately step back from the content, analyze the preceding interaction, and find a posture that will create a more comfortable alliance with the client. The therapist needs to use questioning to help the client identify the source of his or her uncomfortable feelings. It is also vital to obtain the client's perceptions of the therapist's attitudes toward the relationship in question. Knowledge of such perceptions on the part of the client allows the therapist subsequently to clarify his or her position in a powerful way, as the case vignettes presented below will illustrate.

It is helpful for the therapist to reassure the client from the outset of treatment that examination of family of origin dynamics need not culminate in destructive confrontations or alienation from loved ones. The therapist should emphasize that the first task of therapy is to understand the inner mechanisms of the client, not to produce immediate changes in his or her behavior, particularly in long-term familial or marital relationships. The therapist should stress that successful treatment can produce a wide spectrum of effects ranging from complete restructuring of existing relationships to a complete absence of outward changes in those relationships. It will be reassuring to point out that many clients have worked on significant psychological issues successfully without ever having any *discussions* of the treatment content with significant others, let alone *confrontations*. The therapist should also explicitly disavow any investment in promoting relationship outcomes that seem to be particularly threatening to the individual, such as confronting elderly parents or divorcing an alcoholic spouse. As we discussed in an earlier chapter, it may be reassuring for the therapist to make a comment that expresses a positive attitude toward the family member about whom the client seems most concerned, such as "I can hear in what you've already told me that even though your mother has some significant limitations, she is still very concerned in her own way about the welfare of her children, just as any parent would be."

On the other hand, the therapist does need to forewarn clients that an intensification of negative feelings toward certain significant others could very well occur as a direct result of therapeutic work. Raising this issue gives the therapist an opportunity to do some teaching about denial, the nature of affect, as well as the relationship between emotions and cognitions. The therapist should also make a very clear distinction for the client between *feelings* and *behaviors*, perhaps by presenting multiple examples that illustrate instances in which common powerful emotions never lead to actions. Finally, the therapist may also give the client explicit permission to avoid, at least temporarily, interactions with family members that are simply too threatening to consider at the present time.

Except for occasions when ineptness or unresolved personal issues on the part of the therapist have stimulated an adversarial interchange, the client's resistance to discussions about significant others nearly always reflects the operation of key cognitive mechanisms. The therapist will generally encourage the client to examine the sources of his or her concerns about discussing significant others. If the client is in a receptive state, the therapist can use the individual's reactions to discussions of significant others to illustrate the operation of issues such as denial, overvigilance, loyalty, worthlessness, fear of intense affect, and so on. Note that the therapist can label such mechanisms explicitly and in considerable detail while still honoring the client's desire to limit discussion of the family member in question. By naming relevant issues and integrating them with material disclosed in prior sessions, the therapist can keep treatment moving forward without expanding the current content. In the meantime, the client feels respected, validated, and safe.

We want to see our clients learn to protect themselves effectively. If treatment progresses successfully, then we assume that our clients will begin to confront *ongoing* victimization, wherever it might occur in their lives. We find that clients who confront significant others with *past* abuse often come away disappointed. Although clients may claim that they only want to unload their concerns, they usually do have hopes or expectations for the kind of reactions they might receive from the other person. These clients seldom receive support or validation in response to their confrontations. Instead, the client may meet with denial and/or anger on the part of the other individual. Additional family conflicts and scapegoating of the client may result, all of which may simply serve as a distraction from more significant issues that need to be addressed in treatment.

MARIA: WORKING ISSUES IN SEQUENCE AND IN TANDEM

The following case involved serial treatment contacts, usually with sessions spaced 2 to 3 weeks apart, spanning several years. The recovery process included several different phases of work targeting ongoing relationships with significant others. The therapist utilized a number of elements from the client's current relationships to identify the connections between historical material and her presenting complaints. The client first benefited from trauma-oriented work that traced the links between the client's present anxiety and her exposure to family violence in childhood. The client was able to identify and correct some significant relationship patterns that replicated features of her relationship with her abusive father. The client also learned to resist certain biases in information processing as she recognized ongoing victimization in her life, and at the same time reined in obsessive thoughts of self-blame. In the course of her recovery, the client needed to address the link between her core issue of worthlessness and the chronic rejection she had experienced with her mother. Before she could accomplish such a task however, she also needed to know that she could control her anger, since she was fearful of poisoning the positive relationship she now had with the mother. To complicate matters further, the client's fear of her affect stemmed from her identification with her physically abusive father, an identification which also posed other significant implications. Consequently, the therapist needed to untangle and confront several issues, some in tandem and others in sequence. All the while, the clinician sought to help the client to feel in control of her emotions and her behavior, particularly when she interacted with her mother.

Maria, a 35-year-old divorced mother of two, had sought treatment for chronic feelings of depression. She saw herself as having a basic deficiency that rendered her unable to sustain constructive relationships, particularly with men. The intense anxiety the client often felt around others, and the relief she felt once she was alone, only served to strengthen the idea that she would never be able to have normal relationships. Plagued by a sense of hopelessness about her interpersonal prospects, and tortured by the worthless feelings that resulted from her relentless self-criticism, Maria often viewed suicide as her best option.

Maria grew up with an authoritarian father who physically abused her mother and her older brother. As a child, she recalled feeling particularly anxious whenever she saw signs of conflict between her parents, since such disputes often culminated in violence on the father's part. Consequently, Maria learned from a young age to monitor ongoing interactions between members of her family, so that she always seemed to know where everyone was in the house and what they were doing.

Maria told the therapist that as an adult she still monitored everything that went on at family gatherings, which now included spouses and many children. Whenever she attended family functions, she would feel anxious, overwhelmed, and ultimately exhausted, so that she often found it necessary to leave earlier than everyone else. Although she experienced relief on returning home, she also would feel deficient and damaged, ashamed of her inability to relate to others, and more convinced than ever that remaining completely alone was her only option. Suicidal thoughts were then likely to result.

It is noteworthy that Maria never connected her inability to tolerate long periods of contact with her family to her need to monitor all the interactions going on around her. Likewise, she never identified any relationship between her exhaustion after family functions and the stressful conditions she experienced in her household when she was growing up. During the initial stages of treatment, the therapist enabled the client to increase her awareness of several mechanisms that had developed in response to the abusive events of her childhood. Maria now realized why she felt so drained after family gatherings and other social functions. She recognized the powerful tendency to be over-vigilant to signs of anger or conflict in others, particularly males. Maria could see more clearly some of the other ongoing effects of such over-vigilance, for example, tension and behavioral constriction on her part. She was able to let down her guard somewhat in her interactions with others and to avoid berating herself when she did feel anxious around people. Maria began to understand how growing up in an abusive situation primed her to blame herself when others treated her badly. She began to recognize that one of her closest friends often behaved in a demanding and manipulative manner toward her. The friend's be-havior had always caused Maria to obsess about her own inadequacies. The client now learned to resist such ruminations in favor of limiting her exposure to the individual in question.

Despite the gains she had made in treatment, Maria still struggled with an underlying sense of worthlessness. The client tended to blame Catholicism for her intense feelings of shame and guilt, but the therapist continued to suspect that the true source of the problem was much closer to home. In discussing the family conflicts her father had pre-cipitated, Maria did also acknowledge that, as a child, she had fanta-sized herself as her mother's protector. She used to imagine encourag-ing her mother to leave her father and helping to make it possible. Maria described her mother as a somewhat remote, nondemonstrative in-dividual. Although the mother sounded quite cold and withdrawn to him, the therapist remained unable to interest the client in elaborating on the negative aspects of that relationship. The clinician suspected that Maria as an adult was again protecting her mother, this time by refusing to examine the relationship with her in a sustained manner.

The therapist had learned long before to be cautious with Maria, who could easily feel threatened or overpowered by him. The client physically drew back on several occasions when the therapist raised his voice somewhat to emphasize a point. Likewise, Maria also found it uncomfortable when the therapist once rolled his chair forward in her direction, again while trying to punctuate a statement. The client's skittish quality in the presence of a male authority figure was entirely understandable given her aggressive father. The therapist learned to inhibit his body language , and to maintain a softer, slower demeanor with Maria. The clinician had also processed most of the events in the therapeutic relationship with the client, who seemed to have benefited from the information. Given the anxiety Maria had already experienced with him, however, the therapist had no great inclination to push fur-ther on the issue of her mother. Moreover, the client was highly committed to her recovery process and had already gained a great deal from treatment. The therapist was confident that at some point Maria would present him with an opportunity to approach the relationship with her mother in an effective manner.

Maria's difficulties with a female supervisor ultimately led her to examine the relationship with her mother in greater detail. The supervisor had many qualities that caused the client to feel inadequate by comparison. Maria found herself on a treadmill trying to please the supervisor, who appeared to withhold praise as a means of manipulating the client. Any significant admonishment or criticism from the supervisor was enough to drive the client into a symptomatic period, usually involving prolonged rumination, high anxiety, feelings of worthlessness, and at times, suicidal ideation. To complicate matters further, Maria had slipped into disclosing very personal information about herself during periods when the supervisor had seemed more approving and supportive. It now seemed as though the supervisor was willing to use the personal information against her in a very manipulative manner.

The therapist consistently validated Maria's perceptions of the supervisory relationship. The client presented such a detailed picture of her interactions with the supervisor and was so circumspect coming to her own conclusions that the therapist knew a subtle but insidiously victimizing process was occurring in the workplace. Maria realized that she could no longer work so desperately for the supervisor's approval. Moreover, she recognized that she needed to guard personal information much more carefully whenever she spoke with the supervisor. Once she fully appreciated the dangers associated with self-disclosure to the supervisor, Maria was extremely effective in suppressing the behavior. The more the client recognized the victimizing components of the relationship, the more anxious she began to feel in the supervisor's presence. She became worried that she would lose her composure in front of the supervisor. As Maria took steps to leave her position, she began to anticipate angry or vindictive reactions on the part of the supervisor.

The therapist took two paths in response to the client's mounting anxiety. The first involved reframing her anxiety as a natural outgrowth of good reality testing. The therapist repeatedly stated that, unlike other times in her life, Maria had now recognized victimization for what it was, without becoming distracted by concerns about her own inadequacy. Moreover, the therapist emphasized that Maria now fully recognized the *continuing* danger that existed in the relationship with the supervisor. As a consequence, she could no longer feel comforted when the supervisor chose to be charming or superficially supportive. The therapist's second path involved directing the client's attention toward the *trauma-driven* elements of her anxiety. He underscored the connections between the client's reactions to her abusive father and her fears about the supervisor's potential retaliation. He encouraged the client to analyze the validity of her most fearful thoughts about the supervisor. Maria was able to acknowledge some of the distortions in her predictions about the supervisor, thereby reducing the intensity of her panicky feelings as a result.

The therapist believed that the source of the supervisor's power over the client rested not only in her ability to provoke fear, but also in her power to stimulate feelings of worthlessness. Except for her final weeks on the job, Maria's behavior with the supervisor most closely resembled her style of relating to her *mother*, rather than her father. The client could recognize that she strove valiantly for affirmation from her supervisor, just as she had endeavored to please her mother. The therapist began to encourage Maria more consistently to think about the impact of her relationship with her mother, particularly in light of what they had already learned from the interactions with the supervisor.

As the client began to open up a bit more, it became clear to the therapist that Maria's mother had exerted a destructive influence on her emerging sense of self in childhood and adolescence. The mother often treated Maria in an extremely critical, rejecting manner, and in fact, continued to do so on occasion. In the therapist's opinion, the client had always internalized blame for her mother's rejecting behaviors. From a young age, Maria had devoted herself to identifying and attempting to change the personal imperfections she felt were responsible for the lack of approval and affection she experienced. The client remembered that in childhood she could never feel comfortable sitting down in her mother's presence. If she happened to be seated and idle when her mother entered the room, the client would jump up and immediately occupy herself with some household task.

The therapist pointed out repeatedly that it was unlikely a mother who was *simply* quiet or withdrawn would have elicited such a powerful response from her daughter. The client began to agree somewhat uneasily with the therapist's contention that intense disapproval or rejection from her mother was the likely source of her need to appear busy. At times, she could also recognize her mother's critical and hostile tendencies, particularly when the therapist underscored rejecting behavior shown by the mother toward others. Maria also began to acknowledge that she had internalized the responsibility for her mother's negative attitudes toward her, assuming that, if she had been a more worthwhile daughter, she would not have been rejected. She even started to understand how these experiences set up a lifetime of obsessing over her own defects.

However, it was extremely difficult for the therapist to keep Maria's attention focused on the relationship with her mother and its effects on her self-image. As Maria started to process the rejection from her mother and its many implications, she began to feel angry. Maria reported that she was growing ever more irritable and impatient when she had to interact with her mother, who still lived nearby. The client had always equated her own anger with the violent rage of her father, considering herself just as capable of engaging in destructive behavior as he had been. She was particularly fearful of behaving in a hostile or abusive manner toward her mother, who was now widowed and elderly. Consequently, Maria would generally become quite anxious during dialogue with the therapist about her mother, often to the point of being unable to concentrate any longer on the discussion.

The therapist repeatedly assured the client it would serve no purpose for Maria to upset her mother during her declining years when each day with her was so precious. He frequently reiterated that it was predictable the client would experience more angry feelings, since she was beginning to process important features of her family background that she had not examined in any depth previously. The therapist noted often that since Maria, as a parentified child, had always idealized and protected her mother, such angry feelings might be particularly threatening for her. Despite the client's fears, the therapist would say, he remained confident that she had the ability to keep their discussions from poisoning the current relationship with her mother. However, the clinician also reminded Maria that he could easily accept it if she wanted to postpone addressing the issue of her mother for now. The therapist also regularly expressed his desire to *keep Maria in charge* of all future discussions involving her mother. He also added parenthetically at times that it was natural for all the children of elderly parents *he* knew to become cross or irritable from time to time.

The therapist believed that chronic maternal rejection was a major source of Maria's long-standing sense of worthlessness. He suspected that her self-esteem would improve enormously as she began to understand the relationship between her current feelings of worthlessness and the constant rejecting messages she had received from her mother during childhood. On the other hand, Maria's fear of her own anger, itself a legacy of her formative years, held her back from processing information regarding the relationship with her mother. If she were less afraid of her own affect, she would probably find the discussions about her mother much less threatening and, ultimately, more helpful. Consequently, the therapist had to approach the issues of maternal rejection and fear of anger in *tandem* for the time being. If Maria believed she would be able to control her anger, then she might be more willing to think about distressing aspects of the relationship with her mother. Likewise, if Maria could distinguish more clearly between her current relationship with her mother and the nature of their interactions during her formative years, then she might also be less fearful of examining the latter.

When Maria behaved in an angry manner as a child, her mother would tell her how much she resembled her father. Indeed, the client *had* perceived herself as capable of the same kind of violence that the father had exhibited toward the rest of the family. Maria also reported that she had been identified in the family as her father's "favorite." This piece of information made the therapist wonder about the source and intensity of the mother's negative attitudes toward the client. If the client had resembled her father so much and had been identified as his favorite, perhaps she had also been singled out as a scapegoat by her mother. For the time being however, the clinician decided that it would be unproductive to share such speculations with the client.

The therapist told Maria he understood why she would be so frightened by her anger, particularly in light of the comparisons she made between herself and her father. He then asked a series of very specific questions designed to elicit the basis for Maria's concerns about her anger. Could she recall two or three episodes in her life when her anger had been most intense? What thoughts and feelings had she experienced on those occasions? How had she behaved? Was she physically aggressive? Was she verbally aggressive? Had she controlled any impulses to behave more aggressively on those occasions? This particular line of exploration, which the therapist repeated a number of times, was only partially successful. Although Maria reported that she had seldom if ever engaged in aggressive behavior of any significance, she still strongly believed that she had the *potential* to be abusive. Nonetheless, she did agree that thus far her track record revealed consistently good control over her anger. She also conceded that "in general" a person's past behavior was probably the best predictor of their future behavior.

Since it was important to give the client a strong sense of control over her sessions, the therapist would remind Maria whenever the subject of her mother came up that the choice to continue the discussion was entirely hers. In a low-key manner, the therapist would utilize whatever content Maria presented as a means of illustrating the probable effects of the mother's rejecting behaviors on the self-image of a developing child. He did not attempt to amplify the affective intensity of the material the client volunteered about her mother but tried, instead to stick closely to both the content and the actual phraseology she employed. Similarly, the therapist was careful to keep his own affective tone during such discussions closely attuned to Maria's level of emotional intensity at the time.

Despite the therapist's cautious approach, he was able to elicit considerable historical material that illustrated the powerful negative impact of the mother's behaviors on Maria's self-image. On the other hand, the clinician sought to emphasize the differences between the client's experiences in childhood and her *current* relationship with her mother. In fact, the therapist continually underscored the loving concern Maria continued to demonstrate toward her mother. He also repeatedly highlighted evidence of the connection between Maria's abusive father and the fears she experienced about her own anger. Moreover, he would frequently review how she had identified many angry *feelings* on her part, but very few *actions*, in connection with various relationships in the past. He remained on guard for any new indications that she could control anger or any other emotions, particularly when the feelings were most intense, and he tried to bring all such occurrences to Maria's attention. In order to encourage further differentiation on Maria's part, the therapist also asked her repeatedly to review the differences between her angry feelings and behaviors and those that had been exhibited by her abusive father.

Although she still felt as if she had to control herself carefully in her mother's presence, Maria did reach the point where she was no longer fearful of discussing that relationship in treatment. By examining the relationship with her mother more closely, the client was able to gain a better understanding of how her self-image had been formed. Similarly, Maria was now able to see more clearly than ever how some of her symptoms, such as perfectionism and obsessive thoughts about her deficiencies, had developed as *coping strategies* in response to feelings of worthlessness. As a consequence, she was able to achieve even greater control over her compulsive work habits and her relentless self-criticism. Maria reported substantial gains in self-acceptance but knew that she still obsessed too much about her own defects. She continues on in treatment as this volume is being prepared, although a lack of funds and shrinking insurance coverage have severely curtailed the frequency of her sessions.

LOIS: STRENGTHENING BOUNDARIES

Although our clients may harbor fantasies to the contrary, no magical healing takes place just because an individual "goes public" with traumatic material. In fact, some clients may stir up a hornet's nest of unnecessary trouble when they attempt to confront family members about childhood abuse and other potentially explosive subjects. By disclosing highly personal information under unsafe conditions, these individuals may thereby set themselves up to be abused and/or scapegoated anew. In the following case example, the therapist assumed a supportive, investigatory posture, while encouraging close scrutiny of the expectations underlying the client's self-defeating actions. Rather than offer behavioral prescriptions, the therapist encouraged the client to define more clearly her priorities in dealing with her family and then helped her strategize accordingly. With the therapist's assistance, the client did learn how to maintain her personal boundaries in a more effective manner. In discussing the ongoing family conflicts, the therapist used a variety of strategies to redirect the client's attention toward her own issues, particularly worthlessness. As a result of subsequent treatment, the client did learn to confront interpersonal conflict more effectively and without experiencing a crippling loss of self-esteem in the process.

After reading a book on dysfunctional families, Lois had recognized that, as a child, she had been physically abused by her father and her older brother. Within a week or two, she had confronted her two abusers, neither of whom would acknowledge his past behaviors. Around the same time, Lois also berated her mother for having failed to protect her and demanded her support in the conflicts with the father and the brother. Soon two other siblings and an aunt were also drawn into the ever-widening dispute. In the meantime, Lois had not yet even discussed the subject of physical abuse with the therapist she had been seeing for several months.

At her next session, Lois complained to the therapist that instead of confronting the perpetrators of the abuse, everyone in the family seemed to be attacking *her*, the victim. The reverberating family conflicts, which she had precipitated, now became a major preoccupation for Lois, thereby crowding out other important agenda items in treatment. Needless to say, the client had never clearly spelled out for herself the long-range effects of the physical abuse, nor had she expended much time or energy trying to understand the connections between her stressful childhood and her current problems, which included both eating difficulties and self-defeating sexual behaviors.

The therapist believed that Lois had very little insight into her own psychological makeup, including the aftereffects of having grown up in an abusive household. These high-intensity conflicts with her family had the capacity to overwhelm the client and to distract her from the vital task of building self-awareness. The therapist knew from the history that Lois had a tendency to act out impulsively, without an adequate understanding of her own motivations or the potential consequences. At this point, he assumed that she was not likely to admit she had made an error by confronting her family. In fact, Lois was so preoccupied with issues of right and wrong, that she felt blamed any time the therapist attempted to discuss the family friction from the perspective of her own issues. Consequently, she often behaved in a highly defensive manner in her sessions. Helping the client to restrain herself from acting out any further with her family, without eliciting a hostile, defensive response from her in the process, would be a delicate task for the therapist.

Despite her defensiveness, Lois also seemed overly impressed by the authority and education of the therapist. She was prone to make inappropriate demands for advice from him and had difficulty understanding his reasons for declining such requests. Her attitude toward the therapist seemed to be a legacy of her experiences with abusive, domineering older males in her family of origin, particularly her father. For the time being, however, the therapist thought that he might put some of the authority she had vested in him to positive use, by speaking as an authority on the *recovery process*.

The therapist reviewed briefly the responses of various family members to Lois' recent disclosures. He especially underscored the rejection and the lack of validation the client had experienced as well as the similarities between the family members' current responses and the behaviors she had witnessed as a child. He also stressed that *as Lois progressed in her own recovery*, she would find that other survivors of dysfunctional families also had experienced similar reactions when they attempted to share their new insights. In fact, he added, the preponderance of such negative experiences had led him to discourage his clients from confronting members of their families of origin, except in cases of ongoing victimization. Using a mild, nonaccusatory tone of voice, the therapist said that had Lois discussed the matter with him in advance, he almost certainly would have advised against speaking to her family, since he viewed such an action as a setup for disappointment and conflict.

The therapist asked Lois to think about what she had expected to achieve by confronting her family members. Her response was typical of other clients who undertake (or think about undertaking) similar actions, in that she had difficulty identifying the *real* motives for her behavior. Initially, Lois replied that she did not have *any* expectations about how her family might respond to her disclosures. She maintained that her purpose in discussing the abuse had been solely to "dump my bucket," that is, to express herself in a cathartic manner. The therapist persevered in his gentle questioning of the client's motives, however. Was she sure, he asked, that she had *absolutely* no expectations for how her family members would react? As the therapist continued to challenge her, the client was able to acknowledge that she had envisioned a number of more positive outcomes resulting from her discussions with family members. She *had* hoped on some level that her father and her brother might have acknowledged and perhaps apologized for their abusive actions in the past. Moreover, she *had* hoped that her mother would have validated her disclosures, even to the point of confronting the father and brother on her behalf. Like other clients who are challenged to examine their motivations in similar situations, Lois was surprised to find her expectations regarding confrontations with her family were by no means modest or simple.

The therapist asked Lois whether there had been any concrete basis to think that the members of her family had changed since the days of her childhood. Had her father or brother seemed less critical or aggressive toward her in recent years? Had her mother shown any more backbone in dealing with the angry men in the family? Lois replied that there had not been any signs of dramatic changes on anyone's part. To her knowledge, she was the only member of the family who was involved in treatment of any sort. She said that, to her, the recent interactions with her family all seemed like a replay of her childhood. The therapist agreed strongly, reminding Lois that then, as now, she was utterly powerless to change her family system and the individuals in it. However, he stated that fortunately there *was* one important difference between her situation today and her plight as a child, namely that she no longer had to be a helpless victim. At least *now*, as an adult, she could protect herself, the therapist told her. Since it was unlikely that her family members were going to change their attitudes or behaviors, the therapist said, it was up to Lois to protect *herself*, by avoiding further disclosures or discussions of the material she would be working on in treatment. The therapist also told the client that over time she could learn how to recognize and fend off the unrealistic hopes for change that had fueled the desire to confront her family. Using several case examples that involved similar situations, the therapist explained to Lois how denial helped to keep such unrealistic expectations alive.

The therapist did not want to tell Lois how to behave with her family, as he suspected she might have wanted. He wanted to keep the client in a competent position as much as possible during treatment. However, the therapist also recognized that the client did have a legitimate need for his support and guidance in order to learn how to set more appropriate boundaries with her family. Consequently, he told her, "I don't know how you're going to do it exactly, but I'm confident that you're going to learn how to avoid discussing these subjects in the future with your family. I'll be glad to help you any way I can, of course." The therapist then asked Lois to think about which family members might initiate more discussions with her and under what kind of conditions. As the client saw it, her mother and brother were apt to be the most intrusive, perhaps even to the point of *insisting* that she address certain topics with them. Since Lois generally experienced both individuals as aggressive and controlling, she quickly became frustrated when the therapist asked her to think about how to handle them. With an exasperated sigh, she folded her arms across her chest and demanded of the clinician, "So tell me what to do with them!"

The therapist replied that not knowing the individuals involved, he would have no idea what to recommend to her. He said he could understand, however, that Lois could easily feel helpless when she thought of defending herself against two people who had always overpowered her. The therapist reminded the client that although she might resent him saying so, short of engaging in actual torture, no one could really *make* her talk about something against her wishes. He predicted that although she saw herself as powerless, if she were willing to experiment, she might find that she was more capable of resisting than she had realized.

The therapist asked Lois to anticipate some of the things her family members might say or do in order to induce her to talk. As she enumerated the possibilities, it became clear to her that she *would* be able to deflect some of the attempts to initiate a discussion with her. The therapist stated that Lois had just recognized, in the course of their conversation, that she *did* have some ability to defend herself against the intrusive behaviors of her family, contrary to what she had told herself, and him, just a few minutes earlier. Later the therapist would review this exchange repeatedly, whenever the client described herself as helpless. In the meantime, he encouraged Lois to imagine the potential behaviors of her mother and brother that might be most difficult for her to handle.

The client's worst fears centered on being criticized and potentially rejected by her mother. Lois reported that her typical response to such behaviors on the mother's part was to become overwhelmed by a sense of guilt and worthlessness. It seemed to the client that, regardless of the actual validity of her position, the mother could always make her feel as if she had done something wrong. Noting again that Lois might not like what he had to say, the therapist indicated that it might require additional work on her own issues before she could withstand her mother's guilt-inducing messages more successfully. He also suggested that it might help the client to remember that the point of withholding information was to *protect herself*—not to harm anyone else.

The therapist summarized the main points covered in the discussion thus far. He asked Lois to write the following affirmative statements on a file card: "I am not ready yet to discuss my treatment with anyone else in my family. I have no reason to expect them to change. I don't want to hurt anyone; I just want to protect myself from being hurt. All I am asking is that people respect my privacy and my feelings." The therapist suggested that Lois carry the file card in her purse at all times, so that she might read it over during times when she was subjected to external pressure from her family or when she began to feel a self-induced sense of obligation to disclose further information to them. The reader should note that a list of pat reassurances from the therapist would not have been helpful to the client. All the statements written on the file card reflected ideas that Lois had previously either expressed spontaneously or acknowledged with the therapist's assistance.

Although she showed steady improvement, Lois did not have an easy time creating more secure boundaries between herself and her family. On occasion, she still found herself caving in to pressure and disclosing more personal information to them than was prudent. Lois could still easily fall into the old trap of looking to her family, particularly her mother, for nurturance and validation. Every time the client made herself vulnerable in such a fashion, the results were consistently negative in that she would experience rejection, disappointment, and eventually a deep sense of worthlessness as a result. Lois also continued to become overly involved in the psychological problems of her siblings. On the other hand, she would sometimes attempt to protect herself by avoiding her family for months at a time, a strategy that inevitably caused her to feel guilty. Not surprisingly, Lois also experienced similar boundary problems, with the same repetitive cycles of overinvolvement and angry disengagement, in some of her friendships as well.

Throughout his subsequent work with Lois, which continued sporadically over the next 2 years, the therapist consistently resisted her requests for behavioral prescriptions. Despite her initial frustrations, the client began to relate to him in a more mature manner, soliciting his *feedback on her issues* rather than his advice. Many of her "needy," demanding behaviors during the sessions disappeared. After each incident of disappointment or rejection in a relationship, the therapist allowed Lois plenty of time to tell her side of the story and achieve a more stable emotional state before he attempted to focus on the role her own issues had played in the upsetting outcomes. Often Lois was so upset and defensive regarding a particular interaction that it was necessary for the therapist to wait until a later session to explore how she might have set herself up again for relationship difficulties.

In his discussions, the therapist never defended or excused the actions of others, nor did he ever imply that Lois *deserved* any of the mistreatment that she received. Nonetheless, he repeatedly drew her attention to the implicit, unrealistic expectations for nurturance and approval that she carried into many of her close relationships. The client began to recognize how she had unwittingly replicated the relationship patterns from her family of origin in her subsequent friendships as an adult. She started to guard her privacy more consistently and to temper her expectations of the people in her life. Although Lois learned to protect herself from potential mistreatment more effectively, she also became more tolerant of the limitations associated with various relationships.

Over the next 2 years of intermittent treatment, Lois was able to focus intensively on the issue of worthlessness and its effects on her daily life. She understood with increasing clarity how the need to establish a basic sense of self-worth often led her to work compulsively and perfectionistically. Lois recognized that she had become badly overextended because she found it difficult to turn down any opportunity to prove herself. As her self-esteem improved, the client began to take better care of herself by resisting the urge to tackle just one more project or assume just one more responsibility. And, as she felt better about herself, Lois learned to resist the tendency to view every relationship disappointment as a reflection of her personal worth. Moreover, since the client generally felt less threatened in her interpersonal interactions, she no longer engaged in many of the acting out behaviors that had once undermined both her relationships and her self-esteem on a regular basis. As she became less defensive, Lois found that she could tolerate negative feedback from others far better than she had ever imagined.

Although she had been able to achieve more comfortable and satisfying interactions with her friends and acquaintances, Lois gradually accepted the fact that there would always be a potentially painful component in the relationships with her parents and siblings. She did maintain regular contact with all the members of her family of origin, but she did so increasingly on her own terms, and in situations that provided her with a sense of safety. Lois learned to rely more on her husband for support and validation during and after difficult interactions with her family. She also discovered that her mother *could* be a warm and nurturant figure for her at times, particularly when the subject matter under discussion did not involve the family.

INGRID: SHIFTING THE TARGET CONTENT

As we discussed in Chapter 2, each idea we express has a degree of belief attached to it. Moreover, we are all capable of holding mutually contradictory ideas on a variety of subjects of great personal importance. Degree of belief in a particular cognition can vary as a function of a variety of organismic and contextual influences. As individuals become threatened, their attentional processes become narrower, and their beliefs become more rigid. Certain clients have the capacity to become so upset or agitated in response to life events that they simply cannot process new data until they calm down. Moreover, clients also may experience wide fluctuations in both degree of belief and ideational content across situations. Consequently, the therapist always needs to be sensitive to the *timing* of interventions.

The therapist must learn to back away gracefully from ideas on the part of the client that are so strongly held as to be impervious to change. Hammering away with impunity at ideas that are associated with very high degrees of belief is likely to antagonize or alienate clients. Likewise, as we recommended earlier, the therapist should also generally beat a hasty retreat at the first signs of psychological reactance on the part of the client. The therapist can always wait for another time to address the beliefs in question, perhaps when the client is less upset or when the individual seems to have achieved a clearer understanding of some related material. Similarly, the clinician should postpone certain discussions until those moments when the client spontaneously disavows the beliefs involved, or seems to be coping more successfully with the issues in question. In the meantime, the therapist might produce more positive results by concentrating on less threatening material and/or less rigidly held beliefs.

In some cases, the therapist can identify similar cognitive distortions and self-defeating coping strategies recurring across a *range* of situations in the client's life. The therapist may approach the issues that are central to the client's distress through a somewhat circuitous route, by examining situations that are less threatening to the individual. In the following case example, the client, Ingrid, presented with significant marital distress, but was unable to induce her spouse to enter couples treatment. The client also had great difficulty utilizing individual treatment to examine her own role in the marital problems. The therapist recognized that one of the client's friendships seemed similar to her marriage in many respects. Although Ingrid found it hard to focus productively on her marriage in treatment, she was ready to examine the friendship. By changing the "target content" the therapist was able to address the mechanisms that recurred in a number of the client's relationships, including her marriage. In the meantime, Ingrid developed a more trusting and open therapeutic relationship. As a direct result of her work on the troubled friendship, the client was later able to address the subject of her marriage in a nondefensive manner. This case also involved a significant *stress inoculation* component, in that the therapist encouraged Ingrid to rehearse for the full spectrum of hostile dependent behaviors as she attempted to separate from her deeply disturbed friend.

Ingrid sought treatment for mounting feelings of depression, stimulated by a number of factors, including chronic marital dissatisfaction and the pressure of having to care for her disabled, elderly father. She was particularly virulent in her antagonism toward her husband, who sounded distant, selfish, sarcastic, and completely uninvolved in the task of parenting their teenage sons. The client repeatedly solicited the therapist's help in attempting to resolve her marital difficulties, but she was unable to tolerate any discussion of *her* contributions to the difficulties. Ingrid saw herself as totally helpless when it came to her marriage. Again and again, she would reach the conclusion that she had only two options regarding the relationship, either to terminate it or to live indefinitely with conditions remaining exactly as they were. Every time she pondered the potential economic ramifications of divorce, as well as the possible psychological impact on her adolescent sons, Ingrid realized that she was not ready or willing to end the marriage.

Even after more than 10 sessions in treatment, Ingrid continued to expect that the therapist would provide her with the answers to her marital problems. In an indirect, but very noticeable way, she expressed her annoyance with the clinician for not being more of a help to her. Ingrid was unable to recognize that her interactions with her sons, siblings, friends, and co-workers also contained similar themes of helplessness and victimization, despite the therapist's repeated attempts to bring such parallels to her attention.

The therapist knew that he could ill afford to block Ingrid's attempts to discuss the relationship with her husband, despite the fact that the material she offered on the marriage almost never provided him with an opportunity to focus on her issues. He decided to maintain an empathic posture whenever the client discussed the marriage, taking pains to let her know that he could readily understand her frustrations with the husband. Whenever Ingrid described her impasse over the matter of divorce, the therapist joined strongly with her, but in a way that allowed him to change the focus somewhat. He would tell the client that given the enormous economic and psychological ramifications of divorce for all concerned, it was entirely appropriate that she approach such a decision with great care and deliberation. He also repeatedly lauded the client's concern for her children, who after all, could feel the most devastating effects of a marital breakup. The therapist made sure to elicit evidence of Ingrid's frustration with her husband during every discussion of the husband. He would empathize with her impatience with treatment, stating that he too felt badly about not being able to provide her with immediate relief, one way or another, on the marital front. However, the therapist also reminded her that she had invested nearly all of her adult life in the relationship with her husband. In his experience, it was not uncommon for individuals in her position to take many months, or perhaps even a year or more, to make such a momentous decision. The therapist told Ingrid repeatedly that he continued to be optimistic that, as she got to know more about herself and her issues, she would be able to reach a decision on the marriage with which she could be truly comfortable.

In the meantime, the therapist tried to learn more about the rest of Ingrid's life. As mentioned earlier, the themes of helplessness and victimization were not confined to the client's marriage. The client was much more open to looking at her own issues when the therapist focused on problems in her relationships outside the family, without attempting to draw parallels to the marriage. When discussing these more peripheral relationships, Ingrid's thinking patterns were much less rigid, so that she was able to process new information and thereby recognize her own cognitive distortions. Moreover, she seemed less obsessed with issues of blame, so that she was more willing to examine the appropriateness of her own behaviors, and the underlying cognitions, without becoming hostile or otherwise defensive.

The therapist was particularly interested in Ingrid's relationship with Roberta, whom she rather charitably described as her "best friend." Roberta thought nothing of demanding chauffeur service from the client when she was too anxious to drive, yet angrily rejected any suggestion that she seek treatment for her many psychological symptoms. She would purchase outlandishly expensive gifts for Ingrid and her children whenever there was the beginning of conflict in the relationship, yet she had never paid back a dime of the thousands of dollars she had borrowed from her friend. Her declarations of undying love for Ingrid were punctuated by unpredictable angry outbursts that grew to frightening proportions at times. Although it sounded to the therapist as if Roberta might be a legitimate candidate for the Axis II Hall of Fame, Ingrid initially downplayed the impact of her friend's manipulative, hostile-dependent behaviors. Although the therapist took a somewhat neutral, detached position regarding the friendship, he made sure to devote a portion of every session to a review of current developments in the relationship. Often the therapist simply summarized the latest problems with Roberta, and elicited the client's reactions to the material.

The more Ingrid discussed the relationship, the more it became clear to her not only that Roberta regularly victimized her but, also, that *she* set herself up for being mistreated again and again. To underscore the power of denial, the therapist repeatedly highlighted the contrast between Ingrid's current view of the friendship and the minimizing of the relationship that had occurred in previous sessions. Now that she could see Roberta's manipulations and underlying motivations more clearly, Ingrid was truly amazed at the way she had made excuses for her friend's behavior in the past. She recognized that she had often felt responsible for improving Roberta's unhappy lot in life, a point of view her friend had consistently encouraged. Moreover, the client acknowledged that she had allowed Roberta's nonstop emotional demands to interfere with the other important relationships in her life. The therapist predicted that, in time, they might find equally dramatic instances of denial operating in other areas of Ingrid's life, but he moved on to other topics without exploring the issue further.

Despite the change in her perspective, Ingrid found that it was not easy to reverse the pattern with her friend. Roberta would respond to her efforts to withdraw from the relationship with hostile attacks and threats of suicide. Fearing harm to herself and her family, and terrified of precipitating a suicide attempt, Ingrid would react by caving in to Roberta's demands. The therapist continued to underscore the themes of loyalty and overresponsibility in the relationship with Roberta, while highlighting the conditions in the client's family of origin that had primed her to assume such a parentified role in the friendship. He tried to sensitize Ingrid to Roberta's uncanny ability to externalize blame and induce guilt, noting that the client's alcoholic mother had behaved in much the same way during her childhood. The therapist also repeatedly expressed his belief that some of the same themes also occurred in the client's marriage, but he never elaborated upon the potential implications. However, whenever Ingrid spoke about how difficult it was to change her modus operandi with Roberta, the therapist invited her to think about how hard it would be for her to implement changes in her marriage, where the stakes were so much greater. Eventually, the client was able to process the full implications of the therapist's feedback. After recognizing in the course of a session that she had allowed Roberta yet again to take advantage of her, Ingrid finally exclaimed, "I know I'm never going to do anything about my marriage if I can't straighten this thing out with Roberta."

Ingrid was now much more willing to put the issue of her marriage on hold, while she tried to pull away from the destructive relationship with Roberta. Previously, the therapist had resisted Ingrid's attempts to have him advise her about what to do with Roberta. Instead, he had kept her attention focused on the negative *consequences* associated with the friendship and the personal issues that had made her vulnerable to participating in such a relationship. The clinician assumed that unless Ingrid could sustain a more realistic view of the relationship, she would be unable to stick with any plan to disengage from Roberta. Now that the client truly recognized the toxic nature of the relationship, she was more likely to risk facing the inevitable wrath of her friend.

Since Ingrid was strongly committed to disengagement now, the therapist was able to utilize a stress inoculation approach with her. The clinician had heard enough about Roberta's behaviors to envision how she might respond to the client's attempts at disengagement. He encouraged Ingrid to assume that a "worst case scenario," such as a serious suicide attempt, might well occur in reaction to her efforts to end the friendship. He cautioned her not to make any dramatic moves with Roberta until she felt fully capable of withstanding an escalation in her friend's destructive behavior. Ingrid stated that she knew that Roberta would do and say all she could to make her feel guilty if their relationship ended. The therapist asked Ingrid to prepare for the conflicts ahead by anticipating some of the self-defeating thoughts she might have, and rehearsing alternative cognitions, particularly regarding themes of responsibility and self-blame.

The more convinced she was that she needed to protect herself, the less Ingrid concerned herself with her supposed obligations to Roberta. After a false start or two, she was able to erect a firm protective barrier between herself and her onetime friend. Even the therapist was surprised in the end at how little guilt the client felt when the predictable hysterics occurred on Roberta's part. He reviewed the friendship and its termination several times with Ingrid, carefully underlining all the changes that had taken place in her thinking and her behavior. He also underscored the connections between the relationship with Roberta and Ingrid's victimization in her abusive family of origin. Reminding her how powerless she had felt originally with Roberta, the therapist pointed out emphatically that Ingrid's success in ending the relationship proved that she did not need to remain a helpless victim, as she once had believed. He told her that he would remind her of the experience with Roberta whenever she began to see herself in helpless terms in any other situation.

With Roberta finally out of her life, Ingrid was able to appreciate fully how costly the relationship had been, in physical, financial, psychological, and emotional terms. The therapist emphasized that as a result of the operation of denial, the client had lost contact with the toll Roberta had taken on her. Ingrid began to concentrate on improving the relationship she had with her children. As she began to see herself as more competent and powerful, she found herself becoming less threatened by the minor power struggles with her sons. Consequently, Ingrid was also able to behave in a much less petty and destructive way when conflicts with the children did occur. The client did begin to see, however, that the boys suffered directly from the constant tensions between their parents. Predictably, Ingrid began to feel more distress over the state of her marriage.

Earlier in treatment, Ingrid had often spoken of her children in a resentful, rather self-centered way, that had caused the therapist to entertain private questions regarding both her effectiveness as a parent and her overall level of maturity. Consequently, at times he had feared that Ingrid's level of functioning and her capacity to change would turn out to be more limited than he had assumed. The therapist was enormously reassured and encouraged by the renewal which had occurred in Ingrid's parenting once she had settled matters with Roberta. As a result, he was able to dismiss once and for all any reservations he might have entertained regarding her prognosis.

Ingrid's marriage once again occupied center stage in her treatment. This time, however, she was armed with considerable insight into her own issues, a greater sense of self-worth, and a much stronger working alliance with the therapist. The therapist now also had the benefit of a better understanding of the client. The clinician was often able to use data from Ingrid's relationship with Roberta, and other topics previously discussed in treatment, to illustrate key features of her functioning in the marriage. The more Ingrid looked at the relationship with her husband, the more distressed she became about the state of her marriage and its impact on her children. Although she was now more assertive and communicative than at any time in the past, her husband remained as intransigent as ever. On the other hand, the client also found herself reacting to her husband in an angry, belittling manner, sometimes in front of her sons. Feeling just as annoyed and disgusted with her own behavior as she was with that of her husband, Ingrid redoubled her efforts to confront the difficulties in the marriage.

Despite his professed desire to save the marriage at all costs, her husband persistently refused to become involved in couples therapy, even when Ingrid insisted on joint counseling as a condition for remaining in the relationship. Although Ingrid grew more skillful at resisting the tendency to become ensnared by her husband's blaming messages, it appeared that her husband was unable and/or unwilling to communicate with her in a less destructive way. In similar fashion, he continued to avoid taking responsibility for the problems in the marriage. She eventually came to the conclusion that the effort of keeping the marriage together was too costly for everyone concerned. Despite a heavy heart, a deep sense of loss, and a lingering sense of protectiveness toward her husband, Ingrid was able to sustain faith in herself and her chosen course during the lengthy process of separation and divorce which followed. To her surprise, her husband was extremely cooperative about his financial obligations and his parental responsibilities after the divorce. Ironically enough, although her sons expressed considerable anguish over the divorce, they became much more involved with their father after he left the house than they had ever been in the past. Moreover, after an extremely brief period of friction during the legal negotiations, the couple was able to develop an unusually open and supportive relationship following the divorce.

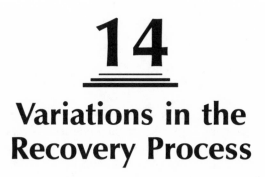

14

Variations in the Recovery Process

TREATMENT FORMAT ISSUES

We encourage therapists to consider using a *range* of formats in treating any given case. Resources such as group therapy, psychoeducational "workshops," and self-help groups all have much to offer clients who are motivated to participate in such experiences. Likewise, as we discuss below, even when treating an individual client, the therapist should also consider the use of interventions that will directly improve family or marital system functioning.

A "PLUG" FOR COUPLES TREATMENT

For the sake of simplicity, we have devoted much of this volume to accounts of individual treatment. As we have noted, however, the cognitive treatment of family of origin material need not be restricted to an individual therapy format. The majority of our cases typically involve family or marital treatment at some point. In many instances, effective individual therapy will result in empowering the client, to the point where he or she is able to convince a previously resistant partner into becoming involved in treatment. Given the proper circumstances (for example, partners who are willing to examine their own issues, a fairly low degree of blaming, minimal triangulation of the therapist, and so on), we find that couples treatment can serve as an especially powerful vehicle for changing individual schemas and coping strategies, while simultaneously strengthening the base of the marriage. Spouses who develop an awareness of how their dysfunctional schema interlock and trigger problematic interactions can then experience more empathy for one another and achieve a greater sense of control over potentially destructive behaviors in their relationship.

TERMINATION ISSUES

Like most clinicians who work with adult children of dysfunctional families, we have grown to respect the benefits associated with long-term therapy. Many of the clients described in this volume were in treatment over a period of *years*, not months. In most instances, we typically see our long-term clients every two or three weeks rather than weekly, once a degree of symptom stabilization has occurred. In the best of all possible worlds, at least as the authors might view it, our clients should stay in treatment as long as one or more of the following statements were true:

1. The client experiences significant ongoing emotional distress or problems in living that can traced directly to psychological issues.
2. The client continues to work at treatment, while avoiding an unhealthy dependency upon the therapist.
3. Direct benefits for the client continue to accrue as a result of therapy.
4. The client sees the projected future benefits of continuing treatment as worth the time and money involved.

As a result of both the depressed economy in our area and the increasing reluctance of health insurers to pay for mental health services, it seems that an ever-smaller number of individuals will have an opportunity to become involved in long-term treatment. There is reason to believe that, in the end, society will pay a direct price for the shrinkage of mental health services, in the form of increased domestic violence, reduced academic performance and vocational productivity, escalating illegitimacy rates, and all the other costs associated with impaired individual and family functioning. Perhaps eventually there will be a proper accounting of the comprehensive long-term benefits associated with effective psychotherapy, so that our services will receive the support they deserve.

Since the influence exerted by family of origin issues can unfold throughout the lifespan of the individual, we view every termination as provisional and perhaps temporary. We generally expect to see our clients again in the future, and most typically do, with increasing levels of influence and effectiveness in each successive period of contact. The role of the therapist can be analogous to that of a family doctor, in that he or she may help to usher the individual and/or family through various life cycle crises. Individual clients and/or families who maintain long-term relationships with a therapist generally are not always in treatment *continuously*, however. In fact, many individuals and families seen in our practice engage in *serial therapeutic contacts* spread over lengthy time spans (for example, 5–10 years or more). The authors find the serial therapeutic pattern to be so common, that they find it useful to assume that any given case will follow such a path. Consequently, we believe that there is a need to include *the seeding of future therapeutic contacts* as an integral, routine part of termination.

Although we certainly recommend that the clinician take a highly permissive attitude toward the client who wants to terminate, it is vital for the therapist to determine the *real* reasons behind the desire to end treatment. Needless to say, the therapist should conduct such an inquiry carefully, without appearing to invalidate the client's position, all the while knowing that in some cases it may not be possible for the individual either to identify or to disclose the true motives for discontinuing. However, as a result of dialogue with the therapist, certain clients may well conclude that the concerns that stimulated the wish to terminate (e.g., expecting to be rejected by the therapist if one continues treatment, fears about becoming overly reliant on the clinician, pressure from significant others to discontinue, and so on) need to be addressed in another manner.

As part of the termination process, the therapist should conduct a detailed review of treatment to date, beginning with the client's presenting symptoms. The therapist should underscore the positive changes in the client's functioning, while also acknowledging in a matter of fact manner any significant difficulties that persist in the individual's life. Every termination is a test of the hypothesis that the client needs no further therapeutic work. Since many of our clients think in all-or-nothing terms to begin with, they are not apt to view termination in such a manner. They are also likely to see the cessation (or the eventual resumption) of treatment as a measure of self-worth. In congratulating the client for past therapeutic accomplishments, the therapist should be careful not to support the idea inadvertently that the individual is somehow a better person because he or she has reached the point of termination. It is important for the therapist to praise the client, not only for actual therapeutic gains, but also for having embarked on a long-term process of personal growth, a process which does not end with the cessation of treatment. The therapist can then raise the possibility of further treatment contacts as a part of the *growth* process and not as another manifestation of pathology or "badness."

The therapist and the client should try to anticipate potential stressors that might cause difficulty for the individual in the future (e.g., the arrival of children, an escalation in a partner's substance abuse, and so on). Since the influence exerted by family of origin issues can unfold throughout the lifespan of the individual, the therapist's feedback should underscore future developmental transitions or crises the client may experience. Likewise, the therapist and the client ought jointly to specify the "early warning signs" (e.g., dysphoric moods, desire to drink, increased marital friction, and so on) that would indicate the desirability of further treatment in the future.

Ideally, the therapist should customize the termination procedure in consultation with the client, so that the unique needs of the individual can shape the disengagement process. Many long-term clients (for example, more than a year in treatment) seem to prefer a gradual weaning process spread over a number of months. For the most part, such a graded approach to termination seems to proceed smoothly, but the therapist needs to be careful about sending mixed messages as treatment winds down, particularly with individuals who might have a tendency to cling. Clients who have difficulties with dependency on the therapist will need to have the details of the termination process very clearly spelled out; such clients will probably do best if a definite endpoint to treatment is determined well in advance. Moreover, in such instances, the therapist should help the client prepare for the possibility that dysphoric affect and other symptoms may escalate as the departure date begins to loom on the horizon.

Finally, the clinician should encourage the client to explore what the loss of the therapeutic relationship will mean. The therapist should take the position that despite the positive changes in the client's functioning and sense of well-being, it would be entirely *normal* and *appropriate* to grieve over the loss of contact with the clinician. Nonetheless, despite the clinician's invitation to discuss the matter, there will still be clients who are unable to acknowledge feelings of attachment to the therapist. Similarly, there are those clients who will be unable to process termination *at all*. These individuals may opt to avoid the whole process by avoiding their final sessions. In such instances, the therapist should at least acknowledge the termination in a letter, making sure to include a clear statement that the client is welcome to return to treatment at any time.

As treatment nears its close, the therapist needs to assume an increasingly passive, detached posture in order to promote disengagement and to support more independent functioning on the part of the client. Consequently, the clinician will no longer address content raised during sessions in the same way. No longer can the therapist attack each instance of denial or question every cognitive distortion. Instead the therapist's emphasis will now be on integrating information *already* gleaned during treatment, not on exploring new material (except when disclosures by the client clearly indicate that termination is no longer appropriate).

In the authors' experience, when the client's distress is based on learning experiences in a dysfunctional family of origin, it will take considerable time to achieve durable changes in thinking and behavior. However, the recovery process can still continue even when the individual is not involved in ongoing psychotherapy. Although the personal growth that occurs in response to treatment has the capacity to produce miraculous results in the lives of many clients, individuals must be allowed to change when they are ready and in the manner of their own choosing. Moreover, therapy is not the only way to address one's issues. There are times when the client must simply become absorbed in the challenges of day-to-day living, perhaps returning to the therapist at some point in the future to discuss the results.

In our experience, clients can be victimized by clinicians who resist termination. We are aware of therapists who have responded to what they considered to be premature termination by making all sorts of dire predictions about the client's future should treatment not continue. Although some individuals may remain in treatment simply because they are unwilling to hurt or displease the clinician in some manner, the therapist who strongarms a client into continuing treatment may end up with a very reluctant collaborator during subsequent sessions. The client may start to cancel or fail to show up for appointments. The clinician may begin to have difficulty setting a meaningful agenda with the client, or may feel as if he or she is the only one really working in the room. In such instances, the therapist's best course of action is to allow the client to terminate in a constructive, self-affirming manner.

Unless safety to life and limb is involved, it is almost always desirable for the therapist to let go gracefully when a client expresses a consistently strong wish to leave treatment. Even when the main impetus for termination is truly the client's resistance, the therapist's strategy should be to support long-term growth, by joining with the client and "seeding" further treatment contacts, not by applying various forms of persuasion, pressure, or psychological coercion. The therapist must avoid setting up the client who terminates "prematurely" to experience a loss of face if he or she experiences difficulties in the future. Even when the therapist explicitly identifies areas of the client's life in which problems might arise, he or she also needs to affirm strongly any positive changes experienced by the individual. The clinician should stress that the client should feel free to return to treatment at any time without expecting to hear "I told you so." Therapists must also make it clear that they would view subsequent treatment involvement as a positive opportunity to assist in the individual's recovery process.

Often clients who enter treatment for the first time will manifest a sharp drop in motivation as soon as they experience symptom relief. They may move to terminate long before they have the slightest awareness of the basic issues that triggered their difficulties. The following case example illustrates how the therapist can terminate in a constructive manner with the client, while carefully sowing the seeds of future treatment contacts.

Ray was a middle-aged married man who drove a delivery truck for a soft drink company. Although the client lacked formal education, he had no fear of working hard and sticking to his commitments. Ray felt fearful and embarrassed about being in a psychologist's office for the first time and pointed out twice during the initial interview that only a sense of complete desperation had brought him there. The symptoms of anxiety he had begun to experience lately were making him afraid that soon he would be totally unable to function.

Ray became visibly upset when the therapist asked him a few questions about his background during the initial interview, but he did manage to acknowledge that his father had been a physically abusive alcoholic. He also alluded to an older brother who was an active alcoholic and a younger sister who had been involved in two violent marriages; he appeared clearly anguished disclosing even these kernels of information. "I don't think we need to go into all of that to solve my problems," he said. Given the man's discomfort and his clearly tenuous commitment to treatment, the therapist quickly stopped trying to elicit additional family history from the client. The clinician did tell Ray that it might become necessary for him to return to family of origin material at a later point.

The therapist then picked up the historical assessment, but this time he began when Ray left home in his late teens. Like other young adults from dysfunctional families, Ray had flourished in the armed forces, which provided him with a safe, predictable environment, free of the stresses associated with his abusive home life. Quite by accident in the course of his service in the Navy, he became the chief cook on a small ship. For the first time in his life, Ray felt competent and appreciated. He acquired a lifelong interest in the culinary arts, an interest that was to serve him very well in later years.

At 21, Ray returned to civilian life with a greater sense of ambition and purpose. Shortly after his return, he met and married his wife. An evidently competent, warm woman, the wife came from a close-knit, loving family, which Ray adopted as his own. Lacking other marketable skills, Ray took a job as a union truck driver, because of the job security and employee benefits. By the time he was 28, Ray had three small children to support.

Since his return from the service, Ray had hoped to use his cooking skills in some sort of business. In his characteristic manner, he made no move to realize his dreams without intensive preparation beforehand. When he was 35, Ray finally began his own catering business, with considerable help from his wife. Ray had decided that in order to be successful in such a highly competitive field, he needed to develop a specific niche for himself. His specialty was catering home wedding receptions. Working a limited number of engagements a year, Ray made every wedding a memorable event, by interviewing the bride and groom extensively beforehand. Predictably, the public appreciated the results of such personalized service, and Ray's reputation spread. His business showed steady growth over a 10-year period, to the point where he needed to hire a number of assistants to help him. A person less fearful of taking risks (indeed, a person who had not been raised in an abusive family) would have long ago left a full-time job to pursue the growing business full-time, but Ray was reluctant to sacrifice the security and the benefits of his "day job." Consequently, as the demand for his services increased, he increasingly began to burn the candle at both ends. In addition to the many hours he worked at his salaried position, Ray's typical weekly schedule involved several nights devoted to food preparation, interviews with prospective customers, paperwork, and 1 or 2 days of the weekend spent on the catering jobs themselves.

Ray called his family physician after he had experienced two panic attacks over a 10-day period. Both episodes had occurred while he was working, one while he was driving a truck during the day and the other while he was catering a wedding reception at night. Since the first attack, he had experienced nearly constant anxiety and agitation, with an accompanying sleep loss, which only exacerbated his difficulties. Ray was desperately afraid that he would stop functioning, and his catering business would be adversely affected as a result.

In addition to the symptoms of anxiety and panic, Ray's presenting complaints also included a depressive component. He reported feeling more and more frequently like a failure and seemed particularly distressed about a number of household projects (for example, painting and papering) that he had neglected to complete "in his spare time." Looking back over the past few months, he was able to identify a pattern of declining energy and enthusiasm about these projects, but he saw the loss of motivation as a manifestation of a personal defect or weakness, not as a natural outcome of such a frantic work schedule.

Ray only remembered one other time in his life when he experienced symptoms similar to the ones that were currently occurring. Unfortunately, he described the episode as a "nervous breakdown." Six years previously, he had served as chairperson of a major fund-raising event for a local charity. Then, as now, he had been saddled with a very high level of responsibility, coupled with enormous time pressures. He also had slept very poorly as the fund raiser approached and recalled only taking cat naps during the actual weekend on which it had occurred. When it came time for him to speak to the assembled volunteers at the conclusion of the successful affair, fatigue and anxiety had evidently rendered Ray speechless. As Ray remembered it, one minute he was being handed the microphone to speak to the group, and the next minute he was asking to have his wife take him home. After resting for a few days, Ray was able to return to his normal activities. However, although he had not experienced similar symptoms again during the intervening years, Ray did believe that in some unspecified way he had never been the same after his "nervous breakdown."

Although Ray certainly seemed like a typical workaholic in most respects, he told the therapist that he lived for the 3 weeks of vacation he and his wife would take, usually a week at a time, during the course of the year. Several years before, the couple had invested in a time-share condominium arrangement that enabled them to plan vacations all over the world. During their excursions, Ray reported feeling relaxed and enjoying himself without the compulsive level of activity that characterized his life the rest of the year. He clearly took great delight in planning the vacations and, later, in poring over the many photographs he invariably would take.

In the therapist's opinion, Ray was a man who had many areas of competency, despite his evident lack of insight. He seemed to require a very respectful approach on the part of therapist, one which avoided identifying deficits, in favor of building on preexisting competencies. Given Ray's concerns over loss of control, and the fearfulness he expressed about even being present in a psychologist's office, the therapist wanted to help him normalize his experiences as much as possible. On the other hand, the therapist also thought it would be important to lay the foundation for exploring the apparently traumatic family of origin material, in the event that it should prove necessary in the future.

The therapist presented Ray with a fairly standard explanation of the functioning of the autonomic nervous system and manner in which symptoms of anxiety and panic are produced. The therapist's demeanor during this discussion could best be described as "scientific," "objective," "bottom-line oriented." He maintained a supportive, but somewhat detached position vis à vis Ray, while carefully avoiding references to inner psychological dynamics. He recommended that Ray read a book by Claire Weekes, again in order to help him see his symptoms in a less threatening light. Somehow the printed word seems to have more credibility in our clients' eyes than the words of their therapists, probably because what an author writes cannot be dismissed as readily as mere "reassurance." The therapist also expressed the suspicion that Ray's previous "nervous breakdown" actually had been a panic attack brought on by the effects of fatigue, but he embedded the suggestion in other comments about anxiety so that Ray would not be able to reject the idea immediately.

The therapist told Ray there were three levels on which they could address the symptoms of anxiety and panic: medical, symptomatic, and psychological. The therapist first reviewed the medical situation with the client. Ray's family physician, who had made the original referral for psychotherapy, had already ruled out the presence of other health problems that might have triggered the anxiety. Moreover, the physician had also prescribed antianxiety medication for use on an as-needed basis. Ray was about as pleased over taking medication as he was about being involved in psychotherapy. Although he found it somewhat comforting to know that the medication was available for use in a dire emergency, he also felt stigmatized by having to keep it around, let alone take it. Perhaps predictably, Ray was extremely intolerant of the side effects, such as sedation, which like the anxiety symptoms themselves, threatened him with a loss of self-control. Clearly then, medication was not going to be the answer for Ray.

Over the four sessions he saw Ray, the clinician placed his primary emphasis on the symptomatic level. The therapist wanted the client to view him as having a logical, concrete, step-by-step plan for reducing the severity of his presenting symptoms. However, the therapist did warn the client,

"You're not going to like this, but if our efforts to help you control your symptoms don't succeed, then we are going to need to look at some broader psychological issues. That might require us discussing some things that will make you uncomfortable. However, I want you to know that I won't sneak into those areas without your permission and will only discuss them if I think it's absolutely necessary."

Note that although the therapist gave no ground on his expert status, indicating clearly that he still thought that the traumatic family of origin material might be at the root of the presenting symptoms, he helped Ray preserve a sense of *control* over what was to transpire in treatment. Moreover, the clinician set up the beginning stages of treatment as an *experiment*, the outcome of which would determine the content of future interventions. Objective data regarding Ray's symptoms and level of distress, not the therapist's prejudices or presuppositions, would dictate the future direction of treatment.

At the intake interview, the therapist urged Ray to remove all sources of caffeine from his diet. Ray grasped the therapist's explanation about the effects of caffeine on arousal level and immediately stopped using foods and beverages that contained it. The therapist taught Ray progressive muscle relaxation (Jacobson, 1938), simultaneously recording the procedure on a cassette tape for the client's use at home. As part of the relaxation training, the therapist asked Ray to visualize some memorable scenes of natural beauty from his previous vacations. Ray responded well on his first exposure to the relaxation training and reported that he was able to produce vivid, soothing images of past vacations. Despite his hectic schedule, the client practiced the relaxation exercises faithfully before bedtime and used the soothing imagery several times a day while at work. Ray quickly learned to induce a rather deep state of relaxation with the exercises and with the imagery. By the third session, he reported that he had successfully used the imagery to fight off the initial twinges of panic he had experienced one day while he was stuck in traffic.

At the second session, the therapist had asked the client to describe his typical weekly schedule. Along with the clinician, Ray himself was quite surprised at how busy and productive he was. He took seriously the therapist's suggestion that he prioritize his personal and professional projects. Between the third and fourth sessions, the client suspended several household projects, and hired a carpenter to complete a particularly troublesome remodeling job he had been unable to finish previously.

The fact that Ray left for a week's vacation between the second and third sessions turned out to be a serendipitous development. The client reported that he was symptom-free for the entire week, until the drive home, when he began to feel increasingly depressed. The therapist pointed out the contrasts between Ray's frenetic everyday lifestyle and his relaxed approach to vacationing. The client seemed much less panicky about the recurrence of his symptoms once he recognized the connection with returning to the weekly grind. He agreed with the therapist's comment that although he seemed perfectly capable of enjoying himself to the fullest in the right situation, he only allowed himself to relax during the 3 weeks of "official" vacation he received each year. Ray began thinking about all the social events and leisure-time activities he had dropped over the years because of the increasing demands of his schedule and resolved to pursue some of the interests and relationships he had allowed to disappear from his life.

As a result of his evident fatigue, and his discussions with the therapist, Ray decided to farm out some of his upcoming business to other caterers. Although the commissions he earned by brokering catering jobs in such a fashion was considerably less than what he would have received had he performed the work himself, Ray was not particularly distressed or guilt-ridden in response to the loss of income. In fact, he felt relieved of a tremendous burden. However, Ray did take a close second look at the fact that he was now generating more business than he could handle. At his final session, he reported that he was now considering moving up the timetable for leaving his full-time job, just as his wife and a close friend had been recommending for some time. Moreover, viewing his business in a different light led to Ray seeing himself as much more successful. As he said to the therapist "I've accomplished a hell of a lot. I *deserve* to feel good. I don't have to be doing something every minute of the day."

The therapist carefully underscored and reinforced every positive change that had occurred in Ray's outlook and his behavior. The clinician added that Ray seemed to have accomplished a successful midlife career change, a goal many other clients of his found extremely difficult, and in some cases impossible, to achieve. The therapist praised Ray for being willing to listen carefully to feedback and then building on it in so many powerful ways. Indeed, the therapist was quite impressed with the thorough manner in which Ray had regained control over his life. He freely admitted that although he had been sure that Ray's symptoms were going to improve, he never would have predicted from the initial interview that such a dramatic turnaround was going to occur. The therapist also praised Ray for being willing to become involved in treatment at all, given how difficult it had been for him even to come to a mental health professional's office. In an offhand way, the therapist mentioned that although the occurrence of future difficulties might require Ray to address some additional psychological issues, particularly those of a historical nature, there was no need at all to speak of such matters at the present time.

The clinician asked Ray to call him immediately if he experienced any similar problems in the future. The client seemed to have no difficulty whatsoever in making such a commitment to the therapist. In fact, Ray stated that he would have no hesitation in contacting the therapist in the future, emphasizing how comfortable he had come to feel in their discussions.

The therapist's nonthreatening, supportive posture enabled Ray to terminate treatment feeling competent and validated. There had been no reason for the therapist to pressure the client in any way. After all, the therapist's suspicion that family of origin issues had played a role in the client's distress had been only a hypothesis, nothing more. Although he started out feeling resistant and threatened, almost to the point of appearing hostile, Ray left treatment with good feelings about the therapist and the process. Six months later, the therapist heard from a third party that Ray was still doing well. The informant also told the therapist that the client had been extremely pleased with the treatment he had received.

References

Allport, G. (1961). *Pattern and growth in personality.* New York: Holt, Rinehart, & Winston.

Barkley, R. A. (1990). *Attention deficit hyperactivity disorder: A handbook for diagnosis and treatment.* New York: Guilford Press.

Barlow, D. H. (Ed.). (1985). *Clinical handbook of psychological disorders: A step-by-step treatment manual.* New York: Guilford Press.

Barlow, D. H. (1988). *Anxiety and its disorders: The nature and treatment of anxiety and panic.* New York: Guilford Press.

Bass, E., & Davis, L. (1988). *The courage to heal: A guide for women survivors of child sexual abuse.* New York: Harper & Row.

Bateson, G., Jackson, D. D., Haley, J., & Weakland, J. (1956). Toward a theory of schizophrenia. *Behavioral Science, 1,* 251–264.

Beck, A. T. (1963). Thinking and depression: 1, Idiosyncratic content and cognitive distortions. *Archives of General Psychiatry, 9,* 324–333.

Beck, A. T. (1964). Thinking and depression: 2, Theory and therapy. *Archives of General Psychiatry, 10,* 561–571.

Beck, A. T. (1967). *Depression: Clinical, experimental, and theoretical aspects.* New York: Hoeber. (Republished as *Depression: Causes and treatment.* Philadelphia: University of Pennsylvania Press, 1972.)

Beck, A. T. (1976). *Cognitive therapy and the emotional disorders.* New York: International Universities Press.

Beck, A. T., & Emery, G. (1985). *Anxiety disorders and phobias: A cognitive perspective.* New York: Basic Books.

Beck, A. T., & Freeman, A. (1990). *Cognitive therapy of personality disorders.* New York: Guilford Press.

Beck, A. T., Kovacs, M., & Weissman, A. (1975). Hopelessness and suicidal behavior: An overview. *Journal of the American Medical Association, 234,* 1146–1149.

Beck, A. T., Kovacs, M., & Weissman, A. (1979). Assessment of suicidal intention: The Scale for Suicidal Ideation. *Journal of Consulting and Clinical Psychology, 47,* 343–352.

Beck, A. T., Rush, A. J., Shaw, B. F., & Emery, G. (1979). *Cognitive therapy of depression.* New York: Guilford Press.

Bedrosian, R. C. (1982). Using cognitive and systems intervention in the treatment of marital violence. In J. C. Hanson & L. R. Barnhill (Eds.), *Clinical approaches to family violence* (pp. 117–138). Rockville, MD: Aspen Press Systems Corp.

Bedrosian, R. C. (1986). Cognitive and family interventions for suicidal patients. *Journal of Psychotherapy and the Family, 2*(3/4), 129–152.

Bedrosian, R. C. (1988). Treating depression and suicidal wishes within the family context. In N. Epstein, S. Schlesinger, & W. Dryden (Eds.), *Cognitive-behavioral therapy with families* (pp. 292–324). New York: Brunner/Mazel.

Bedrosian, R. C., & Beck, A. T. (1979). Cognitive aspects of suicidal behavior. *Suicide and Life Threatening Behavior, 9,* 87–96.

Bedrosian, R. C., & Beck, A. T. (1980). Principles of cognitive therapy. In M. J. Mahoney (Ed.), *Psychotherapy process: Current issues and future directions* (pp. 127–152). New York: Plenum Press.

Bedrosian, R. C., & Epstein, N. (1984). Cognitive therapy with depressed and suicidal adolescents. In H. Sudak, A. Ford, & N. Rushworth (Eds.), *Suicide in the young* (pp. 345–366). Boston: John Wright.

Black, C. (1981). *It will never happen to me.* New York: Ballantine Books.

Black, C. (1985). *Repeat after me.* Denver, CO: M. A. C. Printing and Publications.

Boszormenyi-Nagy, I., & Spark, G. (1973). *Invisible loyalties: Reciprocity in intergenerational family therapy.* New York: Harper & Row.

Bouhoutsos, J. C., Holroyd, J., Lerman, H., Forer, B. R., & Greenberg, M. (1983). Sexual intimacy between psychotherapists and patients. *Professional Psychology: Research & Practice, 14,* 185–196.

Bourne, E. J. (1990). *The anxiety and phobia workbook.* Oakland, CA: New Harbinger Publications.

Bowen, M. (1966). The use of family theory in clinical practice. *Comprehensive Psychiatry, 7,* 345–374.

Brehm, J. W. (1966). *A theory of psychological reactance.* New York: Academic Press.

Brown, D. P., & Fromm, E. (1986). *Hypnotherapy and hypnoanalysis.* Hillsdale, NJ: Lawrence Erlbaum.

Brown, S. (1988). *Treating adult children of alcoholics: A developmental perspective.* New York: Wiley.

Browne, A., & Finkelhor, D. (1986). Impact of child sexual abuse: A review of the research. *Psychological Bulletin, 99,* 66–77.

Buck, R. (1985). Prime theory: An integrated view of motivation and emotion. *Psychological Review, 92,* 389–413.

Burns, D. (1980). *Feeling good.* New York: Morrow.

Calof, D. (1987, March). *Treating adult survivors of incest and child abuse.* Workshop presented at The Family Network Symposium, Washington, DC.

Courtois, C. A. (1988). *Healing the incest wound: Adult survivors in therapy.* New York: W. W. Norton.

Dohrenwend, B. S. (1973). Social status and stressful life events. *Journal of Personality and Social Psychology, 28,* 225–235.

Easterbrook, J. A. (1959). The effect of emotion on cue utilization and the organization of behavior. *Psychological Review, 66,* 183–201.

Elkind, D. (1974). *Children and adolescents: Interpretive essays on Jean Piaget* (2nd ed.). New York: Oxford University Press.

Forward, S. (1989). *Toxic parents: Overcoming their hurtful legacy and reclaiming your life.* New York: Bantam Books.

Fussell, F. W., & Bonney, W. C. (1990). A comparative study of childhood experiences of psychotherapists and physicists: Implications for clinical practice. *Psychotherapy, 27,* 505–512.

Garner, D. M., & Bemis, K. M. (1982). A cognitive–behavioral approach to anorexia nervosa. *Cognitive Therapy and Research, 6,* 123–150.

Glass, D. D. (1985). Onset of disability in a parent: Impact on child and family. In S. K. Thurman (Ed.), *Children of handicapped parents: Research and clinical perspectives* (pp. 145–153). Orlando: Academic Press.

Glass, D., & Singer, J. (1972). *Urban stress.* New York: Academic Press.

Goldfried, M. R., & Davison, G. C. (1976). *Clinical behavior therapy.* New York: Holt, Rinehart, & Winston.

Goldman, C., & Babior, S. (1991). *Coping with anxiety and panic.* New York: Simon & Schuster.

Greenberg, L. S., & Safran, J. D. (1989). Emotion in psychotherapy. *American Psychologist, 44,* 19–29.

Guerin, P. J., & Pendagast, E. G. (1976). Evaluation of family system and genogram. In P. J. Guerin (Ed.), *Family therapy: Theory and practice.* New York: Gardner Press.

Guidano, V. F., & Liotti, G. (1983). *Cognitive processes and emotional disorders.* New York: Guilford Press.

Guy, J. D. (1987). *The personal life of the psychotherapist: The impact of clinical practice on the therapist's intimate relationships and emotional well-being.* New York: Wiley.

Haley, J. (1967). *Advanced techniques of hypnosis and therapy: Selected papers of Milton H. Erickson, M.D.* New York: Grune & Stratton.

Haley, J. (1971). *Uncommon therapy.* New York: W. W. Norton.

Haley, J. (1976). *Problem-solving therapy.* San Francisco: Jossey-Bass.

Herman, J. L. (1992). *Trauma and recovery.* New York: Basic Books.

Hollon, S. D., & Beck, A. T. (1979). Cognitive therapy of depression. In P. C. Kendall & S. D. Hollon (Eds.), *Cognitive-behavioral interventions: Theory, research, and procedures* (pp. 153–203). New York: Academic Press.

Ingersoll, B. (1988). *Your hyperactive child: A parent's guide to coping with attention deficit disorder.* New York: Doubleday.

Jacobson, E. (1938). *Progressive relaxation.* Chicago: University of Chicago Press.

Johnson, V. (1973). *I'll quit tomorrow.* New York: Harper & Row.

Korchin, S. (1964). Anxiety and cognition. In C. Scheerer (Ed.), *Cognition: Theory, research, and practice.* New York: Harper & Row.

Kovacs, M., & Beck, A. T. (1977). The wish to live and the wish to die in attempted suicides. *Journal of Clinical Psychology, 33,* 361–365.

Lang, P. J. (1985). The cognitive psychophysiology of emotion: Fear and anxiety. In A. H. Tuma & J. D. Maser (Eds.), *Anxiety and the anxiety disorders* (pp. 130–170). Hillsdale, NJ: Lawrence Erlbaum.

Lazarus, R. S. (1991). Cognition and motivation in emotion. *American Psychologist, 46,* 352–367.

Leventhal, H. (1979). A perceptual–motor processing model of emotion. In P. Pliner, K. Blankstein, & I. M. Spigel, (Eds.), *Perception of emotion in self and others* (Vol. 5, pp. 1–46). New York: Plenum Press.

Leventhal, H. (1984). A perceptual–motor theory of emotion. In L. Berkowitz (Ed.), *Advances in experimental social psychology* (pp. 117–182). New York: Academic Press.

Maltz, W., & Holman, B. (1987). *Incest and sexuality.* Lexington, MA: Lexington Books.

Maslow, A. H. (1962). *Toward a psychology of being.* New York: Van Nostrand.

McGoldrick, M., Pearce, J. K., & Giordano, J. (Eds.). (1982). *Ethnicity and family therapy.* New York: Guilford Press.

McMullin, R. E. (1986). *Handbook of cognitive therapy techniques.* New York: W. W. Norton.

Minuchin, S. (1974). *Families and family therapy.* Cambridge: Harvard University Press.

Ochberg, F. M. (1988). *Post-traumatic therapy and victims of violence.* New York: Brunner/Mazel.

Piaget, J. (1962). *Play, dreams, and imitation in childhood* (C. Gattegno & F. M. Hodgson, trans.). New York: W. W. Norton.

Piaget, J. (1970). Piaget's theory (G. Gellerier & J. Langer, trans.). In P. H. Mussen (Ed.), *Carmichael's manual of child psychology* (3rd ed., Vol. 1). New York: Wiley.

Pope, K. S. (1988). How clients are harmed by sexual contact with mental health professionals: The syndrome and its prevalence. *Journal of Counseling and Development, 67,* 222–226.

Prochaska, J. & DiClemente, C. (1984). *The transtheoretical approach: Crossing the traditional boundaries of therapy.* Homewood, IL: Dow Jones-Irwin.

Propst, L. R. (1988). *Psychotherapy in a religious framework.* New York: Human Sciences Press.

Putnam, F. W. (1989). *Diagnosis and treatment of multiple personality disorder.* New York: Guilford Press.

Rogers, C. (1951). *Client-centered therapy.* Boston: Houghton Mifflin.

Ross, C. A. (1989). *Multiple personality disorder.* New York: Wiley.

Russell, D. E. H. (1986). *The secret trauma: Incest in the lives of girls and women.* New York: Basic Books.

Safran, J. D., & Segal, Z. V. (1990). *Interpersonal process in cognitive therapy.* New York: Basic Books.

Safran, J. D., Vallis, T. M., Segal, Z. V., & Shaw, B. F. (1986). Assessment of core cognitive processes in cognitive therapy. *Cognitive Therapy and Research, 10,* 509–526.

Satir, V. (1967). *Conjoint family therapy.* Palo Alto, CA: Science and Behavior Books.

Satir, V. (1972). *Peoplemaking.* Palo Alto, CA: Science and Behavior Books.

Seligman, M. E. P. (1971). Phobias and preparedness. *Behavior Therapy, 2,* 307–320.

Solomon, R. L. (1964). Punishment. *American Psychologist, 19,* 239–253.

Solomon, R. L., Kamin, L. J., & Wynne, L. C. (1953). Traumatic avoidance learning: The outcomes of several extinction procedures with dogs. *Journal of Abnormal and Social Psychology, 48,* 291–302.

Stiles, W. B., Elliott, R., Llewelyn, S. P., Firth-Cozens, J. A., Margison, F. R., Shapiro, D. A., & Hardy, G. (1990). Assimilation of problematic experiences by clients in psychotherapy. *Psychotherapy, 27,* 411–420.

Sue, D. W. (1981). *Counseling the culturally different: Theory and practice.* New York: Wiley.

Tennov, D. (1980). *Love and limerance: The experience of being in love.* New York: Stein & Day.

Thurman, S. K., Whaley, A., & Weinraub, M. (1985). Studying families with handicapped parents: A rationale. In S. K. Thurman (Ed.), *Children of handicapped parents: Research and clinical perspectives* (pp. 1–8). Orlando: Academic Press.

Treadway, D. C. (1989). *Before it's too late: Working with substance abuse in the family.* New York: W. W. Norton.

Walen, S. R., DiGiuseppe, R., & Wessler, R .L. (1980). *A practitioners guide to rational-emotive therapy.* New York: Oxford University Press.

Walker, L. E. (1991). Post-traumatic stress disorder in women: Diagnosis and treatment of battered woman syndrome. *Psychotherapy, 28,* 21–29.

Watzlawick, P., Beavin, J. H., & Jackson, D. D. (1967). *Pragmatics of human communication: A study of interactional patterns, pathologies, and paradoxes.* New York: W. W. Norton.

Watzlawick, P., Weakland, J., & Fisch, R. (1974). *Change: Principles of problem formation and problem resolution.* New York: W. W. Norton.

Weekes, C. (1968). *Hope and help for your nerves.* New York: Hawthorne.

Weekes, C. (1972). *Peace from nervous suffering.* New York: Hawthorne.

Weekes, C. (1976). *Simple, effective treatment of agoraphobia.* New York: Hawthorne.

Whitfield, C. L. (1987). *Healing the child within: Discovery and recovery for adult children of dysfunctional families.* Pompano Beach, FL: Health Communications.

Wilson, R. R. (1986). *Don't panic: Taking control of anxiety attacks.* New York: Harper & Row.

Woititz, J. G. (1983). *Adult children of alcoholics.* Pompano Beach, FL: Health Communications.

Wynne, L. C., Jones, J. E., & Al-Khayyal, M. (1982). Healthy family communication patterns: Observations in families "at risk" for psychopathology. In F. Walsh (Ed.), *Normal family processes* (1st ed., pp. 142–164). New York: Guilford Press.

Young, J. E. (1990). *Cognitive therapy for personality disorders: A schema-focused approach.* New York: Professional Resource Exchange.

Zajonc, R. B. (1980). Feeling and thinking: Preferences need no inferences. *American Psychologist, 35,* 151-175.

Zajonc, R. B. (1984). On the primacy of affect. *American Psychologist, 39,* 117–123.

Index